In this book, the term "hypoallergenic" is frequently used in descriptions of Carnation® GOOD START H.A.™ infant formula. There should be no confusion among medical professionals regarding the use of this terminology. It does not imply that no allergic reaction to the product is possible.

No whole protein or protein hydrolysate formula is nonallergenic. However, to prevent any risk of misunderstanding, Carnation Company has made some changes in the labeling of its GOOD START formula subsequent to the conference upon which this volume is based. The term hypoallergenic has been removed from the formula label and the letters "H.A." have been dropped from the formula name. It is now simply called Carnation GOOD START infant formula. The composition and other attributes of the product are unchanged. GOOD START contains cow's-milk whey protein that has been heat-treated and partially broken down to reduce the potential for intolerance or sensitivity associated with standard cow's-milk or soy proteins. It should not be confused with highly processed casein-based formulas advertised for the treatment of cow's-milk allergy.

This volume on Food Intolerance in Infancy is intended to provide medical professionals with the most useful and current information available on this topic. In addition to Carnation Company's sponsorship of the conference on which this volume is based, infant formula and/or funding has been supplied by Carnation Company to several of the investigators whose work is cited in this book.

FOOD INTOLERANCE IN INFANCY
ALLERGOLOGY, IMMUNOLOGY, AND GASTROENTEROLOGY

Carnation Nutrition Education Series

Food Intolerance in Infancy
Allergology, Immunology, and Gastroenterology

Editor

Robert N. Hamburger, M.D.

Pediatric Immunology and Allergy Division
Pediatric Department
School of Medicine
University of California, San Diego
La Jolla, California

Carnation Nutrition
Education Series
Volume 1

CARNATION EDUCATION

RAVEN PRESS ■ NEW YORK

The Carnation Co., 5045 Wilshire Boulevard, Los Angeles, California 90036
Raven Press, Ltd., 1185 Avenue of the Americas, New York, New York 10036

Library of Congress Cataloging-in-Publication Data
Food intolerance in infancy.

    (Carnation nutrition education series ; v. 1)
    Based on the Food Allergy Symposium held in New York City, Sept. 29–30, 1988.
    Includes bibliographies and index.
    1. Infant formula intolerance—Congresses.
2. Hypoallergenic infant formulas—Congresses.   3. Food allergy in infants—Congresses.   I. Hamburger, Robert N.
II. Food Allergy Symposium (1988: New York, N.Y.)
III. Series: [DNLM: 1. Food Hypersensitivity—in infancy & childhood—congresses.   2. Infant Food—adverse effects—congresses.   3. Milk—adverse effects—congresses.   WD 310 F68685 1988]
RJ399.I53F66   1989   618.92'975   89-10575
ISBN 0-88167-545-8

Preface

In my "Bela Schick Memorial Lecture" to the American College of Allergists (1) on the subject of food allergy, I presented some of the results of our studies on the consequences of feeding cow's milk formulas instead of human breast milk to human babies and the problems created by the too-early introduction of solid foods, especially to infants from allergic families. One of the titles of the talk was "Food Allergy in Children and Adults: Overt to Covert," since we, pediatricians, see twice as much disease owing to allergy as do the internists and perhaps ten times more food allergy than they do. As a result, there is a tendency for internists and family physicians to overlook the not so rare adult with symptoms caused by the ingestion of a food.

This book is modeled after a European effort on a related topic, which is an invaluable reference work (2). We have addressed five topics within the text of *Food Intolerance in Infancy: Allergology, Immunology, and Gastroenterology*. In order to better understand the clinical aspects, we examined the biology and physiology of both the digestive and immune systems; we explored the various types of food intolerance; we discussed the diagnosis, prevention, amelioration, and treatment of milk intolerance; and we introduced to the United States a new hypoallergenic infant formula.

You will note that each section of this book is introduced, not necessarily by a worker in the field, but by an experienced and critical academic physician, each of whom briefly introduces the subject of the section. Each was responsible for seeing to it that none of the authors told you "more than you ever wanted to know about 'X'." I have rigorously edited the discussions which follow each section and therefore take full responsibility for any errors of omission or commission.

The Carnation Company provided me with the opportunity to organize a symposium and to assemble world-class authorities on food intolerance, including food allergy, many of whom are friends. Thus, we had the added pleasure of working with friends in the presentation of our studies and the discussion of our ideas. My hope is that you enjoy the book based upon the Food Allergy Symposium held in New York City, September 29 and 30, 1988, as much as we did preparing it.

This book will be of interest to all those who care for infants and children, especially pediatricians, family physicians, general practitioners, allergists, nutritionists, and nurses, as well as gastroenterologists and immunologists.

REFERENCES

1. Hamburger RN. Bela Schick Lecture: Food Allergy: confessions of an agnostic; or, Food allergy in children and adults: overt to covert. *Ann Allergy* 1988;60:454–8.
2. Schmidt E, ed. *Food Allergy*. Nestlé Nutrition Workshop Series, Vol. 17. Vevey: Nestlé/New York: Raven Press, 1988.

ROBERT N. HAMBURGER

Acknowledgments

This work was partially supported by grants from The Carnation Company, the Elizabeth and Carroll Boutell Fund, and the Pediatric Immunology and Allergy Foundation. The assistance of Janice R. Turner, Linda Galbreath, Jill Gilbert, and Maria Ware at the University of California in San Diego and the people at Raven Press, especially Erin Thomas, Natasha Kurchanova, and Rita Scheman is very much appreciated.

The encouragement of my wife, Sonia, my daughters Hilary and Lisa, and my granddaughter, Toya, has made working nights and weekends tolerable. Ernie Strapazon and Laurie MacDonald at Carnation Company provided the enthusiasm to keep me at the onerous task of editing and proofreading this book. Being associated with my co-authors of *Food Intolerance in Infancy* has made it all worthwhile and has produced a text that is, in my opinion, well worth the reader's time.

CONTENTS

Section IV

Section V

Contributors

Kjell Aas, M.D.
Voksentoppen Allergy and Asthma
Institute
Rikshospitalet University Hospital
Oslo, Norway

David J. Atherton, M.D., M.B.,
F.R.C.P.
Consultant in Pediatric Dermatology
The Hospital for Sick Children
Great Ormond Street
LondonWC1N 3JH, Great Britain

Sami L. Bahna, M.D., Ph.D.
Chairman, Department of Allergy and
Immunology
The Cleveland Clinic Foundation
Cleveland, Ohio 44195-5305

Lewis A. Barness, M.D.
Professor and Chairman
Department of Pediatrics
University of South Florida
College of Medicine
Tampa, Florida 33162

B. Björkstén
Professor and Chairman
Department of Pediatrics
University Hospital and Faculty of Health
Sciences
S-581 85 Linköping, Sweden

Jean Bousquet, M.D., Ph.D.
Clinique des Maladies Respiratoires
Centre Hospitalier Universitaire
34059 Montpellier, France

G. Casimir
Pediatric Sleep Unit
University Children's Hospital
Free University of Brussels
Brussels, Belgium

Ranjit Kumar Chandra, M.D.,
F.R.C.P.C., Ph.D., D.Sc.
Professor of Pediatric Research,
Medicine, and Biochemistry
Memorial University of Newfoundland
St. John's, Newfoundland, Canada

Cecil Collins-Williams, M.D.
University of Toronto
Toronto, Ontario, Canada M5P IN5

Robert J. Dockhorn, M.D.
University of Missouri School of Medicine
Kansas City, Missouri 64108

J. Duchâteau
Pediatric Sleep Unit
University Children's Hospital
Free University of Brussels
Brussels, Belgium

Edmund J. Eastham, M.D., M.B.,
B.S., F.R.C.P.
Consultant Pediatric Gastroenterologist
Department of Child Health
Royal Victoria Infirmary
Newcastle upon Tyne
NE1 4LP, England

J. Eden-Köhler
Children's Hospital of the University of
Düsseldorf
Düsseldorf, Federal Republic of Germany

K. Fälth-Magnusson
Department of Pediatrics
University Hospital and Faculty of Health
Sciences
S-581 85 Linköping, Sweden

Laurence Finberg, M.D.
Professor and Chairman
Department of Pediatrics
State University of New York
Health Sciences Center at Brooklyn
450 Clarkson Avenue
Brooklyn, New York 11203

Samuel J. Fomon, M.D.
Professor, Department of Pediatrics
Division of Pediatric Nutrition
College of Medicine
University of Iowa
Iowa City, Iowa 52242

Pierre R. Guesry, M.D.
Medical and Scientific Director
Nestlé Technical Assistance Company
Avenue Nestlé
CH-1800 Vevey, Switzerland

Robert N. Hamburger, M.D.
Professor of Pediatrics
University of California San Diego
Pediatric Immunology and Allergy
Division M-009-D
La Jolla, California 92093

G. Hattevig
Head, Immunology and Allergy Division
Department of Pediatrics
University Hospital and Faculty of Health
Sciences
S-581 85 Linköping, Sweden

William C. Heird, M.D.
Associate Professor of Pediatrics
College of Physicians and Surgeons of
Columbia University
630 West 168th Street
New York, New York 10032

David J. Hill, M.D., F.R.A.C.P.
Head, Allergy-Clinical Immunology Unit
Royal Children's Hospital
Melbourne 3052, Australia

C.S. Hosking, M.D., F.R.A.C.P.,
F.R.C.P.A.
Director of Immunology
Royal Children's Hospital
Melbourne 3052, Australia

Iréne Jakobsson, M.D.
Department of Pediatrics
Malmö General Hospital
S-214 01, Malmö, Sweden

R. Jost
Nestlé Technical Assistance Company
Avenue Nestlé
CH-1800 Vevey, Switzerland

A. Kahn, M.D.
Pediatric Sleep Unit
University Children's Hospital
Free University of Brussels
Brussels, Belgium

N-I.Max Kjellman, M.D.
Associate Professor of Pediatrics
Department of Pediatrics
University Hospital and Faculty of Health
Sciences
S-581 85 Linköping, Sweden

Tor Lindberg, M.D.
University of Omeå
Omeå, Sweden S-90185

Helmuth Loeb, M.D.
Academic Children's Hospital
Free University of Brussels
Laarbeeklaan 101
1090 Brussels, Belgium

Lasse Lothe, M.D.
Department of Pediatrics
Malmö General Hospital
S-214 01, Malmö, Sweden

Steven Machtinger, M.D.
Chairman
Department of Pediatrics
Redwood Medical Clinic
2900 Whipple Avenue
Redwood City, California 94061

François-Bernard Michel, M.D.
Clinique des Maladies Respiratoires
Centre Hospitalier Universitaire
34059 Montpellier, France

J.C. Monti
Nestlé Technical Assistance Company
Avenue Nestlé
CH-1800 Vevey, Switzerland

M.J. Mozin
Pediatric Sleep Unit
University Children's Hospital
Free University of Brussels
Brussels, Belgium

M.F. Muller
Clinique Universitaire Erasme
Av. JJ Crocq 15,
Brussels, Belgium

Buford Lee Nichols, Jr., M.D.
Children's Nutrition Research Center
Baylor College of Medicine
Medical Tower Building
6608 Fannin, Suite 601
Houston, Texas 77019

Richard D. O'Connor, M.D.
Clinical Professor of Pediatrics,
University of California, San Diego
Chief, Division of Asthma, Allergy and
   Clinical Immunology
Sharp Rees-Stealy Medical Group
San Diego, California 92101

J.J. Pahud
Nestlé Technical Assistance Company
Avenue Nestlé
CH-1800 Vevey, Switzerland

E. Rebuffat
Pediatric Sleep Unit
University Children's Hospital
Free University of Brussels
Brussels, Belgium

Eberhard Schmidt, M.D.
Professor and Chairman
Children's Hospital of the University of
   Düsseldorf
Düsseldorf, Federal Republic of Germany

Richard A. Schreiber, M.D.
Fellow, Combined Program in Pediatric
   Gastroenterology and Nutrition
Massachusetts General Hospital and
   Children's Hospital
Boston, Massachusetts 02114

M.C. Secretin
Nestlé Technical Assistance Company
Avenue Nestlé
CH-1800 Vevey, Switzerland

M. Sottiaux
Pediatric Sleep Unit
University Children's Hospital
Free University of Brussels
Brussels, Belgium

Ernie Strapazon, Ph.D.
Carnation Company
5045 Wilshire Boulevard
Los Angeles, California 90036

Yvan Vandenplas, M.D.
Academic Children's Hospital
Free University of Brussels
Laarbeeklaan 101
1090 Brussels, Belgium

Ulrich Wahn, M.D.
Children's Hospital
Free University of Berlin
Fachbereich 3
Heubnerweg 6
D-1000 Berlin 19, Federal Republic of
   Germany

W. Allan Walker, M.D.
Professor in Pediatrics, Harvard Medical
   School; and Chairman, Combined
   Program in Pediatric Gastroenterology
   and Nutrition
Massachusetts General Hospital and
   Children's Hospital
Boston, Massachusetts 02114

John A. Walker-Smith, M.D.
Head, Department of Pediatric
   Gastroenterology
Queen Elizabeth Hospital for Children
Hackney Road
London E2 8PS, Great Britain

Ekhard E. Ziegler, M.D.
Department of Pediatrics
College of Medicine
University of Iowa
Iowa City, Iowa 52242

FOOD INTOLERANCE IN INFANCY
ALLERGOLOGY, IMMUNOLOGY,
AND GASTROENTEROLOGY

Food Intolerance in Infancy: Allergology, Immunology, and Gastroenterology, edited by Robert N. Hamburger. Carnation Nutrition Education Series, Vol. 1. The Carnation Co., Los Angeles/Raven Press, Ltd., New York © 1989.

Introduction: A Brief History of Food Allergy with Definitions of Terminology in Food Intolerance

Robert N. Hamburger

Pediatric Department, School of Medicine, University of California San Diego M-009-D, La Jolla, CA 92093

As Lessof (1) indicated in 1983, food allergy is regarded in England as "fringe medicine" or a "cult subject." One reason for that is fadism, but more importantly, as the head of pediatric genetics in my department said recently,"We all must eat food . . . why would mother nature permit such an abnormality as food allergy to persist in man?" The question appeared to have an answer years ago in the Federico Gomez Memorial Lecture of the Hospital Infantil (2). Whenever a deleterious recessive genetic trait persists in more than a very small percent of the population, a search for some heterozygous advantage should be made. In the case of immunoglobulin E (IgE) production and allergic disease, it was hypothesized that the homozygous low IgE producer would be very susceptible to overwhelming intestinal worm infestations; the homozygous high IgE producer, although resistant to worms, would be at increased risk for potentially lethal anaphylactic reactions. The heterozygote would have a modest risk for allergic disease (estimated at 20%), which was thought might have been a fair price to pay for good resistance to worms. In fact, the figures observed fit very well with the Hardy-Weinberg prediction. In Western Europe, Canada, and the United States where there is clean water and good hygiene, the heterozygous advantages are no longer obvious. But for those who came here from Southeast Asia or the Philippines, it has been evident that they have been selected for the ability to produce high levels of IgE; and data showed that they have four times higher IgE levels and twice as much allergy as age-, sex-, and socioeconomically matched controls (3).

Bahna and Heiner (4) indicated in their treatise devoted exclusively to *Allergies to Milk:* " . . . (some) clinicians do not believe the condition exists . . . (there are those) who overzealously label infants milk sensitive" with almost any upset. Somewhat surprising for a disease that has been medically described for more than 2,258 years (Hippocrates is said to have noted that cow's milk could cause gastric upset and urticaria prior to 370 B.C. (5)). Five hundred years later, Galen described a case of milk allergy (6). In 1901 Dr. F. Hamburger (7) (no known relation to the author) gave a modern description of milk allergy and Schlossman (8) reported ana-phylactic shock owing to milk ingestion. That same year (1905) Finkelstein pub-lished the first recorded death caused by milk ingestion. By 1916 the American pediatrician, F.B. Talbot (9), clarified that what was being called an "idiosyncratic reaction" to cow's milk was, in fact, anaphylaxis or as we would term it today, "atopic allergic reaction" to cow's milk.

Our studies show that egg and peanut proteins are much more commonly aller-genic than cow's milk or soy proteins. Why, then, is the occurrence of cow's milk allergy so much more frequent? The answer, no doubt, is at what age these foods are conventionally fed. The incidence of cow's milk allergy increased astronomi-cally when safe commercial production of cow's milk-based infant formulas was ac-complished and soy allergy followed with the production of soy-based formulas. It has taken 50 years to get new mothers (of all social and economic groups) in Amer-ica to value breast-feeding once again after seeing a decline to under 15% breast-feeding 15 or 20 years ago. Why does it take so much effort and education to rees-tablish breast-feeding as the method of choice for American women? A recent im-portant observation in primates that my daughter, Lisa, brought to my attention is that breast-feeding is not an instinctive inborn phenomenon in higher primates like nest building is in birds. Breast-feeding has to be taught. It is customarily learned by young females observing their mother or other close relatives breast-feeding. Thus, if a family goes two or three generations without breast-feeding, the new mother's success rate, without personal instruction, is very low.

That is one reason why we, in the early 1970s, began investigating the apparent increase in early-onset allergic disease and the possibility of prophylactic interven-tion. Because we had recently shown the strong genetic influence (10–12) on the regulation of serum IgE levels, we were not too certain of how much effect a pro-phylactic regimen might have on the incidence of atopic allergic diseases in infancy. We were much encouraged by our preliminary study (13–15), but also chastened by the difficulty of getting an unselected study population. As we discovered, the only mothers willing to enroll in this rather arduous regimen were those with a lot of seri-ous allergic disease in one or both parents' families. Results that were impressive, despite the valid criticisms, included a strongly positive correlation between the length and exclusivity of breast-feeding and the infant's serum IgE level at 4 months and 1 year of age. The longer the exclusive breast-feeding (with no formula and no solid foods added) the lower the IgE level and the less clinical symptoms of allergy during the first 2 years of life.

The results of the preliminary study encouraged us to embark on a 5-year (com-pleted in 1988, 10 years after writing our proposal) collaborative study with the Kaiser-Permanente Allergy group in San Diego (16–19). The design of this study was meant to avoid many of the criticisms of almost all of the prior prophylaxis studies. Random assignment was difficult enough to accomplish, but maintaining blindness, as to category assignment, by both the patients and the physicians was al-most impossible. In addition, patients compared protocols, regimens, and instructions, altered theirs, and during the years of the study period (1980–88), the incidence of successful breast-feeding in San Diego County increased enormously—thereby reducing the expected difference between the prophylaxis study group and the control group(s). Nevertheless, in our recently submitted first paper since the actual completion of the study (20), it is apparent that breast-feeding plays the major role in the prevention of cow's milk allergy. Smoking by the nursing mother is seen to be a serious risk factor, apparently nonspecifically stimulating the infant to turn on the production of IgE.

In closing this brief historical overview, I want to touch on some other problem areas with respect to food allergy, which were emphasized in my "Bela Schick Memorial Lecture" at the American College of Allergy meeting in Boston, November 1987 (21). First is the problem of the lack of a definitive test or a gold standard for the diagnosis of food allergy. As I stated, even with a careful history and physical examination and skin tests, radioallergosorbent tests (RASTs), and food challenges, conflicting results may be seen:

> In a double-blind food challenge study (22) they stated that "The majority of foods were replaced in the diet within nine months of their incrimination" and " . . . rechallenge at regular intervals has shown that the food can be reintroduced into the diet by the third year (of life) without risk." Whereas a publication (23) the same year " . . . indicated that 30% of food-allergic children become clinically tolerant before three years of evolution, 40% before six years . . . (only) 53% before 12 years" in children with proven IgE sensitization. In addition, they noted that oral tolerance varied significantly with the specific food: " . . . tolerance to cow's milk seems to be far earlier and easier to reach than to egg and fish (p <0.001 at nine years)." They also reported that levels of specific IgE at the onset of disease were significantly higher (p <0.01) in those with *persistence* of clinical sensitivity. The disagreement as to whether food allergy is outgrown in nine months or nine years is based on serious scientific studies, whereas most of the other food allergy controversies are based on differing opinions and clinical impressions, not scientific data.

The second problem that many physicians have not appreciated in food allergy is cross-reactivity. Again quoting from my paper (21):

> One frequent example for which we have learned to be on guard is the infant with a positive RAST or skin test to a grass pollen, which in fact, is really a cross-reaction with a strongly positive test to wheat (or rice). The converse is seen in older children and adults who are highly allergic to several grasses (some of which may be cross-reactions as well) who have more weakly positive reactions (by RAST and/or skin tests) to one or more of the grains. I remind my students that it is not too surprising since all of our eatable grains originally derived from grasses.

The words food allergy, properly used, mean IgE-mediated disease. Food allergy, in fact, is one type of food intolerance, along with others such as enzyme defects (e.g., lactose intolerance caused by lactase deficiency), absorption defects, enteritis, idiosyncratic reactions, and other immunologic reactions to foods, such as the formation of immune complexes. But recently, even these categories have become confused with the description of immune complexes containing both IgE and IgG and the description of an IgE rheumatoid factor. To add to the problem, even in pure IgE-mediated food allergy, two additional variables often confound us; they are the dose and the additive effects. That is not the problem of chemical additives which can produce both a true IgE-mediated allergy and a chemically induced histamine release in the rare susceptible individual. The dose and additive effects in food allergy are based on clinical observations that individuals with IgE cow's milk antibody may tolerate 1 ounce of cow's milk orally but not 4 ounces. The other observation is that some patients can tolerate a small amount of egg or wheat in a meal but not both at the same time without having a reaction. There may also be a priming effect in food allergy, as has been clearly described in allergic rhinitis; such that once the intestinal lining has been damaged by a local allergic reaction, other food allergens may cross the mucosal barrier. Following an acute gastroenteritis, old food allergies may briefly recur and chronic enteritis may produce food intolerance. The production of new allergens during the digestive process has been well described (24). Finally, parasitosis and its enormous stimulation of IgE production concomitant with ingestion of a food in some animals is known to produce a bystander IgE response to the food. Data and clinical observations on many of the foregoing topics will be presented in this volume and I will save my comments and conclusions for the end. To conclude, there follows a definition of terms commonly used (or misused) in discussion of food allergy. The definitions are modified from the text (25) provided by the American Academy of Allergy and Immunology Committee on Adverse Reactions to Food and the National Institute of Allergy and Infectious Diseases.

DEFINITION OF TERMS

Adverse reaction (sensitivity) to a food. A general term that is applied to a clinically abnormal response to an ingested food, additive, or contaminant.

Food allergy (hypersensitivity). An immunologic reaction (IgE mediated) to a food or a food additive. In Europe the term is more broadly defined as "any immunologic reaction to a food." Among some persons it is a frequently misused term when adverse reaction to a food is meant.

Food anaphylaxis. The classic allergic, hypersensitivity, IgE-mediated reaction to a food or food additive.

Food intolerance. A general term used to describe any abnormal physiologic response to an ingested food. The mechanism is not known and may include: idiosyncratic, metabolic, enzymic, pharmacologic, emotional, or toxic reactions.

Food toxicity (poisoning). An adverse effect caused by a toxin or bacterial product in the food. Food toxicity may mimic anaphylaxis and is then termed anaphylactoid.

Anaphylactoid reaction to a food. An anaphylaxislike reaction to a food as a result of a nonimmune (chemical) release of inflammatory mediators.

Pharmacologic food reaction. An adverse reaction to an ingested food or food additive that results from a naturally derived or added chemical that produces a druglike or pharmacological effect.

Metabolic food reaction. An adverse reaction to an ingested food as a result of an effect on the metabolism of the host.

Food idiosyncrasy. A quantitatively rare, nonimmunologic, abnormal response to a food resembling a hypersensitivity reaction (anaphylactoid) and may involve a familial or genetic predisposition.

REFERENCES

1. Lessof MH, ed. *Clinical Reactions to Food.* New York, Chichester: John Wiley & Sons, 1983.
2. Hamburger RN: Niveles de inmunoglobulina E., herencia a la alergia e inmunidad a los helmintos. (Levels of immunoglobulin E, inheritance of allergy and immunity to intestinal parasites.) *Bol Méd Hosp Infant Mex* 1973;20:309–23.
3. Orgel HA, Lenoir MA, and Bazaral M. Serum IgG, IgA, IgM, and IgE levels and allergy in Filipino children in the United States. *J Allergy Clin Immunol* 1974;53:213–22.
4. Bahna SL, Heiner DC. *Allergies to Milk.* New York: Grune & Stratton, 1980.
5. Chabot R. *Pediatric Allergy.* New York: McGraw-Hill, 1951.
6. O'Keefe ES. The history of infant feeding. II. Seventeenth and eighteenth centuries. *Arch Dis Child* 1953;28:232–40.
7. Hamburger F. Biologisches Uber die Eiweisskorper der Kuhmilch und Uber Sauglingernahrung. *Wien Klin Wochenschr* 1901;14:1202–4.
8. Schlossman A. Uber die Giftwirkung des Artfremden Eiweisses in der Milch auf den Organismus des Sauglings. *Arch Kinderheilk D* 1905;41:99–103.
9. Talbot FB. Idiosyncrasy to cow's milk: its relation to anaphylaxis. *Boston Med Surg J* 1916;175:409–10.
10. Bazaral M, Orgel HA, Hamburger RN. IgE levels in normal infants and mothers and an inheritance hypothesis. *J Immunol* 1971;107:794–801.
11. Hamburger RN, Bazaral M. IgE levels in twins confirm genetic control in human beings. *J Allergy Clin Immunol* 1972;49:91 (Abstr).
12. Bazaral M, Orgel HA, Hamburger RN. Genetics of IgE and allergy: serum IgE levels in twins. *J Allergy Clin Immunol* 1974;54:288–304.
13. Hamburger RN, Orgel HA.The prophylaxis of allergy in infants debate. *Pediatr Res* 1976;10:387 (Abstr).
14. Hamburger RN, Orgel HA. Prophylaxis of allergy. *West J Med* 1976;125:215 (Epitome).
15. Ziering RW, O'Connor RD, Mellon M, Cook DA, Tomaszewski, M, Street DH, Hamburger RN. University of California San Diego prophylaxis in infancy study: an interim report. *J Allergy Clin Immunol* 1979;63:199 (Abstr).
16. Hamburger RN. Prophylaxis of atopic asthma in the first two years of life. *Allergol Immunopathol* 1979;6:71–3.
17. Hamburger RN, Heller S, Mellon MH, O'Connor RD, Zeiger RS. Current status of the clinical and immunological consequences of a prototype allergic disease prevention program. *Ann Allergy* 1983;51:281–9.
18. Hamburger RN. Diagnosis of food allergies and intolerance in the study of prophylaxis and control groups in infants. *Ann Allergy* 1984;53:673–7.
19. Zeiger RS, Heller S, Mellon M, O'Connor RD, Hamburger RN. Effectiveness of dietary manipulation in the prevention of food allergy. *J Allergy Clin Immunol* 1986;78:224–38.
20. Zeiger RS, Heller S, Mellon MH, Forsythe AB, O'Connor RD, Hamburger RN, Schatz M. Effect of prenatal and postnatal dietary prophylaxis on development of atopy in early infancy: a randomized study. *J Allergy Clin Immunol (in press).*
21. Hamburger RN. Bela Schick Lecture: Food Allergy: confessions of an agnostic; or, Food allergy in children and adults: overt to covert. *Ann Allergy* 1988;60:454–8.

22. Bock SA. Prospective appraisal of complaints of adverse reactions to foods in children during the first three years of life. *Pediatrics* 1987;79:683–8.
23. Boyano MT, Martin EM, Pascual C, Ojeda JA. Food allergy in children. II. Prognostic factors and long-term development. *An Esp Pediatr* 1987;26:241–5.
24. Vanella LM, Gonzalez AM, Miguez V. Antigenos incompletos derivados de las proteinas lácteas en el suero de lactantes alérgicos a la leche. (Partially digested milk protein [peptide antigens] in the serum of infants allergic to cow's milk.) *Allergol Immunopathol* 1978;6:507–18.
25. Anderson JA, Sogn DD, eds. *Adverse Reactions to Foods*. U.S. NIH Publication 1984;84–2442.

ACKNOWLEDGMENTS

This work was partially supported by grants from the Carnation Company, the Elizabeth and Carroll Boutell Fund, and the Pediatric Immunology and Allergy Foundation. The assistance of Janice R. Turner, Linda Galbreath, Jill Gilbert, and Maria Ware is very much appreciated.

Food Intolerance in Infancy: Allergology, Immunology, and Gastroenterology, edited by Robert N. Hamburger. Carnation Nutrition Education Series, Vol. 1. The Carnation Co., Los Angeles/Raven Press, Ltd., New York © 1989.

Introduction to Section I

Buford Lee Nichols, Jr.

Children's Nutrition Research Center, Baylor College of Medicine, Houston, TX 77019

The immunologic aspects of the adverse reactions of some infants to the feeding of cow's milk continue to arouse concern among pediatricians. As early as 1901, F. Hamburger (1) clearly described an anaphylactic reaction in an infant fed cow's milk. Four years later, Schlossmann and Finkelstein identified the specificity of milk proteins in this immune reaction. Schlossmann (2) demonstrated the presence of precipitating antibodies to cow's milk in these infants. In 1906, Pirquet (3) recognized the immunologic basis of systemic reactions to the administration of antisera for the management of bacterial diseases. He described the ''serum sickness'' response as one of ''allergy,'' meaning to work against a foreign substance.

The fundamental work on the nature of the immune response to dietary proteins was continued in the United States at Cornell Medical School by Oscar Menderson Schloss, M.D. (1882–1953) (4). He was professor and head of the Department of Pediatrics at Cornell Medical School, and served 2 years as chairman of Pediatrics at Harvard University. His chairmanship at Cornell ended in 1934.

Schloss' work is best summarized in his ''Harvey Lecture'' delivered in 1924 (5). During his career, he demonstrated that young normal infants absorb foreign proteins for a transient period of time after new foods are introduced into their diets. Antigen absorption was increased in children with acute and chronic diarrhea. Malnourished children absorbed the antigen, but did not develop antibodies until their nutritional recovery was under way. Schloss was unable to differentiate the role of the absorbed antigen in the development of toxic symptoms during infantile diarrhea. This problem continues to confound researchers. Schloss used sensitive immunologic techniques to identify precipitating antibodies (immunoglobulin G [IgG]) and anaphylactoid antibodies (IgE) and demonstrated correlations with skin hypersensitivity (delayed hypersensitivity). He reported the presence of the same immunological process which occurs in marasmus in normal infants, but in abbreviated forms. He further demonstrated that intact proteins appeared to be absorbed through the oropharyngeal mucosa, as well as through the gastrointestinal tract, in infants with cleft palate.

Schloss envisioned three lines of defense against immune hypersensitivity to ingested proteins:

1. Hydrolysis of ingested proteins by digestive enzymes.
2. Impermeability of the intestine to protein fragments insufficiently degraded to lose their antigenicity.
3. Production of dietary antigen-specific antibodies which divert absorbed protein from body cells to prevent their harmful effects.

   The field of immunology has expanded since Schloss delivered the "Harvey Lecture" in 1924. The issues addressed in his meticulous clinical investigations remain relevant to the pediatrician of today.

1. What is the clinical significance of the enteral absorption of antigenic protein by infants? Does it bear any resemblance to the spectacular symptoms developed by the sensitized animal reinjected with a sensitizing protein?
2. What are the mechanisms by which the body clears and neutralizes the normally absorbed antigen?
3. What are the mechanisms of antigen absorption and clearance modified during maturation?

REFERENCES

1. Hamburger F. Biologisches Uber die Eiweisskorper der Kuhmilch und Uber Sauglingernahrung. *Wien Klin Wochenschr* 1901;14:1202–4.
2. Dees SC. Allergy to cow's milk. *Pediatr Clin North Am* 1959;6:881–900.
3. Pirquet C. Allergie. *Muench Med Wochenschr* 1906;53:1457–8.
4. Schloss OM. The intestinal absorption of antigenic protein. The Harvey Society. 1924;2156–87.
5. Gordon HH. Oscar Menderson Schloss. In: *Pediatric Profiles*. BS Veeder, ed. St. Louis: CV Mosby, 1957;202–10.

*Food Intolerance in Infancy: Allergology,
Immunology, and Gastroenterology,* edited by
Robert N. Hamburger. Carnation Nutrition
Education Series, Vol. 1. The Carnation Co., Los
Angeles/Raven Press, Ltd., New York © 1989.

Chemistry of Food Allergens

Kjell Aas

*Voksentoppen Allergy and Asthma Institute, Rikshospitalet University Hospital,
Oslo, Norway*

DEFINITION OF TERMS

Scientific as well as clinical work in allergy must satisfy strict criteria as to specificity and precision. Specificity and precision are particularly important with respect to terms used in communications about food allergy. Failures as to this have added unnecessary confusion to this field. I find it appropriate to begin this review with some descriptive definitions; others will be given later.

Allergy. Hypersensitivity reactions caused by immune reactions that are harmful to the tissues or disruptive of the physiology of the host. The immune reaction triggers complex biochemical and/or inflammatory sequences that result in clinical symptoms. The symptoms depend on the degree of reactivity of the involved tissue receptors and of the effector cells.

Allergen. The antigenic molecule that takes part in the immune reaction that results in allergy. Food allergen indicates an allergen found in food, and in this discussion, is restricted to those reacting with immunoglobulin E (IgE) antibodies.

Allergenic source. The material or food that contains allergens.

Immunogen. The molecule or part of it that is able to initiate proliferation of immunocompetent lymphocytes or trigger the synthesis of specific antibodies.

SCOPE OF PRESENTATION

Any food item may provoke allergic symptoms in predisposed individuals but may also trigger similar symptoms caused by nonimmunologic biological effects. This discussion is concerned only with natural allergens found in food with particular emphasis on information achieved from studies of the codfish allergens as a model. There is not much new information because a similar presentation was published (1). In food allergy, the role of antibodies other than those of IgE is poorly understood, so in this presentation, I will discuss only allergens reacting with IgE.

FOOD ALLERGENS ARE (MOSTLY) PROTEINS

All natural allergens that react with IgE antibodies have, so far, been shown to be proteins. Many of them are glycoproteins, which means that they contain one or more sugar molecules in addition to the amino acids (1–7). A protein is mainly made up of a number of amino acids bound together in peptide linkages with or without a few additional carbohydrate residues in the primary structure. Each amino acid is characterized by its side chain. The side chains represent chemically active sites with a certain physiochemical power. They contribute to the final shape and the power field of the molecule and so does any carbohydrate residue present. The chain or sequence of amino acids is twisted and is given its final shape through conformational changes caused by the chemical forces between the side chains. These forces fold the molecule into its tertiary structure. Chemical forces from outside also influence the final shape and the net chemical power of the molecule.

The amino acids can in a way be said to act as letters in a chemical alphabet containing 20 different letters. Carbohydrate molecules within the amino acid chain act as additional letters. Combination of the chemical letters in different ways creates a multitude of words (peptide fragments) and phrases (proteins) in the language of protein chemistry. Some of the words are made by the amino acid letters as found in the original sequence of the chain. They are sequential denominators. Others are made when amino acid letters, which are remote in the primary sequence chain, are brought close together through the folding of the chain. The latter are conformational denominators.

ANTIGENS AND IMMUNOGENS IN FOOD

Each food item contains a number of different proteins and many other substances. Each protein has a number of different antigenic traits. When absorbed, the antigenic molecules trigger antibody production. The immunogenicity and antigenicity differ from protein to protein and seem to depend on host factors as well as a combination of genetic, environmental, and adjuvant factors. Part of the antigenicity is destroyed and a few more antigenic characteristics may arise or become unmasked in food items caused by structural changes following digestion during the intestinal passage. Increased absorption results in more prominent immune response and higher serum concentration of antibodies. This is well known for cow's milk, for example. Increased serum concentrations of antibodies to cow's milk are common in diseases with flattened intestinal epithelium, such as celiac disease. Most of these antibodies do no harm. They are only innocent waste products.

The complexity of the mixture of proteins found in allergen sources and in extracts of allergenic foods can be demonstrated by a number of techniques: Sodium dodecyl sulfate polyacrylamide gel electrophoresis (SDS-PAGE), isoelectrofocusing (IEF), PAGE or starch gel electrophoresis with immunoprinting, and crossed radioimmunoelectrophoresis (CRIE). A wide variety of modifications of these and similar methods have been used. New methods are invented. We can rightly speak about immunoacrobatics in this connection.

Progress in protein separation methods has been an important propagator in this field of immunology, and immunology has propagated progress in protein separation and characterization. Many possibilities for scientific progress have been opened for those interested.

MAJOR, INTERMEDIATE, AND MINOR ALLERGENS

Only a proportion of the several proteins found in a given allergen source act as offenders in the majority of patients allergic to the matter. The most important ones are called major allergens. Less important allergens, statistically speaking, are called intermediate and minor allergens, respectively.

CRIE can be used to define this more precisely. If so, a CRIE reference system has to be included in order to promote meaningful communication (8).

A *major allergen* is defined as one that binds IgE antibodies in at least 50% of serums from all the patients allergic to the substance and that shows strong binding in at least 25% of the serums. A *minor allergen* binds IgE antibodies in not more than 10% of the serums from the same patient population. It should be kept in mind that a so-called minor allergen may play a major role in rare individual patients. *Intermediate allergens* have binding capacities between these two.

Most food items seem to contain several distinct allergens of major, intermediate, or minor importance, respectively. They also contain an additional number of antigens which have not (yet) been shown to bind IgE antibodies. Egg white in hen's egg, for example, is a complex mixture of at least 20 distinct proteins but only 4 or 5 of them are said to be allergenic (9,10). It is possible and even likely that any one of the so-called non-IgE-binding antigens does bind IgE antibody in the serum of one or another rare individual who has not yet been studied in this respect.

Blands et al. (11) demonstrated 40 antigens in wheat flour. Eighteen of them were able to bind IgE and 3 were considered to be major allergens. Theobald et al. (12), in a study of the serums from patients with baker's asthma, concluded that IgE and IgG antibodies seemed to react with the same components in wheat. A clear-cut distinction between antigens and allergens was not obtained in their study.

These studies were concerned with inhalant allergies to flour, however, and the results are not necessarily applicable to cereals in food. The majority of individuals reacting to wheat dust tolerate wheat in the food because the most important allergens are destroyed through the process of making food from the flour. This represents a diagnostic pitfall which may result in meaningless elimination diets for a number of patients suffering only from the inhalant form of allergy to the flour.

Cow's milk contains more than 25 distinct proteins that may act as antigens in man. According to several investigators the most important allergens are found in β-lactoglobulin (60 to 80% of cow's milk-allergic patients), casein (60%), lactalbumin (50%), and bovine serum albumin (50%). Others claim that bovine serum albumin, casein, and bovine gamma globulin rank the highest.

WHAT MAKES A PROTEIN AN ALLERGEN?

During the past several years, many allergen sources have been studied. A wide variety of allergens have been isolated and characterized at least in part. However, most of this work has been concerned with inhalant allergens (13). One may ask why some proteins act as strong allergens whereas others in the same food do not. For some allergen sources, one may get the impression that the proteins found in the highest concentration are most likely to become allergens, but this is not consistently so. Casein, for instance, is by far the most prominent protein in cow's milk but it is not as important in allergy as β-lactoglobulin that represents approximately 10% of the total protein. Ovalbumin in hen's egg constitutes more than half of the total protein in the egg white, and is the most important allergen. Lysozyme, however, is a very weak allergen although it represents as much as 3.5 to 10% of the total protein.

Theoretically, there may be special physicochemical traits that are important for the transport of the molecule through living membranes, for passage of biochemical barriers, or for phagocyte handling without being directly related to antigenicity. Host factors are probably as important as the molecular structure (4). Features allowing the molecules to be absorbed from the intestinal lumen in active allergenic forms seem to be important for food allergens that elicit symptoms distant from the intestines. This depends not on the whole molecule, but on antigenic substructures, as shall be discussed later.

It has not been possible to point out any physicochemical feature that is characteristic for major allergens apart from being proteins with a molecular weight usually between 10,000 and 100,000 daltons. Those who study the classical scientific literature as to this may easily become confused or led astray. As evaluated today, some of the documentation has been confirmed, some has been shown to be only halfway true, and some has been dismissed as wrong. Completely pure allergen systems are mandatory for investigations of this kind. Impurities provide pitfalls that many have fallen into. There is a vast number of papers witnessing the sad fact that much time, resources, and printer's ink have been wasted on crude and impure preparations.

Furthermore, IgE molecules may also become bound to carbohydrate side chains in a nonspecific (nonimmunological) way. This is typical for so-called lectins not to be discussed in detail here. The presence of lectins in a number of food items is, however, of clinical importance because it results in a number of false-positive diagnoses and meaningless dietary restrictions.

DENATURATION AND DIGESTION

Identification of allergens in a given food starts with a crude extract of the matter. This involves the risk that some allergenic components are not represented in the original form or not at all in the extract. Some of them may be insoluble and lost in the sediment. Others may be present in an altered form. Denaturation and inactivation as to IgE binding may occur during the preparation of the extract. This occurs, for example, for some fruit allergens (14).

The molecular folding and charge of proteins are influenced by forces exerted on them from the environmental electrolytes and other proteins. The process of fractionation and isolation of protein molecules implies great risks of inducing alterations in the conformation and charges of some of the molecules in question. Dilution itself may induce marked changes. It is more likely than not that isolation and dilution induce some changes of the allergenic molecules that you purify. In fact, when you have succeeded at last to isolate an allergen with all signs of immunological homogeneity, you may detect that the material may be further separated in an electrical field when you use a medium and buffer of the right kind (or the wrong kind, as you may feel it!). Such so-called isoallergens are antigenically identical molecules that migrate differently in an electrical field. They may well represent the same original molecules but some of them may have been slightly changed as to conformation and charge during the separation manipulations. The changes do not, however, affect the antigenic and allergenic sites in question.

Questions about the degree of resistance to denaturation and digestion are especially important for food allergens. Clinical observations indicate this. Many of the allergens in question may be very susceptible to denaturation during preparation of the food. When it comes to allergens in apples, for instance, inactivation may occur as soon as the apple is cut and crushed. Furthermore, many patients react fiercely to raw but not cooked apples, carrots, and potatoes. A large number of bakers get allergic asthma or allergic rhinitis as an occupational disease from inhaling flour dust, but they tolerate the same cereal grains in the food.

On the other hand, many food items elicit allergic reactions almost irrespective of what you do to the food in question. They provoke allergic reactions even when found as steam droplets from the food being cooked or fried. This applies to hen's eggs, peanuts, nuts, peas, fish, and seafood. In other words, the allergenic epitopes in some food allergens are inactivated by denaturation and digestion; others are not affected. The latter maintain the allergenic activity. Here we have arrived at something essential in the discussion of the chemistry of food allergens.

EPITOPES (ANTIGENIC/ALLERGENIC DETERMINANTS)

The antibody (or the immune receptor of an immunocompetent lymphocyte) binds specifically to a very limited part of the antigenic molecule. This binding site is called an epitope or antigenic determinant. Part of the epitope reacts with the appropriate antibody-binding (Fab) part of the light chain and another part with the heavy chain of the antibody in question.

Allergenic epitope refers to the very limited part of the molecule that is bound to the antibody-binding (Fab_{IgE}) site of an IgE antibody. The number of allergenic epitopes which are accessible for the specific antibodies, and their binding dynamics, may be the factors that determine the potency of the particular allergen.

Most of what we know about epitopes is derived from studies with IgG antibodies. The complete antigenic anatomy with respect to epitopes has been mapped for hen's egg lysozyme, for example (15). This molecule acts as a minor allergen, but it is not known if IgE and IgG antibodies bind to the same epitopes on it. All proteins may be considered to be complex mosaics of epitopes reacting with antibodies of different immunoglobulin classes. Epitopes are in a way comparable to 4 to 20 letter words in the language of protein chemistry. Some features may be decisive, others less so seen from the antibody viewpoint. Some components may act only as necessary spacing elements keeping the essential denominators at an optimal distance from each other, or they may take part through more or less essential binding forces.

CONFORMATIONAL AND SEQUENTIAL EPITOPES

Most epitopes are conformational. They result from the three-dimensional folding of the molecule. The folding brings together amino acids that were originally found at different sites in the primary amino acid sequence chain. Denaturation of the protein will usually alter the folding and break up this kind of epitope. Laboratory manipulation during protein fractionation may have similar effects. This makes it particularly difficult to identify conformational epitopes. It is still more difficult to synthesize such epitopes.

A number of epitopes are sequential. They are organized from a number of amino acids (with or without sugar moieties) as found in the original linear amino acid sequence. This type of epitope often remains unchanged after denaturation of the protein and may be left untouched by enzymes not specific for amino acid bonds present within the epitope itself. Sequential epitopes thus lend themselves much more easily for identification and synthetization.

CROSS-REACTIVITIES

A number of the proteins present in a given food may have some epitopes in common. This accounts for immunological cross-reactivities between different proteins within a given food, and between different related foods. Patients allergic to the major allergen (Allergen M) in codfish, for example, therefore react also to haddock and carp white muscle proteins that also contain Allergen M. In fish allergy, some patients react to all fish species tested for, whereas others exhibit a marked species differentiation (15,16). Mackerel and salmon, for instance, contain some antigens in common with those of codfish and other quite distinct ones (Fig. 1). They do not contain Allergen M and hence do not cross-react with codfish with respect to the major allergen. For some patients, cross-reactivities implying intermediate and minor allergens may, however, be of significance.

Cross-reactivities are also found between eggs of different birds and between egg

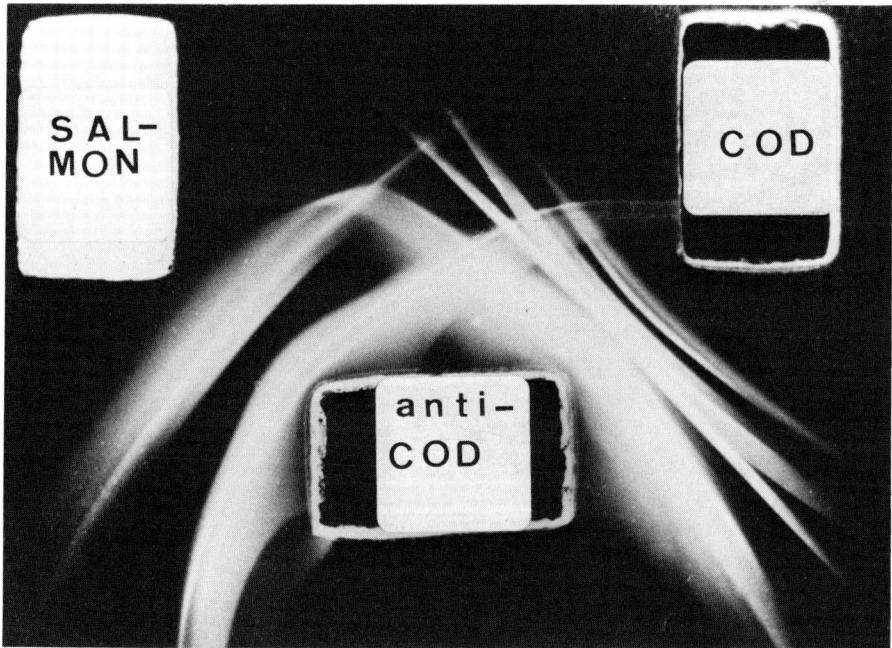

FIG. 1. Immunodiffusion experiment showing antigenic cross-reactivity and species differences, respectively, for salmon and codfish.

and muscle proteins of the bird, between different seafoods (17), and many other foods within the same order. Cross-reactivities are also found between certain pollen, vegetables, and fruits (18).

THE CODFISH ALLERGEN MODEL

Sequential allergenic epitopes representing major allergens are called for as tools in molecular research concerned with the immunology of allergy. This was one of the major concerns for scientists at the time I was myself occupied with this kind of research some years ago. At that time, as today, immunotherapy, for example, was widely practiced but we know nothing essential about the immunology associated with amelioration of allergy—be it through Nature or as a result of the therapy.

One reason for failure is most likely that our thinking and research could not compete with the immunological systems with respect to specificity and precision. Much discussion and research resources have, for example, been concerned with the role of so-called blocking antibodies, in the context of antibodies that bind to the allergenic molecule irrespective of binding sites. In allergy research and communication, however, we ought to be more precise and specific about immunological binding! It is not likely that a blocking antibody may interfere with IgE synthesis unless it affects the distinct IgE-binding epitope in question. The antibody of possible interest in this respect would be an allergenic epitope-blocking antibody.

There were indeed many questions to answer in this connection: Do all antibodies, be it IgG or IgE, bind to the same epitopes on the allergenic molecule? Does IgE react only with certain types of epitopes? What is an allergenic epitope? What makes an allergen an allergen?

A few years ago nobody had answers to these questions. Nothing was known about the composition and structure of allergens—not to mention the tiny fragments called epitopes.

It was a 7-month-old boy who presented me with a suitable model for research as to this. He was admitted to the pediatric department with severe atopic symptoms. The infant was entirely breast-fed and his symptoms occurred when his mother had eaten fish herself.

This observation suggested that the allergenic molecules in question had resisted (a) cooking (denaturation) followed by (b) digestion (proteolysis) in the mother's intestines, (c) passage through several membranes (to the breast milk), (d) a second digestion in the infant's intestines, and (e) new passages through living membranes in the infant. The allergens in question were still active when reaching the specific IgE antibodies in various tissues in the infant. From these observations, it was likely that the epitopes in question had to be associated with sequential units of amino acids and could probably be found in rather short fragments. Here was a model allergen for epitope research!

I selected codfish for the purpose after showing that most of the fish-allergic children seen in my department reacted to this species. Codfish was shown to contain one major allergen (Allergen M) found in the white muscle tissues. We were able to crystallize and isolate this major allergen (Fig. 2). All our codfish-allergic patients reacted to this allergen. In addition, codfish white muscle contains other intermediate and minor allergens and so does the blood serum of the fish.

In the most sensitive patient systems, the purified allergen was extremely potent. It provoked marked local whealing reactions in passive transfer or so-called Prausnitz-Küstner tests (PK tests) in concentrations corresponding to less than 10,000 molecules injected into the sensitized sites.

Double-blind food challenges with microgram quantities given to the PK-test recipients provoked similar reactions. The latter experiments confirmed that the purified allergen or fragments of it were absorbed in an active form also through normal adult intestines.

The material was used in several investigations. We found a good correlation between results of the radioallergosorbent test (RAST) and PK-passive transfer tests (19). Employing RAST we could show that serums from all our codfish-allergic patients contained IgE antibodies to the major allergen in question.

The major allergen is heat-stable and quite resistant to proteolytic digestion and denaturation procedures. This supported the idea that the allergenic activity might be found in a linear sequence. Further investigations confirmed this.

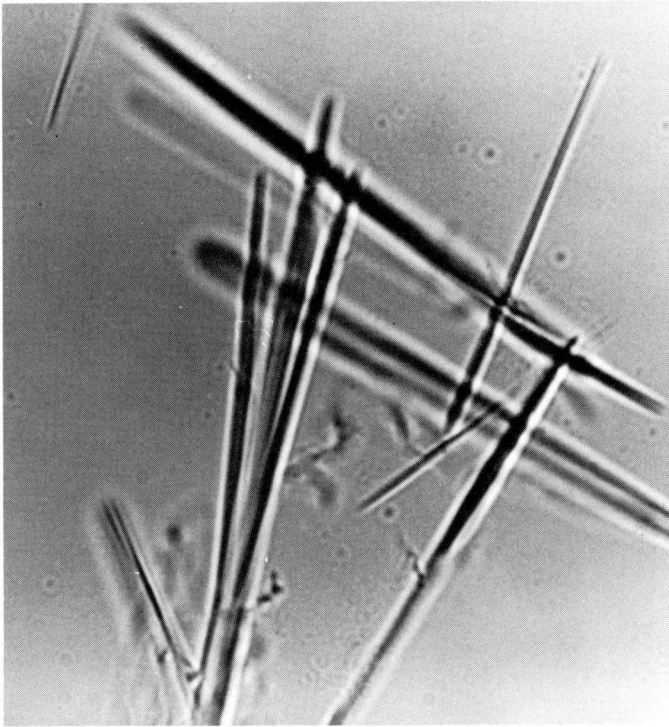

FIG. 2. Protein crystals containing the major allergen in codfish.

The purified allergen turned out to be a valuable tool for further work in basic as well as clinical work within the immunology of allergy. It was therefore shown that a large number of individuals had IgG antibodies to codfish but most of the IgG antibodies to codfish reacted with proteins other than the major allergen in question. Furthermore, some IgG antibodies (rabbit), which bound to the allergenic molecule, reacted with the same epitope as did IgE antibodies (human) but some did not; the latter reacted with quite different parts of the same molecule. This suggests that we have to revisit the role of so-called allergen-binding antibodies and allergenic epitope-blocking antibody.

CHARACTERIZATION OF AN ALLERGENIC EPITOPE

The amino acid sequence of the purified allergen was analyzed fragment by fragment. This provided enough material to propose the hypothetical model for a sequential allergenic determinant (IgE-binding epitope), presented during the 1975 Nobel Symposium in Stockholm (4). The hypothetical model has since then been substantiated and confirmed.

It was based on the assumption that the epitope may be formed by a few critical amino acid side chains found in a sequence. One or several amino acids present in the chain might act only as rather indifferent spacers keeping the important amino acids at an optimal distance from each other.

Furthermore, at that time, it had become evident that the biological reaction in IgE-mediated allergy was brought about when the allergen bound two IgE antibody molecules on the surface of mast cells or basophils. To be allergenically active, the allergen had to have at least two accessible allergenic determinants, probably of identical composition.

Assuming this, the molecule in question could have six (or even more) allergenic determinants (IgE-binding epitopes) composed by two closely connected carboxylic side chains (ASP + GLU) kept at a critical distance from the basic residue (LYS). According to this the sequences (-ASP-GLU-LEU-LYS-), (-ASP-GLU-ASP-LYS-) and possibly (-ASP-ASP-x-LYS-) pointed themselves out as particularly interesting candidates (Fig. 3a). Similar constellations could probably as well occur as conformational units (Fig. 3b). Short enzymatic cleavage products from the native Allergen M resulted in peptides containing ASP-GLU-LEU-LYS and ASP-GLU-ASP-LYS which were allergenically active.

Further investigation of this has been carried out by my former collaborator Said Elsayed, now in a laboratory in another city in Norway. He has shown that the region composed of residues 41–64 of Allergen M encompassed three of the tetrapep-

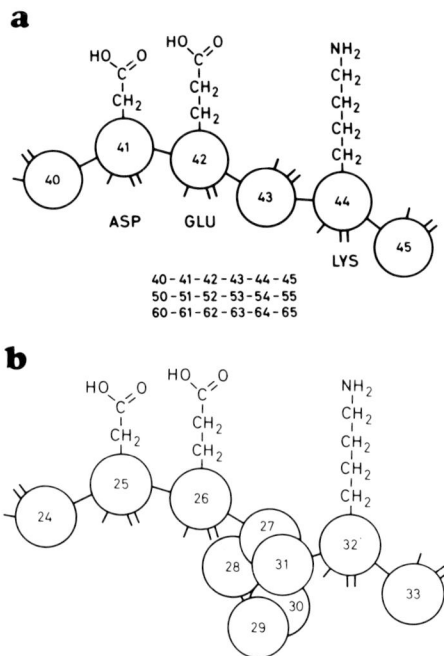

FIG. 3. (a) Sequential and (b) conformational combinations of amino acids thought to form allergenic epitopes in Allergen M of codfish.

tides described, kept apart by two segments of six variable amino acid residues. Initial efforts to block passive transfer tests and of RAST inhibition with a synthetic form of the tetrapeptide in question were not successful (Aas and Carlson, *unpublished observations*, 1977). Elsayed and co-workers (20) produced somewhat longer synthetic peptides corresponding to the allergenic active peptides in question. A synthetic peptide composed of 16 amino acids comprising two of the tetrapeptides bound IgE antibodies in the sera from codfish-allergic patients and was active in PK-transfer tests. The peptide also interfered with rabbit antiserum IgG antibodies to Allergen M (21,22). The nature of the interspacing amino acids appears to be without significance.

The 16-amino acid peptide was very active in inhibition experiments but not impressively active in direct *in vivo* tests. This observation together with the observation that the 4-amino acid peptide (-ASP-GLU-LEU-LYS-) alone did not inhibit the PK-transfer test or RAST (Aas and Carlson, *unpublished observations*, 1977) (20) suggest that the two tetrapeptides present in the 16-amino acid sequence may be mutually critical for the binding of the antibody in question. Perhaps the binding to the IgE antibody in question demands two almost identical tetrapeptides—one for the light-chain Fab and the other for the heavy-chain Fab?

IMPLICATIONS FOR FUTURE RESEARCH

At least two of the epitopes in question are necessary for the binding to IgE antibodies in the biological tests of allergy to codfish. The codfish study has suggested that quite small peptides may carry allergenic activity containing two identical epitopes for IgE antibodies. Peptides of that small size will easily pass into the circulation through normal and intact nonatopic intestines. This explains why even well-hydrolyzed cow's milk substitutes for mother's milk are able to provoke allergic reactions in some infants.

To act as an immunogen for IgE antibody synthesis only one epitope is sufficient. A carrier substance for the epitope structure may be provided by the host itself. In any case, extremely small fragments containing one epitope might suffice for sensitization in a disposed individual. Then it is not likely that sensitization depends only on the degree of permeability of the gut but rather on combinations of genetic and adjuvant factors in the host as well as the type of epitopes.

Furthermore, it is likely that efforts of oral immunotherapy will succeed only for those epitopes that are resistant to denaturation through digestion. Preliminary experimental efforts of oral hyposensitization with codfish allergens appeared effective, but were not extended to any controlled trial caused by difficulties to avoid severe reactions *(unpublished observations)*.

Many food items seem to contain resistant sequential epitopes and should lend themselves to epitope mapping. Among them, ovalbumin from hen's egg points itself out as a particularly suitable model because so much information is already available about ovalbumin. Identification of major allergenic epitopes in ovalbumin could provide important basic information. Availability of the epitopes would make it possible to study many aspects of allergy and tolerance, respectively. Work is in progress as to this (23).

Recently, allergenic epitopes have been identified on the major allergen in ragweed antigen E by using monoclonal antibodies (24). Monoclonal antibodies have also been used for epitope mapping of inhalant allergens found in the larvae of certain nonbiting insects *(Chironomus thummi thummi)*. These larvae are commonly used in a dried form as food for aquarium fishes. The dust from this may provoke allergic rhinitis and asthma in sensitized individuals (25).

These studies suggest that monoclonal antibodies may be powerful tools in the study of epitopes of isolated allergens also found in food for human consumers.

The availability of synthetic peptides that represent the allergenic epitopes of natural allergens may open new fields for studies of IgE-mediated immunology. They may prove valuable in efforts to unveil mechanisms in induction as well as suppression of the immune responses in question. Indeed, we need much more knowledge as to this for all kinds of allergen and particularly so in the confusing field of intolerance and allergy to food.

Patients think about allergy specificity with respect to allergen source. Physicians need to think about allergy specificity with respect to allergens on the molecular level. Scientists have to be concerned with allergen epitope specificity. To make progress, we have to sharpen our minds and be more specific and precise than before—on the same level of precision and specificity as the immunologically competent cells that we want to outmaneuver!

Modern techniques make efforts to isolate and characterize allergenic molecules and allergenic epitopes easier than before. This is not easy work, however! To the contrary, it is a demanding, tedious, and time-consuming process full of challenges, problems, pitfalls, and frustrations. It demands the most of specificity and precision. Any scientific aberration may be destructive for your results and interpretations. But it may also be very yielding—and it is often great fun!

REFERENCES

1. Aas K. The biochemistry of food allergens: what is essential for future research? In: Reinhardt D, Schmidt E, eds. *Food Allergy,* New York: Raven Press, 1988;1–11.
2. Bleumink E. Food allergy. The chemical nature of the substances eliciting symptoms. *World Rev Nutr Diet* 1970;12:505–70.
3. King TP. Chemical and biological properties of some atopic allergens. *Adv Immunol* 1976;23:77–105.
4. Aas K. Common characteristics of major allergens. In: Johansson SGO, Strandberg K, eds. *Molecular and Biological Aspects of the Acute Allergic Reaction*. New York: Plenum, 1976;3–19.
5. Aas K. What makes an allergen an allergen. *Allergy* 1978;33:3–14.
6. Aas K. Die Natur des Allergene. *Die gelben Hefte* 1980;20:77–85.
7. Brostoff J, Challacombe SJ, eds. *Food Allergy and Intolerance*. London: Baillière Tindall, 1987.
8. Aukrust L, Aas, K. A reference system in crossed radioimmunoelectrophoresis. *Scand J Immunol* 1977;6:1093–5.
9. Hoffman DR. Immunochemical identification of the allergens in egg white. *J Allergy Clin Immunol* 1983;71:481–6.

10. Langeland T, Aas K. Allergy to hen's egg white; clinical and immunological aspects. In: *Food Allergy and Intolerance*, Brostoff J, Challacombe SJ, eds. London: Baillière Tindall, 1987;367–74.
11. Blands J, Diamant B, Kallos P, Kallos-Deffner L, Löwenstein, H. Flour allergy in bakers. I. Identification of allergenic fractions in flour and comparison of diagnostic methods. *Int Arch Allergy Appl Immunol* 1976;52:392–406.
12. Theobald K, Thiel H, Kallweit C, Ulmer W, Konig W. Detection of proteins in wheat flour extracts that bind human IgG, IgE, and mouse monoclonal antibodies. *J Allergy Clin Immunol* 1986;78:470–7.
13. Marsh DG, Goodfriend L, King TP, Löwenstein H, Platts-Mills TAE. Allergen nomenclature. *Bull WHO* 1986;64:761–7.
14. Björkstén F, Halmepuro L, Hannuksela M, Lahti A. Extraction and properties of apple allergens. *Allergy* 1980;35:671–7.
15. Aas K. Fish allergy and the codfish allergen model. In: *Food Allergy and Intolerance*, Brostoff J, Challacombe SJ, eds. London: Baillière Tindall, 1987;356–66.
16. Aas K. Studies of hypersensitivity to fish. Allergological and serological differentiation between various species of fish. *Int Arch Allergy Appl Immunol* 1966;30:257–267.
17. Lehrer SB. The complex nature of food antigens: studies of cross-reacting crustacea allergens. *Ann Allergy* 1986;57:267–72.
18. Dreborg S, Foucard T. Allergy to apple, carrot and potato in children with birch allergy. *Allergy* 1983;38:167–72.
19. Foucard T, Johnasson SGO, Aas K. Concentration of IgE antibodies, PK-titers and chopped lung titres in sera from children with hypersensitivity to cod. *J Allergy* 1973;51:39–44.
20. Elsayed S, Titlestad K, Apold J, Aas K. A synthetic hexadecapeptide derived from Allergen M imposing allergenic and antigenic reactivity. *Scand J Immunol* 1980;12:171–5.
21. Elsayed S, Apold J. Immunochemical analysis of codfish Allergen M; locations of the immunoglobulin binding sites as demonstrated by the native and synthetic peptides. *Allergy* 1983;38:449–59.
22. Elsayed S. The native and synthetic peptides of codfish Allergen M. A short review. In: Boström H, Epne H, Ljungstedt N, eds. *Theoretical and Clinical Aspects of Allergic Diseases*. Stockholm: Almqvist & Wiksell, 1983;237–53.
23. Elsayed S, Holen E, Haugstad MB. Antigenic and allergenic determinants of ovalbumin. II. The reactivity of the NH_2 terminal decapeptide. *Scand J Immunol* 1988;27:587–91.
24. Olson JR, Klapper DG. Two major human allergic sites on ragweed pollen allergen antigen E identified by using monoclonal antibodies. *J Immuol* 1986;136:2109–11.
25. Mazur G, Becker W-M, Baur X. Epitope mapping of major insect allergens (chironomid hemoglobins) with monoclonal antibodies. *J Allergy Clin Immunol* 1987;80:876–883.

Food Intolerance in Infancy: Allergology, Immunology, and Gastroenterology, edited by Robert N. Hamburger. Carnation Nutrition Education Series, Vol. 1. The Carnation Co., Los Angeles/Raven Press, Ltd., New York © 1989.

Transfer of Antigens via Breast Milk

Steven Machtinger

Children's Hospital at Stanford, Palo Alto, CA 94304

When one considers that 70 years have passed since Talbot first noted the association between eczema in an exclusively breast-fed infant and chocolate eaten by the nursing mother, it is surprising that the concept of sensitization to food antigens present in breast milk is neither widely accepted nor even widely known. In fact, only 11 years after Talbot's report in the first volume of the *Medical Clinics of North America* (1), Harry Donnally (2) conclusively demonstrated that intact hen's egg antigens gain access to breast milk within 1 to 2 hr following maternal egg ingestion.

Perhaps the landmark study of Grulee and Sanford (3) suggesting a protective effect of breast-feeding over cow's milk-based formula led researchers to view nursing in a different light. Perhaps the rise in the use of proprietary and condensed milk formulas with the subsequent decline of breast-feeding made this line of inquiry seem archaic. Whatever the reason, few articles appeared on the subject between 1930 and 1975.

In the past 15 years, as a result of Western society's rekindled interest in nursing, there has been a burgeoning number of reports of infants whose atopic or adverse symptoms could be attributed to food antigens present in their mother's milk. Armed with new, although not necessarily more powerful, immunologic techniques, researchers have confirmed and extended the work of Donnally.

Many questions remain speculative or at best partly answered. With what frequency and in what amounts do food antigens gain access to breast milk? How soon do food antigens appear in breast milk after maternal ingestion? How long do they persist after dietary restriction? How often is the presence of food antigens in the breast milk associated with adverse reactions in the nursing infant? Is there a relationship between the amount of antigen in the milk and the effect on the infant? Is the amount present sufficient to both sensitize susceptible infants and precipitate symptoms? Are other factors present that modify the effect of antigen upon the infant? Is the presence of food antigen in breast milk an incidental, accidental, or intentional biologic phenomenon? The purpose of this chapter will be to address some of these questions.

DO FOOD ANTIGENS ENTER BREAST MILK?

A number of both direct and indirect methods have been employed to implicate food antigens in breast milk as the cause of adverse reactions in the nursing infant. Indirect methods involve exploiting the effects visited upon the infant. This may be approached clinically by assessing the response of the breast-fed infant's symptoms to manipulation of the maternal diet. Alternatively, measurement of food-specific immunoglobulin E (IgE) antibodies by skin testing or radioallergosorbent test (RAST) in presumably exclusively breast-fed infants could indicate sensitization via the breast.

As will be discussed further, the latter methods depend upon certifying that exposure to specific foods has not occurred by any other route. The former method has often depended upon observation of subjective symptoms such as colic and diarrhea. Such symptoms may be difficult to quantify. Although dramatic and irrefutable symptoms have been recorded in exclusively breast-fed infants, elimination of bias requires blinding, verification by qualified observers, and sometimes repetition of elimination and oral challenge. Hence, direct methods are preferable in the demonstration of food antigens in breast milk.

Within several years after Talbot's description (1), Shannon (4) reported that guinea pigs sensitized to egg proteins, either by injection of egg white or by human breast milk thought to contain egg, could suffer anaphylaxis when later challenged with the opposite substance. His observations could not be duplicated (5) and were called into question (2).

In May 1929, Henry H. Donnally (2) presented the results of an elegant experiment at a meeting of the Society for the Study of Asthma and Allied Conditions. Expanding upon the work of Walzer (6) he used an adaptation of the Prausnitz-Küstner reaction to detect egg antigen in the skin of 14/15 and the breast milk of 3/15 normal lactating women. Having passively sensitized an area of the skin of each woman with reagin-containing serum from a boy highly allergic to egg, he then challenged each mother with a breakfast of two raw eggs over ice. In 93% of the cases, wheal and flare patterns appeared promptly at the site of injected reagin. He thus confirmed Walzer's demonstration that intact food antigens may be readily absorbed from the gastrointestinal tract of normal individuals.

Later, Donnally passively sensitized other areas of skin of these 14 women and rechallenged with raw eggs. Using the wheal and flare reaction as an indication of antigen absorption, he then collected breast milk from these women by electric breast pump. The whey fraction of these milk specimens was injected into the arms of other passive recipients of reagin (Fig. 1). For negative controls, breast milk obtained after an overnight fast but prior to oral egg challenge was injected into adjacent, previously passively, sensitized sites. Donnally was able to demonstrate the presence of egg antigen in 20% of subjects. It has been estimated that this method was sufficiently sensitive to detect egg antigens at concentrations in breast milk ranging from 20 pg to 20 ng/ml (7).

Thus, nearly 60 years ago, Donnally had proven that food antigens could enter breast milk. He did not, however, examine either the persistence of antigen in sub-

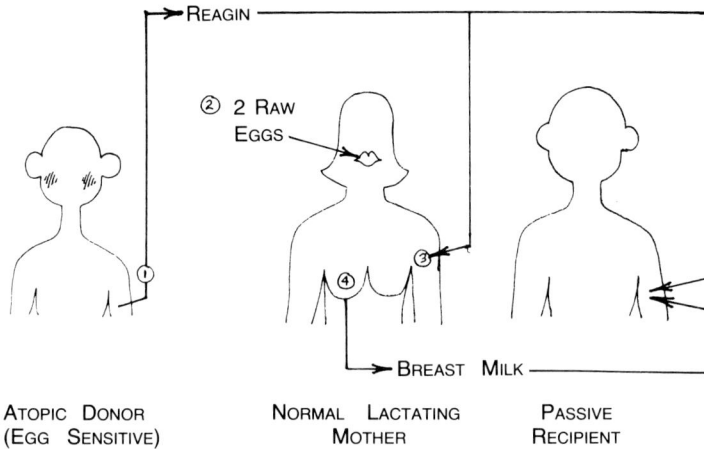

FIG. 1. Detection of food antigens in breast milk by passive sensitization with reagin. **1**: Blood containing Reagin (IgE antibody) is removed from egg-sensitive child with dermatitis and used to sensitize passively the skin of normal nursing mothers and other normal recipients. **2**: Breast milk is collected from nursing women after overnight fast. After ingestion of two raw eggs, additional breast milk is collected after passively sensitized skin develops typical wheal and flare pattern (**3**), indicating intestinal absorption of egg antigens. **4**: Whey fraction of breast milk is ingested into passively sensitized skin of second recipient. If breast milk contains egg antigen, skin develops wheal and flare reaction. (From Donnally, ref. 2, with permission.)

sequent breast milk specimens or the relationship of such antigens to symptoms in nursing infants. Moreover, although he had demonstrated that food antigens may enter breast milk under experimental conditions, raw eggs on an empty stomach do not constitute a typical breakfast.

Almost 50 years later, Jakobsson and Lindberg (8) reported that cow's milk protein should be detected in human breast milk by the relatively insensitive method of Ouchterlony, immunoprecipitation in gel. Their findings were questioned because of the known limits of this method (approximately 1 μg/ml) and because the antiserums used were not shown to be specific to cow's milk (7,9). Others (10) were unable to replicate the results, observing cross-reactivity of antiserums with human milk proteins. Of the major cow's milk proteins, only β-lactoglobulin has no human counterpart and may be used as a marker for cow's milk protein in breast milk. Employing rabbit antiserums against β-lactoglobulin, immunoprecipitation in gel was found to be insufficiently sensitive to detect cow's milk antigens in breast milk (10).

In 1984, Kilshaw and Cant (7) developed a solid-phase, double-antibody, sandwich-type radioimmunoassay to measure several food antigens in breast milk. β-Lactoglobulin as well as ovalbumin and ovomucoid were used as antigens. Utilizing this method, β-lactoglobulin was detected in the breast milk of 53% of 19 women following ingestion of 8 ounces of whole cow's milk. Antigen was seen as late as 6 hr after maternal milk challenge (Table 1).

Jakobsson et al. (11) used a somewhat different radioimmunoassay technique to find β-lactoglobulin in the breast milk of 47% of 38 women. No special diet was prescribed. In a later communication using the same assay, this antigen was de-

TABLE 1. *Presence of β-lactoglobulin in breast milk*

Author/year	Method	N	% Pos.	% >1 ng	High concn.[a] (ng/ml)	Duration	Diet
Kilshaw and Cant, 1984 (7)	RIA[b]	19	53	26	6.4	6 hr	8 oz. milk
Stuart et al., 1984 (13)	ELISA[b]	28	18	18	20	12 hr	Usual
Jakobsson et al., 1985 (11)	RIA	38	47	47	33	9 days	Usual
Machtinger and Moss, 1986 (10)	ELISA	41	70	12	6.4	3 days	Usual

[a]Highest concentration detected.
[b]RIA, radioimmunoassay; ELISA, enzyme-linked immunosorbent assay.

tected on one occasion at levels exceeding 800 ng/ml (12). With a minimum sensitivity of 5 ng/ml, they found β-lactoglobulin in 93 of 232 or 40% of breast-milk specimens from 25 women. Only 5% of the positive specimens contained β-lactoglobulin in excess of 100 ng/ml. These were all collected from the same mother over a period of time. In another mother who abstained from all dairy products because of symptoms of colic in her infant, β-lactoglobulin could still be detected at low levels 9 days after challenge (11).

Double-antibody, sandwich enzyme-linked immunosorbent assay (ELISA) methods have also been used to detect β-lactoglobulin in breast milk. Stuart et al. (13) found β-lactoglobulin in 18% of 28 women at levels as high as 20 ng/ml. The apparent limit of sensitivity of their assay, although not explicitly stated, appeared to be 1 ng/ml. In their subject group, this cow's milk antigen could be detected as late as 12 hr after withholding milk from the maternal diet.

Utilizing a similar technique but with a sensitivity of 10 pg/ml, Machtinger and Moss (10) found β-lactoglobulin in the breast milk of 70% of 41 women at concentrations as high as 6.4 ng/ml. In 12% of the women, levels exceeded 1 ng/ml. In one woman whose diet excluded dairy products because of colic in her nursing infant, β-lactoglobulin at a concentration of 1 ng/ml was detected several hours after a challenge with milk and ice cream. This bovine antigen fell to 340 pg/ml 3 days after the mother once again eliminated dairy products and was undetectable by the 5th postchallenge day. The infant's colicky symptoms resolved within 48 hr (Fig. 2).

Other food antigens have been detected in breast milk (Table 2). Ovalbumin and ovomucoid have been measured by radioimmunoassay (RIA) following a raw egg meal. They were detected in 59 and 78%, respectively, at levels as high as 6.2 and 2.9 ng/ml (7).

Wheat antigens were found by Kulangara (14) in 16 of 17 random breast-milk samples using passive cutaneous anaphylaxis. Recently a double-antibody, sandwich ELISA method with a sensitivity of 1 ng/ml was employed to detect gliadin in 54 of 80 breast-milk samples from 53 women in amounts ranging from 5 to 95 ng/ml

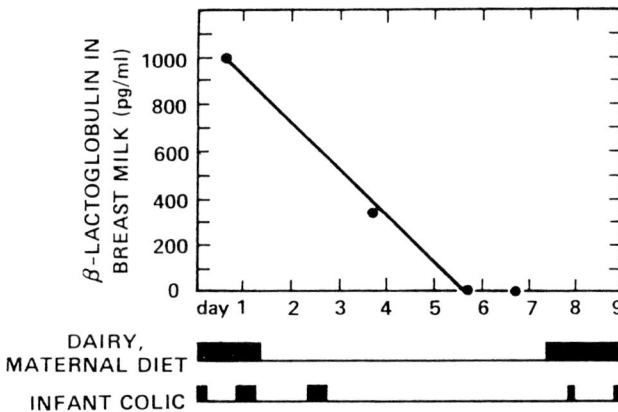

FIG. 2. Persistence of β-lactoglobulin in breast milk for at least 3 days after reintroduction of cow's milk into maternal diet. Note correlation of infantile colic with maternal milk intake and presence of β-lactoglobulin in ingested breast milk. (From Machtinger and Moss, ref. 10, with permission.)

(15). The percentage of breast-milk specimens containing antigen was much higher in the 1st week after parturition than at later times (77% versus approximately 50% at 6, 12, and 20 weeks). Moreover, breast milk specimens containing gliadin at levels in excess of 10 ng/ml were found only during the 1st week of lactation. Gliadin appeared in maximal amounts in milk obtained 2 to 4 hr after maternal challenge.

These studies indicate that food antigens such as cow's milk, egg, and wheat commonly enter breast milk in measurable quantities. Levels in excess of 100 ng/ml are unusual although a few specimens contain individual antigen concentrations in excess of 35 ng/ml. Nevertheless, most breast milk specimens contain various food antigens at levels ranging from several picograms to several nanograms per milliliter. These antigens appear promptly in the breast milk after maternal ingestion but

TABLE 2. *Presence of food antigens in breast milk*

Author/year	Food	Method	N	% Pos.	High concn.[a] (ng/ml)	Duration (hr)	Diet
Donnally, 1930 (2)	Egg	PK[b]	15	20	20		2 Raw eggs
Kilshaw and	OA[b]	RIA[b]	22	59	6.2	6	1 Raw egg
Cant, 1984 (7)	OM[b]	RIA	9	78	2.9	6	1 Raw egg
Troncone et al., 1987 (15)	GLIA[b]	ELISA[b]	53	68	95	6	20 g GLIA

[a]Highest concentration detected.
[b]PK, Prausnitz-Küstner reaction; OA, ovalbumin; RIA, radioimmunoassay; OM, ovomucoid; GLIA, gliadin; ELISA, enzyme-linked immunosorbent assay.

may persist for several days at gradually decreasing levels following maternal abstention.

Given an average feeding of 120 ml of breast milk, a nursing infant might receive several micrograms of antigen to any given food several times each day. This is an amount considered sufficient for sensitization.

A point has been made that care must be taken to avoid cross-contamination of specimens in studies where antigens are measured at levels as low as these (2,7). After all, when one is dealing with substances in amounts not exceeding 0.0003% of an ounce, the methods employed must be scrutinized as meticulously as the results. Kilshaw and Cant (7) report that nanogram quantities of β-lactoglobulin may be detected in washings from the hands of laboratory personnel. Having sounded this note of caution, it is concluded that the presence of food antigens in breast milk may be accepted without further question.

DO FOOD ANTIGENS PRESENT IN BREAST MILK CAUSE ADVERSE REACTIONS IN INFANTS?

The discovery by observant clinicians, that foods present in the maternal diet could adversely influence the nursing infant, created the field of breast milk immunology. The history of the subject has been one of conflicting claims that breast-feeding either protects against or promotes allergic sensitization and related problems in infants. Although protective effects of breast-feeding remain inconclusive, it is well established that food antigens present in breast milk may induce a variety of adverse reactions in nursing infants.

The optimal demonstration of such adverse reactions involves a simple modification of the classical double-blind oral challenge used to diagnose food allergy or intolerance. A suspect food is eliminated from the maternal diet. The infant is observed for resolution of some untoward symptom. If the infant improves, the mother is then challenged with the eliminated food in an attempt to precipitate a return of the infant's symptoms. The challenge is performed under blinded conditions. An alternate method involves challenging the infant directly with the incriminated food antigen.

Surprisingly few double-blind challenges have been reported in the literature. Cow's milk protein has been demonstrated to induce colic (16), colitis (17,18), and anaphylactic shock (17). Eczema has been induced by breast milk containing either egg (19) or soy protein (18). Warner's study (19) is particularly interesting as he was able to demonstrate that breast milk obtained from the mother receiving egg in her diet could cause a classical wheal and flare pattern when injected into the infant's skin. Breast milk obtained while the mother abstained from egg did not cause a reaction by skin testing.

A greater number of reports have not taken the pains to blind the observers, whether parents or clinicians, to the nature of the challenge food. Under such conditions, symptoms such as diarrhea, vomiting, rhinorrhea, wheezing, and urticaria as well as eczema and colic have been attributed to foods such as citrus fruits, wheat, chocolate, coffee, apple, and banana (1,20,21). The reliability of these studies depends upon the severity and consequent unambiguous nature of the infant's symptoms and upon the credibility of the observer. Nevertheless, a sufficient number of double-blind and well-documented unblinded cases have been reported to conclude that food antigens present in breast milk do precipitate adverse effects in infants.

CAN FOOD ANTIGENS PRESENT IN BREAST MILK SENSITIZE NURSING INFANTS?

Having determined that food antigens commonly gain access to breast milk in significant amounts and that typical atopic symptoms may be precipitated by such antigens in breast-fed babies, one would think it an easy exercise to prove that sensitization of the infant is the result. This is not the case. Because exposure to food antigens may occur from other sources, proving that it is antigen in breast milk that is at fault is difficult. A case report is illustrative.

Case report. A 12-month-old female infant developed anaphylaxis following the ingestion of 5 ounces of low-fat milk. The infant had received her first feeding of cow's milk the previous evening when 1 ounce was tolerated without apparent adverse effect. The episode began with uncontrollable sneezing and clear rhinorrhea starting several minutes after the milk ingestion. Within 20 min the infant developed hives of the chest, face, and eyelids and irritability. Fifteen min later, respiratory distress with wheezing became evident. The child became unresponsive and limp. Paramedics were summoned. At a local emergency room, the infant received epinephrine and diphenhydramine. She made an uneventful recovery within 5 hr. Cow's milk RAST drawn on that day was class 4 + (>17.5 Phedebas RAST Units (PRU)).

The infant, a normal full-term product of an uneventful pregnancy, had been exclusively breast-fed until 7 months when selected solid foods were sequentially introduced. The infant was weaned to a proprietary soy protein formula at 10 months without incident. The mother, an immunologist, had taken pains to exclude cow's milk from her child's diet because of her knowledge of the increased risk for cow's milk protein allergy during infancy and because of a history of asthma and eczema in her husband. The mother had no history of atopic disease and did not restrict her own diet during pregnancy nor after her daughter's birth. Feeding of supplemental cow's milk-based formula in the newborn nursery could not be excluded as having occurred.

Following the anaphylactic episode, the infant was placed on a strict exclusion diet. A repeat cow's milk RAST performed 4 months later was still class 3 (12.1 PRU). RAST against casein and β-lactoglobulin were class 0 and class +/− (0.20 PRU), respectively. Total IgE was 74 IU/ml, a significant elevation for a child of 15 months of age. Interestingly, the mother had a class 2 RAST to β-lactoglobulin despite a total IgE of only 4.64 IU/ml and no history of milk intolerance. The mother's breast milk obtained prior to weaning contained 740 pg/ml of β-lactoglobulin determined by double-antibody solid-phase ELISA.

The infant did not receive skin testing or intentional oral challenge. One year after the anaphylactic event, she was inadvertently fed six cheese-containing crackers. Despite receiving syrup of Ipecac and vomiting, urticaria developed within 15 min. A repeat RAST test against cow's milk was once again class 4 (>17.5 PRU). Two and a half years after the initial reaction, this child continues to avoid dairy products.

Other authors have sited similar episodes of anaphylaxis following the first feeding of milk or other common food allergens after a presumed period of exclusive breast-feeding (20,22,23). Confirmation of sensitization has been accomplished by skin testing (20) or RAST (23).

These are dramatic case histories but they do not prove that sensitization occurred via the breast. Other possible routes of food-antigen exposure must be considered and eliminated in order to reach that conclusion. These routes include exposure in the intrauterine environment, and inadvertent or surreptitious feedings of food antigens during the period of exclusive breast-feeding (Table 3).

Even in the case sited above, where cow's milk antigens were measured in the breast milk, sensitization might have occurred by some alternate route. One might argue that mother's milk contained sufficient foreign antigen to sensitize if not to precipitate symptoms. Yet in this case, 1 ounce of milk fed directly to the infant failed to precipitate symptoms. That means that to prove sensitization by means of breast milk, it would be necessary to exclude previous exposure of the infant to at least 1 ounce of cow's milk from other sources.

Intrauterine exposure to substances in the maternal diet has been documented for drugs, viral antigens, helminthic infections, and toxins as well as foods. Evidence that intrauterine sensitization occurs comes from two quarters: clinical reports of infants whose adverse reactions, especially anaphylactic reactions, began after their first feedings of cow's milk formulas in the newborn nursery (17), and the detection of food-specific IgE antibodies in serum of newborn infants. IgE antibodies have been detected in newborns against milk (24), egg (25), and wheat antigens (26). It has been estimated that intrauterine sensitization accounts for 1 to 2% of all infantile food allergy (27).

Exposure of the nursing infant to food antigens during early extrauterine life may

TABLE 3. *Potential vectors of infantile sensitization to foods*

Intrauterine
Breast milk
Adventitial or surreptitious
   Nursery
   Alternate caregivers
   Parental protocol variances
   Ingredients in prepared foods
   Trace amounts contaminating hands, lips, clothes, etc.

occur from many quarters. Infants often receive cow's milk-based formula supplements in the newborn nursery (23). It is possible to eliminate this source of potential sensitization if the nursery adopts a policy of no supplementation other than water (28). From a clinical standpoint, this is impractical as each pediatrician will have a personal approach to supplementation in the immediate postpartum period when breast milk volume is still low.

A source of exogenous food antigens more difficult to control is food fed to the breast-feeding infant by alternate caregivers. Apparently, grandmothers have been found to be notable miscreants in this area of protocol violations. Hamburger et al. (29) found that four exclusively breast-fed infants, followed prospectively from before birth, developed positive skin tests to egg protein at 4 months of age. In three of the four cases, furtive feedings of egg had been given by grandparents. Babysitters and day-care facilities place the parent out of the direct line of supervision of their infant's diet. Such caregivers may feed the child food containing restricted antigens.

Compliance even among highly motivated atopic parents or parents whose previous children have had significant problems with allergic conditions during infancy may falter as the infant matures. Zeiger et al. (27) excluded cow's milk from the diet of infants and nursing mothers from the last trimester through the 1st year of age. This restriction was part of an allergy avoidance protocol designed to test the hypothesis that with appropriate education and support, infants from high-risk atopic families could be shielded from environmental precipitins. Using cow's milk-specific IgG antibodies in the infant as a marker for milk ingestion, they found that by 1 year of age, 30% of the children had received cow's milk in violation of the protocol. Moreover, food allergy or food-specific IgE was found four times more frequently in these infants than in those whose parents had not circumvented the protocol.

It is difficult for caring parents to resist the temptation to give their inquisitive infants just a taste of ice cream or some other delicacy off their own dish. Such a seemingly insignificant morsel consisting of only a gram or so of food represents an exposure at least a thousand times greater than the approximately half a microgram of the same antigen that might be present in a feeding of breast milk.

In all likelihood, sensitization occurs by means of food antigens present in breast milk. The proof that this occurs is elusive and probably irrelevant. A more germane question is, will infants who are exclusively breast-fed become sensitized to common food antigens prior to weaning despite a genuine attempt at prevention? To frame the question in this fashion takes into account the reality of child-rearing, the multiplicity of paths by which food exposure may occur, and the rigors of compliance.

IS BREAST-FEEDING DETRIMENTAL TO INFANTS?

In hopes of preventing, diminishing, or at least delaying the onset of food allergy in high-risk infants, proponents have advocated exclusive breast-feeding as a means of avoiding foreign food proteins during the first few months of life (30–32). This is a period thought to be characterized by increased vulnerability caused by immaturity of the gastrointestinal system (33) and of the immune system (34). Controversy over the advantages of breast-feeding has raged since the time of Grulee and Sanford (3). Although some studies have claimed profound benefits from breast-feeding, others have demonstrated negligible effects. Still others have reported breast milk to be disadvantageous. The subject has been recently and admirably reviewed by Kramer (35).

The realization that food antigens are present in breast milk indicates a fallacy in the hypothesis that breast milk should be advantageous over other forms of nutrition. An exclusive diet of breast milk is not one free of food antigens. Rather it is one which contains a multitude of food antigens although in very small amounts. One may entertain teleological arguments of why such antigen presentation might benefit the immunologically normal infant. Whatever that argument, it may not apply to the infant inclined to allergy by genetic predisposition.

Two theories have been proposed to explain how sensitization occurs in infancy. Taylor et al. (34) suggested that a relative paucity of secretory IgA (sIgA) antibodies in the immature newborn gut permits excessive absorption of undigested food antigens. An otherwise normal IgE system would thus be stimulated by these unimpeded foreign antigens.

It has been suggested that breast milk could benefit infants in two ways. Breast milk contains sIgA antibodies directed against food antigens (36). These passively acquired antibodies could bind to IgA receptors on the luminal surface of intestinal enterocytes helping to limit the absorption of food antigens from the gut (33). It has even been proposed that sIgA facilitates digestion of food antigens (37). Breast milk also contains soluble factors which have been shown to stimulate cord blood lymphocytes to mature and produce IgA (38). Thus, breast milk could provide temporary passive immunity while stimulating active immunity in the nursing infant.

On the other hand, Jarrett (39) proposed that the defect in atopic disease is an inability of suppressor thymus-derived cells (T cells) to inhibit IgE production by plasma cells. In this theory, antigens commonly cross the mucosa of the respiratory and gastrointestinal tract in quantities sufficient to trigger an immunological response. This is thought to occur despite the presence of an intact luminal immunologic barrier that includes sIgA. In both normal and atopic individuals, helper T cells are stimulated at exceedingly low levels of antigen to promote IgE synthesis. With increasing exposure, normal suppressor T cells inhibit IgE synthesis. In the atopic state, this suppressor inhibition is believed to be defective responding only to much higher levels of antigen and resulting in continued IgE synthesis.

Studies of cow's milk protein allergy in infancy have supported the latter theory. Gerrard and Shenassa (20) have contrasted cow's milk allergy in infants fed either formula or breast milk. They found that although positive skin tests were uncommon in the allergic formula-fed group, they were prominent in breast-fed infants and often associated with large wheals. Reactions to oral challenge were striking in the breast-fed group as opposed to their formula-fed counterparts. They concluded that food allergies in formula-fed infants might not be IgE-mediated although those in breast-fed infants certainly are. Similar findings have been noted by others (40).

In a prospective study, Björkstén and Saarinen (41) found that cow's milk RASTs were elevated only in infants who had been assigned to the exclusively breast-fed group. Interestingly, although they felt that sensitization had occurred in the newborn nursery, positive RASTs were not detected until 4 to 6 months of age, suggesting later exposure. Total IgE has also been found to be higher at 12 months of age among infants who were weaned later than their counterparts (42). These findings have been reproduced by others (43).

In a recent prospective study, Lindfors and Enocksson (44) reported that breast-fed infants who received significant amounts of cow's milk-based formula in the newborn nursery were less likely to develop atopic disease by 18 months of age than similar infants who had not received supplementation. The difference was confined to infants with a biparental history of atopy. In these subgroups, atopic disease was six times more likely if the infant was exclusively breast-fed than if they had received cow's milk supplements (44).

Such studies would appear to support Jarrett's contention (39) that sensitization is promoted by exposure to small amounts of antigen and overcome by larger quantities. Donnally's observations (2), that food antigen is readily absorbed across the intact intestinal mucosal lining, lend support to the concept that gut-associated sIgA can never completely exclude foreign antigens and further substantiates this line of evidence.

On the other hand, there is some evidence in support of transient sIgA deficiency as a cause of atopic disease in infancy. sIgA antibodies directed against cow's milk proteins have been detected in breast milk (30,36). An association has been found between low levels of anti-cow's milk sIgA in the breast milk of mothers and high allergy symptom scores in their exclusively breast-fed infants (Fig. 3). This report, however, was retrospective in design and awaits confirmation through a prospective study now in progress (10).

Contrarily, despite the presence of sIgA in breast milk, researchers have been unable to demonstrate a significant difference between breast-fed and formula-fed infants in salivary content of either total IgA (45) or specific sIgA directed against casein or β-lactoglobulin (46).

Thus, there is little compelling evidence to recommend exclusive breast-feeding over alternate forms of nutrition as a means to prevent allergic sensitization.

Breast-feeding may be beneficial when it is part of an ambitious program of allergen avoidance including complete elimination of allergenic foods from the maternal diet and delayed introduction of weaning foods coupled to additional environmental control measures in the home. Such a program is difficult to implement and even more difficult to maintain (27). Moreover, when infractions of the protocol regimen occur, the infant may become sensitized. Infants sensitized in such a fashion may later experience profound allergic symptoms at the time of weaning.

In conclusion, food antigens commonly enter breast milk and may cause adverse reactions in nursing infants. Sensitization to food antigens probably occurs via

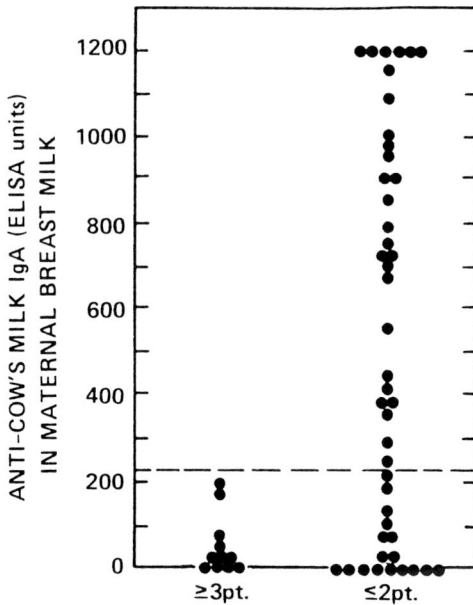

FIG. 3. Breast-milk immunoglobulin A (IgA) antibody levels (in enzyme-linked immunosorbent assay (ELISA) units) in infant groups of high and low symptom scores. Each point represents average antibody content of multiple samples from an individual mother's breast milk (mean 3.5). All 11 of the high-score symptom group received milk with antibody levels below the median value (220 ELISA units, *dashed line*) versus 17 of 26 in the low-score symptom group (chi-square = 13.7; $p < 0.001$). (From Machtinger and Moss, ref. 10, with permission.)

breast milk but is difficult to prove because infants may be exposed to foods from a variety of sources. Little advantage has been demonstrated from exclusive breast-feeding as a means to delay the onset of allergic sensitization in infants at risk for atopy unless as part of a more universal program of allergen avoidance. Such a program is difficult to maintain and thus prone to failure.

REFERENCES

1. Talbot FB. Eczema in childhood. *Med Clin North Am* 1918;1:985–6.
2. Donnally HH. The question of the elimination of foreign protein (egg-white) in woman's milk. *J Immunol* 1930;19:15–40.
3. Grulee CG, Sanford HN. The influence of breast and artificial feeding on food antigen infantile eczema. *J Pediatr* 1936;8:223–5.
4. Shannon WR. Demonstration of food proteins in human breast milk by anaphylactic experiments in guinea pigs. *Am J Dis Child* 1921;22;223–31.
5. Stuart HC. The excretion of foreign protein in human milk. *Am J Dis Child* 1923;25:135–56.
6. Walzer M. Studies in absorption of undigested proteins in human beings. *J Immunol* 1927;14:143–74.
7. Kilshaw PJ, Cant AJ. The passage of maternal dietary proteins into human breast milk. *Int Arch Allergy Appl Immunol* 1984;75:8–15.
8. Jakobsson I, Lindberg T. Cow's milk as a cause of infantile colic in breast-fed infants. *Lancet* 1978;2:437–9.
9. Shacks SJ, Heiner DC. Allergy to breast milk. *Clin Immunol Allergy* 1982;2:121–36.
10. Machtinger S, Moss R. Cow's milk allergy in breast-fed infants: the role of antigen and maternal secretory IgA antibody. *J Allergy Clin Immunol* 1986;77:341–7.

11. Jakobsson I, Lindberg T, Benediktsson B, Hansson BG. Dietary bovine β-lactoglobulin is transferred to human milk. *Acta Paediatr Scand* 1985;74:342–5.
12. Axelsson I, Jakobsson I, Lindsberg T, Benediktsson B. Bovine β-lactoglobulin in the human milk. *Acta Paediatr Scand* 1986;75:702–7.
13. Stuart CA, Twiselton R, Nicholas MK, Hide DW. Passage of cow's milk protein in breast milk. *Clin Allergy* 1984;14:533–5.
14. Kulangara AC. The demonstration of ingested wheat antigens in human breast milk. *IRCS (Int Res Commun Syst) Med Sci Libr Compend* 1980;8:19.
15. Troncone R, Scarella A, Donatiello A, Cannataro P, Tarabuso A, Auricchio S. Passage of gliadin into human breast milk. *Acta Paediatr Scand* 1987;76:453–6.
16. Jakobsson I, Lindberg T. Cow's milk proteins cause infantile colic in breast-fed infants: a double-blind crossover study. *Pediatrics* 1983;71:268–71.
17. Lifschitz CH, Hawkins HK, Guerra C, Byrd N. Anaphylactic shock due to cow's milk protein hypersensitivity in a breast-fed infant. *J Pediatr Gastroenterol Nutr* 1988;7:141–4.
18. Cant A, Balles JA, Marsden RA. Cow's milk, soya milk, and goat's milk in a mother's diet causing eczema and diarrhoea in her breast-fed infant. *Acta Paediatr Scand* 1985;74:467–8.
19. Warner JO. Food allergy in fully breast-fed infants. *Clin Allergy* 1980;10:133–6.
20. Gerrard JW, Shenassa M. Food allergy: two common types as seen in breast and formula fed babies. *Ann Allergy* 1983;50:375–9.
21. Gerrard JW. Allergy in breast-fed babies to ingredients in breast milk. *Ann Allergy* 1979;42:69–72.
22. Park EA. A case of hypersensitiveness to cow's milk. *Am J Dis Child* 1920;19:46–54.
23. Schwartz RH, Kubicka M, Dreyfuss EM, Nikaein A. Acute urticarial reactions to cow's milk in infants previously fed breast milk or soy milk. *Pediatr Asthma Allergy Immunol* 1987;1:81–93.
24. Michel FB, Bousquet J, Greillier P, Robinet-Levy M, Coulomb Y. Comparison of cord blood immunoglobulin E and maternal allergy for the prediction of atopic diseases in infancy. *J Allergy Clin Immunol* 1980;65:422–30.
25. Businco L, Marchetti F, Pelligrini G, Berlini R. Predictive value of cord blood IgE levels in "at-risk" newborn babies and influence of type of feeding. *Clin Allergy* 1983;13:503–8.
26. Kaufman HS. Allergy in the newborn: skin test reactions confirmed by the Prausnitz-Kustner test at birth. *Clin Allergy* 1971;1:363–7.
27. Zeiger RS, Heller S, Mellon M, O'Connor R, Hamburger RN. Effectiveness of dietary manipulation in the prevention of food allergy in infants. *J Allergy Clin Immunol* 1986;78:224–38.
28. Hide DW, Guyer BM. Clinical manifestations of allergy related to breast- and cow's milk-feeding. *Pediatrics* 1985;76:973–5.
29. Hamburger RN, Heller S, Mellon M, O'Connor RD, Zeiger RS. Current status of the clinical and immunologic consequences of a prototype allergic disease prevention program. *Ann Allergy* 1983;51:281–90.
30. McClelland DBL, McDonald TT. Antibodies to cow's milk proteins in human colostrum. *Lancet* 1976;2:1251–2.
31. Chandra RK. Prospective studies of the effect of breast feeding on incidence of infection and allergy. *Acta Paediatr Scand* 1979;68:691–4.
32. Saarinen UM, Kajosaari M, Backman A, Siimes MA. Prolonged breast-feeding as prophylaxis for atopic disease. *Lancet* 1979;2:163–6.
33. Walker WA. Antigen penetration across the immature gut: effect of immunologic and maturational factors in colostrum. In: Ogra PL, Dayton D, eds. *Immunology of Breast Milk,* New York: Raven Press, 1979;227–35.
34. Taylor B, Norman AP, Orgel HA, Stokes CR, Turner MW, Soothill JF. Transient IgA deficiency and pathogenesis of infantile atopy. *Lancet* 1973;2:111–3.
35. Kramer MS. Does breast feeding help protect against atopic disease? Biology, methodology, and a golden jubilee of controversy. *J Pediatr* 1988;112:181–90.
36. Hanson LA, Ahlstedt S, Carlsson B, Fallstrom SP. Secretory IgA antibodies against cow's milk proteins in human milk and the possible effect on mixed feeding. *Int Arch Allergy Appl Immunol* 1977;54:457–62.
37. Green FHY, Freed DLJ. Antibody-facilitated digestion and the consequences of its failure. In: Hemmings WA, ed. *Antigen Absorption by the Gut*. Baltimore: University Park Press, 1978;189–97.
38. Pittard WB, Bill K. Differentiation of cord blood lymphocytes into IgA-producing cells in response to breast milk stimulatory factor. *Clin Immunol Immunopathol* 1979;13:430–4.

39. Jarrett EEE. Activation of IgE regulatory mechanisms by transmucosal absorption of antigen. *Lancet* 1977;2:223–35.
40. Kaplan MS, Solli NJ. Immunoglobulin E to cow's-milk protein in breast-fed atopic children. *J Allergy Clin Immunol* 1979;64:122–6.
41. Björkstén F, Saarinen UM. IgE antibodies to cow's milk in infants fed breast milk and milk formulae. *Lancet* 1978;2:624–5.
42. Juto P, Björkstén B. Serum IgE in infants and influence of type of feeding. *Clin Allergy* 1980;10:593–600.
43. Firer MA, Hosking CS, Hill DJ. Effect of antigen load on development of milk antibodies in infants allergic to milk. *Br Med J* 1981;283:693–6.
44. Lindfors A, Enocksson E. Development of atopic disease after early administration of cow milk formula. *Allergy* 1988;43:11–6.
45. Gross SJ, Buckley RH. IgA in saliva of breast-fed and bottle-fed infants. *Lancet* 1980;2:543.
46. Frick M, Reiger CHL. Local antibodies to α-casein and β-lactoglobulin in the saliva of infants. *Pediatr Res* 1987;22:399–401.

Food Intolerance in Infancy: Allergology,
Immunology, and Gastroenterology, edited by
Robert N. Hamburger. Carnation Nutrition
Education Series, Vol. 1. The Carnation Co., Los
Angeles/Raven Press, Ltd., New York © 1989.

Interim Discussion for Section I

Kjell Aas, Robert N. Hamburger,
Steven B. Machtinger, and Buford Lee Nichols, Jr.

Dr. Nichols: Both Dr. Hamburger and Dr. Aas defined allergy as being strictly mediated by immunoglobulin E. I personally have some difficulty accepting that. I look at this more from a Cartesian point of view and see that there are other mechanisms involved. Dr. Machtinger did point out that controversy exists about understanding tolerance. He pointed to Soothill's view that IgA plays a role and Jarrett's view that suppressor thymus-derived cells (T-cells) play a role. Already we have introduced more than immunoglobulin E (IgE) into the immunological response called allergy. I want to challenge the panel to explain why they feel content to limit the word allergy to IgE-mediated mechanisms.

Dr. Aas: I did not specify allergy as only reacting with IgE. In my definition, I specify allergies as immunologically mediated hypersensitivity in general, but I stated that I, in this paper, restricted myself to discuss IgE. You can't cover the entire field in one paper.

Dr. Hamburger: I would like to make two comments. One, there is in my chapter a set of definitions of terms (Hamburger, *this volume*), and I placed them there for just this purpose and just this reason, because the problem is a semantic one and not an immunologic one. In Britain, in fact throughout all of Europe, they use the word allergy exactly as Dr. Nichols is using it. That is, it is any immunologic reaction that is adverse. Whereas in the United States, the word has almost lost its meaning, but it was conventionally restricted to what is now called, IgE-mediated allergic disease. To get around that, we now have incorporated the word atopic or atopy, and you will hear most academic American speakers talking about atopic allergic reactions, which used to be redundant but is now necessary to clarify the usage. Thus, atopic allergic reactions are solely IgE-mediated. Allergic reactions in general may have any one of the five immunoglobulins involved, and some people think that even IgD does something adverse, but I haven't been convinced of that; and of course, that includes cellular immunologic reactions and complement mediated immunologic reactions as well. I really don't believe there is a controversy on that issue. I think it's simply a semantic problem.

Dr. Machtinger: I think you're being unfair. Certainly colic is a complex of symptoms which have a number of possible mechanisms, many of which may be behavioral or may be interactions between the mother and the infant. Also, colic may at some times be due to allergy, but certainly that is not necessarily an IgE-mediated reaction. At least within the breast-fed group, most of the reactions that we see, certainly the ones that are well characterized, are those that appear to be immediately hypersensitive in nature or defined by IgE antibodies. There are cases of infants who receive cow's milk or cow's milk formula by direct feedings who have chronic gastrointestinal (GI) blood loss and respiratory problems. These may be mediated by protein intolerance or other types of immune reactions. But at least with the breast-fed group, and possibly only because the amount of antigen which the infant is exposed to is small, the reactions appear to be IgE-mediated.

Dr. Nichols: I would like to follow up your comment by asking you a question. If antigens are absorbed, so what? I don't think the question is whether they are absorbed and whether it's harmful to breast feed because antigens can be absorbed by the mother and then absorbed by the baby. I think the miracle is that we tolerate them, and I didn't hear you say anything about mechanisms of tolerance.

Dr. Machtinger: Well, I think the vast majority of infants do tolerate whatever it is that you give them. I think that is the major difference between the atopic individual and the nonatopic individual.

Dr. Nichols: Professor Aas, there is a whole body of information that indicates that the processing of antigens is extremely important in terms of the biological response. This is certainly true for gastrointestinal diseases of a chronic inflammatory nature, and it's certainly true that some people have now shown that there are some tissue types that are more prone to allergic disease of the respiratory tract. I didn't hear you say anything about the tissue typing and the genetics of tissue typing as it might influence response to antigens in this context.

Dr. Aas: Well, you introduce a discussion which is very complex, because until now we haven't yet even mentioned the words immunogens or tolerogens. Your question: "so what with the absorbed antigen?" could be extended with "so what with the absorbed immunogen?" Does it act in a positive way in most of the immune systems, but badly in the IgE system because of some lack of control in that system? In addition, I would remind you that, although we are speaking mostly about the ingestion of food antigens, at the same time we also inhale a lot of food antigens. I have studied commercial house dust extracts from the United States, among others, and in any house dust extract on the market a few years ago, in addition to antigens from mites, animal dandruff, and other things, we found in every extract antigens of cow's milk, egg, fish, pea, peanut, nuts, soy, and wheat. So we have to look at this also.

Dr. Nichols: You would have found more if you had more antibodies. Thank you for making that point, and that probably explains Dr. Machtinger's and Dr. Hamburger's observations that you do see a rise in antibodies in breast-fed infants.

Dr. Hamburger: I would like to comment on your question about transplantation antigens. I know you know that there has been an enormous search by the Hopkins group and others, our own as well, for relationships between proneness to specific responses. In a few families there has been some relationship located, but nothing that is ubiquitous and nothing that runs across family lines or where you can make a general statement, such as if you have DW-8, for example, you're likely to respond to peanut. That just hasn't been found, although it has surely been looked for.

Dr. Jakobsson: I am Dr. Jakobsson from Malmö, Sweden. I have a short comment to Dr. Machtinger. First, I would say I agree with most of the things you told us, but I think it's very important to stress one thing which has to do with tolerance or intolerance. When we discuss advantages, or if we should discuss advantages or disadvantages with breast feeding, I think it's important to stress that we are talking about a very small group of risk infants. Most infants do not develop intolerances, but they do develop tolerances to several of the food antigens, and it might very well be that these small amounts of food antigens that we have in human milk are quite important for tolerance development. I think we should not forget that.

Dr. Machtinger: I think the point I was trying to make is that in recent years, as more and more mothers have returned to breast-feeding, we of course are beginning to see more and more allergic reactions in infants who do breast-feed. There simply weren't many infants breast-feeding and we didn't see many of the allergic reactions. As this has gone on and we have seen these reactions, I think on our part we have said: well, perhaps if we remove the foods from the maternal diet or if we restricted the infant's diet even more, we would somehow prevent allergic sensitization. I think that may be a mistake. I think perhaps what we need to do is recommend breast-feeding with supplementation.

Dr. Nichols: I think that Van Pirquet emphasized that the allergic response was part of a spectrum of immune responses and he implied and stated very clearly that there are benefits as well as liabilities to the response.

Dr. Berger: I am Dr. William Berger. I am an allergist practicing in Mission Viejo, California. Being a pediatric allergist, I very often will see children who have highly allergic problems as a first child, and it's usually the pediatrician who is making the recommendations for breast-feeding. The thing that has always been particularly interesting to me and is a question to me now is that pediatricians for a very long time now recommend breast-feeding to mothers who have a history of an atopic child or an atopic family history. For many years formula-feeding was the mode of treatment and now that breast-feeding is in vogue, breast-feeding seems to be the one that is being recommended very highly. The thing that has always been a question in my mind is that the breast-feeding now is being recommended to mothers to prevent allergy, or at least delay allergy onset in the second or third child who comes from an atopic family. From what you have been saying, it seems that these highly atopic children through breast-feeding are being introduced to the very foods that are being delayed in other children. In other words, there is a delay of onset of introduction of things such as wheat, chocolate, or peanut in other children, but the ones who are the most atopic are getting it now very early through the mother's breast milk. Why aren't we seeing more allergic reactions in this group? Pediatricians may not be aware of it, but from the information that you have been giving us, they are actually being exposed to more allergenic foods at an earlier stage in their life, yet why aren't we seeing more allergic reactions in those children?

Dr. Nichols: To paraphrase that, antigens appear, so what? Now I would ask you again the same question, antigens appear in human milk, so what?

Dr. Machtinger: Well, there are allergic reactions occurring in infants who are exclusively breast-fed, and I tried to make that point.

Dr. Hamburger: Dr. Berger's question is well put, and I think that what really is not being emphasized is the point that Dr. Jakobsson made so clearly, and that is, if you breast-feed and the mother is on a rational hypoallergenic diet, you do indeed cut down the number of sensitized individuals or infants in prone families. But buried in that group is a small group in which there is nothing that can be done to stop them from being sensitized, and those are the ones that Dr. Machtinger is pointing to and saying: see, breast-feeding isn't all that protective. It is in fact, as Dr. Berger indicated, very protective for most prone infants, but as John Gerard pointed out years ago, there are babies who cannot be stopped from making an allergic reaction as far as we know today. And those babies, no matter what you do with them or with their mother's diet or with their breast-feeding, are going to come up with positive radioallergosorbent test (RAST), positive skin tests, and positive reactions to some foods.

Dr. Galant: Stan Galant from California. I have two questions. As you were talking about breast milk and the foods that get into breast milk from what the mother eats, I was thinking, has anyone taken a careful look at the breast milk proteins themselves? In other words, we're making the assumption that breast milk is totally nonimmunogenic. People ask me, ''Doc, is there anything in the breast milk itself that could be allergenic?'' and I have always assumed that there is not. But has anyone taken a careful look with some of the modern techniques to elucidate that? My second question is: Those in the audience that take care of families may be very disturbed by some of the new evidence that raises questions again that supplementing breast milk with cow's milk may actually be good, whereas some of the earlier studies, coming out of Europe particularly, show almost a linear relationship between efficacy of breast-feeding and how much cow's milk was introduced over the first year of life, and now we are saying just the opposite. So, if possible, I think it would be good to get a consensus on how to approach the second child in the family where there is a lot of allergy in terms of recommendation of breast-feeding and how the mother proceeds with that.

Dr. Machtinger: I know of no study where people have actually looked at whether or not proteins native to the breast milk cause allergy in breast-fed infants. I would think that would be a very difficult study to do because you would have to eliminate all foreign proteins from the breast milk. You would have to put the woman on an elemental diet for a period of time and then look for allergy in the infant. I am not aware of any studies of that sort. What I'm trying to say in my presentation today is that it's really time that we took a very close look at the recommendations we make about exclusive breast-feeding. Certainly, in exclusively breast-fed infants and infants whose mothers are on highly restricted diets, there are adverse reactions and some of those are atopic reactions. I certainly have seen that in my clinical practice. One can't be sure from where the sensitization is occurring. Certainly variations in the protocol which we suggest to parents, let's not give your child any cow's milk or any foreign antigens before 6 months and tell the mother let's not eat, my usual line is you can't have any milk, any ice cream, any sour cream, or any pizza. But it's very difficult to completely eliminate these foreign food proteins from the diet. The result is that the infants are going to be exposed. We are fooling ourselves if we think that the average infant we have placed on an exclusive diet of breast milk and whose mother has been told to avoid certain foods is not being exposed to those foods. I believe Dr. Hamburger has shown that in several of his recent publications. So it seems to me that these kids are being exposed.

Dr. Collins-Williams: Collins-Williams from Toronto, Canada. I have not been as despondent as Dr. Machtinger on having the mothers stick to their restricted diet because I don't think you have to eliminate so many of the foods. When I was working with Dr. Bret Ratner in 1949 in this city, we did this experiment you were talking about, the Prausnitz-Küstner (PK) reaction, and showing that it would become positive if the mother ate the food. For example, in one experiment on five people, including myself, we showed that if we took raw egg on an empty stomach, we could get very huge PK reactions. On the other hand, if we repeated that a week later and took the same quantity of well-cooked egg, none of us got positive PK reactions. That would imply that you can do a lot in the way of restricting the mother's diet by cooking foods. Now that doesn't apply to everything. It doesn't apply to fish and it doesn't apply to nuts, but it does apply to a lot of other foods. So, I have never had much trouble in having a mother follow the diet. Now I've never had the opportunity to do a scientific study and prove what it did, but all I'm saying is you can get her to follow that kind of a diet.

Dr. Powell: Geraldine Powell, Galveston, Texas. I have a question to Dr. Machtinger. When you're measuring β-lactoglobulin (BLG) in breast milk, are you measuring it in the presence of antibody to BLG? If so, how can you quantitate it?

Dr. Machtinger: What people have done is that they have used standard references. Some people have added BLG back to breast-milk specimens of women who have been placed on a cow's milk-free diet so that they have a good one-to-one comparison in an attempt to zero out the effect of the antibody that is present. The other thing is that if you look at anti-cow's milk IgA antibodies in breast milk, there are some antibodies against BLG, but I believe the prime antibody is anti-casein. So there is probably less anti-BLG IgA in breast milk. People who have looked at that find a lower frequency and usually lower levels. But, you're right, it may interfere somewhat with your quantification. It's more important to say, is it there rather than just how much is present.

Dr. Powell: I don't think it can be done, and the same applies to the study that you've quoted, which is to try to quantitate antibody to cow's milk if antigen is present in the same breast milk, and then to try to correlate this with the development of atopic sensitivity or with tolerance. You've got the same problem if you've got both antigen and antibody floating around, and I don't think you can quantitate either. You can only say antigen or antibody is present, but you can't make anything of the numbers, such as "it disappeared in 6 days" and such. That's the problem you have with that, and I agree it's demonstrated that antigen is present, but "how much?" is the question. It might be a lot.

Dr. Gluck: Joan Gluck from Miami, Florida. I am a pediatric allergist. What I have observed in the children whom I see with allergy is that the infants that come in with the most severe allergies are the ones that are breast-fed. They have the worst eczema, and the earliest asthma, and have been in the hospital. I feel definitely that breast milk is a factor. However, when you look at the older children that come in who have been breast-fed, those who are just starting to have symptoms when they are 7, 8, or 9 years old, their allergies are mild. They have very few physical symptoms of allergies and the mothers are just there because the child has a little sniffing and has never been sick in his life. So I think you are looking at a tremendous spectrum of reaction to the antigens that are in the breast milk, and there is a very small fraction of babies that will react tremendously to breast milk probably much more than they would to formula, which is what you have really been alluding to in these different presentations. I have a comment for Dr. Hamburger. You mentioned many factors that you have to look at when you consider food allergy, but one that you didn't mention, just to be a nitpicker, is that there is an additive effect of eating the same food every day which also needs to be taken into account, probably in the maternal diet as well as in the child's diet.

Dr. Hamburger: I agree. I want to elaborate on something that Dr. Stan Galant raised. Years ago, we looked at infants who we knew had anti-β-lactoglobulin antibody in their own serum, and we looked at them from the point of view of trying to find other cross-reactions with other milks. We looked at goat and several of the commercial formulas, but we never found any infant's anti-β-lactoglobulin that cross-reacted with mother's milk, and at that time we had a battery of a dozen or more. So I have the impression that if it occurs at all, it must be extremely rare that anybody makes an autoimmune reaction, which that would be, to human breast milk proteins.

Dr. Faygosh: I am Dr. Faygosh from Chicago, Illinois. We have seen that there are allergens present in the breast milk. However, we have also noticed that in spite of those allergens, many of the babies who are breast-fed will show either minimal reactions or no reactions at all, and they are protected. We have also seen that the maturity of the gut and the secretory IgA defects are probably the causes of allergic reactions in babies. Are we now looking at the protective things which are present in the breast milk which might be helping these babies?

Dr. Machtinger: Very possibly there are immunologic constituents of breast milk that we have only touched upon.

Food Intolerance in Infancy: Allergology, Immunology, and Gastroenterology, edited by Robert N. Hamburger. Carnation Nutrition Education Series, Vol. 1. The Carnation Co., Los Angeles/Raven Press, Ltd., New York © 1989.

Gut Immaturity in Neonates

Richard A. Schreiber and W. Allan Walker

Combined Program in Pediatric Gastroenterology and Nutrition, Massachusetts General Hospital and Children's Hospital, Boston, MA 02114

The development of an intestinal mucosal barrier to defend against noxious agents that transit the gut lumen represents an important adaptation of the gastrointestinal tract to the external environment (1–3). That the mature gut mucosa contains quantitatively the largest bone marrow-derived lymphocyte (B-cell) population in the body and that total immunoglobulin A (IgA) production in the intestine is twice that of sytemic IgG production underscores the importance of the intestinal barrier to host defense (4).

At birth, the newborn is confronted with gut colonization, bacterial and viral toxins, and dietary protein antigens. These substances, if permitted to penetrate the intestinal mucosa, can potentially induce inflammatory or allergic reactions, which may result in gastrointestinal and systemic disease states (5). Thus, an extensive system of intestinal mucosal defense, involving both immune and nonimmune mechanisms, must develop to protect the host from its external environment. For example, a complex series of cellular events may induce a local immune response, at the level of the intestinal mucosa, and at the same time suppress a systemic immune response (6). The result of this physiological process is to prevent penetration of antigen across the luminal surface, yet also induce systemic tolerance to that antigen.

The purpose of this review is to describe these and other features of the mature mucosal barrier and outline our current understanding of the factors that contribute to its development in the newborn period. The consequences of antigen penetration across an immature or damaged intestinal mucosa, particularly in infancy, will also be addressed.

THE MUCOSAL BARRIER

Nonimmunological Components of the Mucosal Barrier

Both nonimmunological and immunological determinants contribute to the integrity of the mucosal barrier (7). These processes may operate independently or in concert to generate an effective mucosal defense. Table 1 lists some of the compo-

TABLE 1. *Components of the mucosal barrier*

Nonimmunologic	Immunologic
Saliva	Gut-associated lymphoid tissue (GALT)
Gastric acid	Secretory IgA
Proteolysis	Immune complex-mediated mucous release
Peristalsis	
Mucous coat	
Microvillous membrane	

nents that comprise the intestinal barrier. Generally, the nonimmunological factors limit colonization of the gut, prevent microorganism adherence to the intestinal luminal surface, and regulate the penetration of dietary antigen and protein fragments across the epithelial surface.

Saliva, being rich in secretory IgA, phagosomes, and a variety of lysozymes can modify bacterial colonization of the mouth and potentially inhibit microorganism adherence to the oral mucosa (8). High gastric acidity deters intestinal colonization by gram-positive organisms. For example, it is well documented that patients with achlorhydria are predisposed to bacterial overgrowth (9). Gastric acid may also affect the load of antigen that enters the small intestine. Increased macromolecular transport across the intestinal lumen has been demonstrated following neutralization of gastric acid with bicarbonate (10). At birth, basal gastric output is low and is even lower in prematures (11). Acid output increases until 4 weeks of age when adult levels are reached. Environmental factors probably account for this observation, because the rise in acid output is dependent upon postnatal age and not actual chronological age.

Mucus, synthesized and secreted by intestinal goblet cells, serves as an additional defense to the diffusion, penetration, and attachment of intraluminal microorganisms and antigens across the microvillous surface (12). With increased mucous discharge, the thickness of the mucous coat expands, enhancing the efficacy of the physical barrier. Immunologic, infectious, or chemical agents may affect the amount of mucin released. For example, acetylcholine will stimulate mucin secretion whereas adrenergic agents have no effect (13). IgE-mediated mast cell histamine release has been demonstrated to enhance mucin release (14). Intraluminal IgA immune complexes may also stimulate mucin secretion (15). Mucus contains specific carbohydrate moieties that can interfere with the attachment of bacteria or antigens to the microvillous surface. For example, glycoproteins similar to the mannose receptor for *Escherichia coli* or the fucose receptor for *Vibrio cholerae* may be found in mucus (16). These products can function as receptor inhibitors and allow for trapping of microorganisms before they reach the intestinal epithelial surface and bind to receptors there. In the newborn rat, the ratio of carbohydrate to protein content of mucus is less than that of the adult rat, and there is a decrease in fucose and *n*-acetylgalactosamine moieties (17). The properties of the intestinal cell membrane differ as the intestinal epithelial cell migrates up the villus and as the animal ages (18). These changes may also affect antigen penetration across the mucosal barrier. In the rat, binding of bovine serum albumin and β-lactoglobulin to the microvillous membrane can vary with age (18). For example, 18-day-old animals bind significantly more protein than adult rodents. Bresson et al. (19) have demonstrated, in rabbit intestine, that the microvillous membrane protein-to-lipid ratio is decreased in newborns compared with adults. An increased binding of cholera enterotoxin to newborn microvillous membrane was also observed in this rabbit model. These compositional differences of the immature barrier may influence the likelihood for bacterial or toxin penetration across the mucosal surface. Studies of these ontogenic differences in nonimmune mucosal barrier determinants may enhance our comprehension of antigen transport in early life and help explain the pathophysiology of a number of intestinal diseases.

Immunological Components of the Mucosal Barrier

Secretory IgA (sIgA), the principal immunoglobulin of the mucosal immune system, is present in highest concentration in gastrointestinal secretions (20). Indeed, the intestine secretes more sIgA daily than the total systemic daily IgG production (4). sIgA is a dimeric or polymeric molecule composed of single IgA molecules covalently linked by a peptide or J chain (21). Whereas monomeric serum IgA is produced mainly in the bone marrow, polymeric IgA is synthesized by mucosal plasma cells. There are two isotypes, IgA_1 and IgA_2. In adults, over 90% of serum IgA is of the IgA_1 subclass. The IgA_2 subclass accounts for up to 40% of sIgA (4). IgA_1 is highly susceptible to degradation by bacterial proteases. These structural and functional differences between serum IgA and sIgA support the idea that the mucosal and systemic immune systems are indeed separate. Once synthesized by plasma mucosal cells, sIgA is transported to the intestinal lumen by binding to secretory component. Secretory component is a transmembrane protein seen on the basolateral epithelial cell surface (22). The primary function of secretory component is for the selective transport of sIgA into external secretions. In the intestinal mucosa, secretory component located within the basal aspect of the epithelial cell binds sIgA. The immunoglobulin is carried into the epithelial cell by pinocytosis. The secretory component-sIgA complex transports across the cell in vesicles to the luminal border. There, the polymeric IgA is released by reverse pinocytosis into the intestinal lumen. Because sIgA is less susceptible to proteolytic digestion, it retains most of its functional capacity as it transits the intestinal tract (21).

sIgA likely impedes mucosal penetration of microbes, antigens, or toxins by complexing with them in the lumen or within the mucous coat (23,24). In newborn animals and humans, the concentration of IgA in saliva, stool, and serum is decreased (25,26). It is thought that this transient deficiency may in part account for the increased attachment of antigen to the intestinal surface in this age group. Patients with selective IgA deficiency demonstrate circulating immune complexes and precipitating antibodies to absorbed bovine milk proteins following milk ingestion (27). Three of seven subjects with IgA deficiency had increases in serum antigen-antibody complexes which peaked at 120 to 150 min after milk intake (27). The predisposition of IgA-deficient patients to immune complex diseases such as rheumatoid arthritis or systemic lupus erythematosus (SLE) may be related to this disturbance in intestinal barrier integrity (28,29). Presumably the same process occurs in the transient IgA-deficient newborn, accounting in part for the increased incidence of intestinal allergy that is seen in infancy.

THE IgA CELL CYCLE

sIgA is synthesized by plasma cells that inhabit the intestinal lamina propria. The elaboration of sIgA by this cell population is believed to be regulated by the gut-associated lymphoid tissue (GALT). One of the principal elements of GALT, the Peyer's patch, represents an important site for antigen presentation to intestinal lymphoid tissue—a necessary first step in the sIgA cell cycle (30).

There are specialized membranous epithelial cells or M cells that overlie Peyer's patches, which are specifically designed to facilitate access of luminal antigen to the intestinal lymphoid tissue. These cells differ from other mucosal cells in that they have few microvilli, a poorly developed glycocalyx, and an absence of lysosomal organelles (31). Evidence from histochemical studies has demonstrated that M cells, in contrast to intestinal mucosal cells, will preferentially take up and process horseradish peroxidase after small quantities of this substance are introduced into the intestinal lumen (32). In another study, 1 hr after inoculation of Reovirus type I into mouse ileum, virus particles were present in the layer immediately below the M cells (33). Thus, there is both functional and structural evidence to support the concept that M cells represent a major site for antigen presentation and uptake.

The Peyer's patch consists of a dome region, a lymphoid follicular or B-cell zone, and a parafollicular thymus-derived cell (T-cell) zone (21). The dome region lying immediately below the M cells contains B and T lymphocytes and macrophages. The follicular zone contains germinal centers rich in immature B cells, which ultimately will be committed to IgA production. Adjacent to this zone is the T-cell region composed primarily of helper T_4 cells.

Once antigen is taken up by the M cells and transported through the dome region, specific IgA-committed B cells migrate from the follicular zone to the mesenteric lymph nodes where maturation and proliferation occur. From this site, B cells travel via the thoracic duct to the systemic circulation. These cells may home back to the lamina propria where they become IgA-secreting plasma cells or they may lodge in other tissues including the lactating mammary gland, the uterine cervix, the lungs, or the lacrimal glands. This forms the common mucosal immune system, and the circular route of IgA-committed B cells from GALT back to the lamina propria is termed the IgA cell cycle (34).

THE IMMATURE MUCOSAL BARRIER

Recent studies using immunohistochemical techniques have demonstrated an absence of immunoglobulin-producing cells in fetal intestine (35). By 12 days of age, IgM- and IgA-secreting cells begin to appear in the intestinal mucosa. Up until 1 month of age, however, the majority of these cells express IgM, whereas in the adult intestine, the ratio of IgA:IgM:IgG is 20:3:1 (35). Selnar et al. (36) have shown that salivary sIgA is absent in newborns but appears in over 90% of infants by 1 year of age. Intestinal lymphoid aggregates are seen as early as 14 weeks gestation and by 20 weeks, distinct B- and T-cell zones develop. By the end of the second trimester, intestinal follicles are easily recognized (37).

The immaturity of both the nonimmunological and immunological components of the intestinal barrier favors antigen presentation and uptake primarily by a mechanism that differs from that of the mature barrier (Fig. 1) (7). The initial event in this process is an interaction between large molecules within the intestinal lumen and the microvillous membrane. When a sufficient number of molecules approach the cell membrane, invagination occurs and vesicles are formed. These vesicles migrate to the supranuclear region of the mucosal epithelial cell where they coalesce to form large vacuoles. Here, intracellular digestion occurs. However, small quantities of ingested molecules escape breakdown and migrate to the lateral basal surface of the cell. During periods of barrier immaturity, an excessive quantity of antigens are absorbed (38). In contrast, when the nonimmunological and immunological components of the mucosal barrier mature, the amount of antigen uptake diminishes.

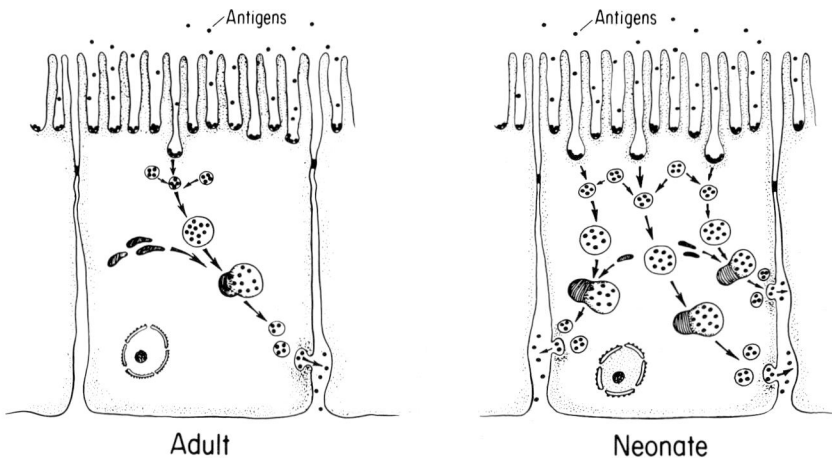

FIG. 1. The surface and enterocyte function of small intestine from adult and neonatal mammals is a determinant to the uptake of intestinal allergies and to the role of allergen uptake in mucosal immune responses. The surface of the adult intestine binds less avidly to allergens and has less uptake of allergic molecules than that of the neonatal intestine.

It is likely that both intrinsic host genetic factors and the extrinsic intraluminal environment contribute to this ontogeny of the mucosal immune barrier (39). That the intestinal barrier is indeed immature and incompletely developed at birth may partly account for the predisposition of the newborn and infant to various clinical disease states (5).

REGULATION OF THE IMMUNE RESPONSE

The mechanism for induction of specific IgA-committed B cells within the follicular zone of the Peyer's patch in response to intraluminal antigen and the subsequent regulation of B-cell migration to specific sites within the common mucosal immune system are an incompletely understood area that is under intense research. Current immunological theory suggests that helper T_4 cells, when presented with antigen in association with molecules of the major histocompatibility complex, can be activated to release various lymphokines. This activation, in turn, can stimulate the proliferation of B cells (40). At the level of the Peyer's patch, evidence for cellular interaction of helper T cells in the parafollicular zone with follicular B cells was presented by Elson et al. (41) who demonstrated that murine Peyer's patch T cells stimulated with concanavalin A led to enhanced IgA expression of intestinal B cells. There are two possible mechanisms to account for the T-cell regulation of the IgA response. Helper T cells may induce follicular B cells to undergo isotypic switch so that IgA production is promoted rather than IgM (42). Alternatively, T cells bearing receptors for IgA can specifically stimulate IgA-secreting B cells resulting in the selection of this isotypic cell population for eventual differentiation into true plasma cells (43).

A significant immunoregulatory feature of GALT is the phenomenon of systemic immune tolerance following ingestion of dietary antigen. As already outlined, intraluminal antigen can induce helper T cells in Peyer's patch to prime B cells for subsequent specific local mucosal IgA responses to that antigen. Yet, at the same time, there is suppression of systemic IgE and IgG immune responses (tolerance) to any dietary antigen that may have penetrated the mucosal barrier (44). It is likely that tolerance arises from Peyer's patch suppressor T cells, which once induced, migrate to peripheral lymphoid tissue and mediate systemic anergy (45). The fine tuning of this intricate balance between IgA helper T cells and IgG suppressor T cells at the level of GALT involves another effector cell, the contrasuppressor T cell. These latter cells prevent T-cell suppression of parafollicular helper T cells, thereby serving to augment the local sIgA immune response (46). Clearly, the regulation of the local intestinal and systemic immune responses to intraluminal antigen involves a complex network of cellular immune events that are still incompletely defined.

HEPATOBILIARY CONTRIBUTION TO THE INTESTINAL MUCOSAL BARRIER

Another recently characterized dimension to the sIgA cell cycle is the liver and biliary tract. Jackson et al. (47) demonstrated a high concentration of sIgA in rodent bile. Interestingly, following biliary duct ligation, there was a 90% reduction in the level of sIgA in the small bowel (47). In a series of elegant experiments by Manning et al. (48), ligation of the thoracic ducts in rats led to a significant drop in biliary sIgA levels despite intact portal blood flow. These studies suggested that biliary sIgA was derived from the systemic and not the portal circulation and that, at least in rodents, large quantities of sIgA were delivered to the intestine via the biliary tract. An important link to this pathway was the finding of secretory component in the sinusoidal plasma membrane border of the hepatic cell (49). It is at this site that polymeric IgA binds to the hepatocyte and then transfers to the bile canaliculus. From there it enters the bile duct and transits into the small intestine. sIgA may also access the hepatocyte through a specific hepatic cell membrane asialoglycoprotein receptor (50). In humans, it has been established that approximately one-third of biliary sIgA is synthesized locally by hepatic plasma cells (51). The contribution of hepatic-derived sIgA to intestinal mucosal defense has not yet been completely defined. However, a recent study observed that following primary mucosal immunization with cholera toxin, specific IgA-secreting plasma cells appear in the liver prior to their appearance in the intestinal lamina propria (52). This suggests that the liver may play an important role in host protection against newly acquired intestinal antigens. Moreover, when other determinants of the mucosal immune defense are absent or immature, as in the newborn infant, hepatic-derived sIgA may be even more important to the integrity of the intestinal barrier.

EFFECT OF IMMUNOLOGICAL AND NONIMMUNOLOGICAL COMPONENTS TO THE MUCOSAL BARRIER

Recent observations have suggested that immunological components of the mucosal barrier can operate in concert with nonimmunological components to augment the overall protective capacity. In earlier work, we reported that the proteolysis of intestinal antigens was considerably greater in immunized animals than in nonimmunized controls and that the enhanced proteolysis most likely resulted from the interaction of immune complexes present in the mucous coat with pancreatic enzymes absorbed onto the surface of the intestine following secretion into the lumen (53). Another example of combined protection is the enhanced discharge of mucin that occurs in intestinal anaphylaxis. Using radiolabeled goblet-cell mucus to quantify release, Lake et al. (54) showed that IgE-mediated mast cell discharge of histamine resulted in enhanced release of goblet-cell mucus into the intestinal tract. Finally, we demonstrated that immune complexes to intestinal antigens formed on the intestinal surface were cleared by Kupffer's cells in the liver more readily than were antigens alone (55). This aspect of mucosal defense may be important in preventing gram-negative bacteria or endotoxins from gaining access to the portal circulation.

DISEASES RELATED TO A DEFICIENT MUCOSAL BARRIER

If the complex process of mucosal barrier defense is disrupted or if specific deficiencies in the components of the mucosal barrier exist, an increased incidence of antigen-induced intestinal diseases may ensue. Clinical conditions that may be associated with pathologic uptake of antigens are listed in Table 2, and a few representative examples will be discussed to illustrate the putative association between intestinal antigen penetration and clinical disease.

Necrotizing Enterocolitis

Necrotizing enterocolitis is an acute acquired gastrointestinal lesion of the newborn that is characterized by focal or diffuse ulceration and necrosis of the lower small bowel and colon (56). It is the most common gastrointestinal emergency in the neonatal intensive care unit, accounting for 1 to 5% of all intensive care admissions (57). Necrotizing enterocolitis most often develops in premature infants who have commenced enteral feeding. Other risk factors include low birth weight, umbilical vein catheterization, hypoxia, and perinatal complications such as C section, low 1-min Apgar scores, or respiratory distress syndrome (58). The pathogenesis of this disease is believed to be multifactorial arising from deficiencies in intestinal blood flow, infection, and enteral feeding. Because this condition primarily occurs in prematures, it has been proposed that necrotizing enterocolitis may be a disease of the immature mucosal barrier (59). A number of observations have supported this theory. Over 90% of cases of necrotizing enterocolitis are associated with enteral feeding with milk formulas. The absence of immunoglobulins in commercial formula, combined with the underdeveloped intestinal barrier of the premature, may be important precipitating factors to the development of necrotizing enterocolitis at this age. Human breast milk contains significant levels of sIgA and other immunoglobulins as well as nonspecific protective agents including lysozyme, complement, and lactoferrin which together can potentiate the efficacy of the intestinal barrier (60). The incidence of necrotizing enterocolitis in breast-fed prematures is less than in infants receiving formula (61). A number of studies have also demonstrated that breast-fed infants have a reduced susceptibility to intestinal infection (62). In animal models, breast milk was found to confer protection against necrotizing enterocolitis (63,64). Breast milk contains factors that not only enhance the intestinal mucosal barrier but may also facilitate intestinal maturation (65). It is quite plausible then that breast milk augments the integrity of the mucosal barrier conferring host protection against development of disease states. More recently Eibl et al. (66) supple-

TABLE 2. *Clinical conditions possibly associated with the immature mucosal barrier*

Necrotizing enterocolitis
Gastrointestinal allergy
Inflammatory bowel disease
Celiac disease
Chronic active hepatitis
Nephritis

mented prematures with an oral immunoglobulin preparation containing IgA and IgG. None of 88 cases receiving oral IgA-IgG developed necrotizing enterocolitis compared with 6 of 91 control infants. Because prematures are transiently deficient in sIgA, these results nicely demonstrate the important contribution of immunoglobulin to the intestinal mucosal barrier and its overall role in host defense and disease prevention.

Allergic Disease

That food hypersensitivity generally or cow's milk allergy specifically is much more common in infants than among adults has led to the idea that immaturity of the gastrointestinal barrier may be an important contributing factor to the pathogenesis of food allergy (5). As described earlier, the mature immune response to antigen involves the stimulation of suppressor T cells and induction of immune tolerance to that antigen (45). However, experimental data in the neonatal mouse suggest that the immature mucosal barrier favors priming of the immune response and enhanced immunoresponsiveness rather than induction of immune tolerance (67,68). These effects are expressed by both cell-mediated and antibody responses including IgG and IgE antibody idiotypes. Investigators have shown that immunoreactive antigen is absorbed in greater amounts from neonatal than from adult intestinal tract, when both are fed under comparable conditions (38). Small or moderate amounts of antigen absorbed from the neonatal gut might be expected to enhance specific immune responsiveness, whereas larger amounts would tend to tolerize them (Fig. 2). In contrast, the mature digestive capacity of adults would be expected to fragment proteins more effectively, which by virtue of their size, could be taken up in significant amounts thus favoring the development of tolerance. Current studies in our laboratories show that acute prefeeding of a trypsin inhibitor to adult mice before a normally tolerizing feeding results in a substantial increase in the concentration of antigen-specific determinants in the serum and a reversal in the usual immunological effect of antigen feeding from tolerance to priming for specific antibody responses (Hanson et al., *manuscript in preparation*). These observations are consistent with the hypotheses that gastrointestinal uptake and processing of protein can profoundly affect the immunological outcome of antigen ingestion (Fig. 3). Although other variables including genetic predisposition, host immunoresponsiveness, and environmental factors likely contribute to the generation of an allergic state, gut permeability to luminal antigens and antigen processing at the mucosal level undoubtedly play an important role in the development of food allergy.

Inflammatory Bowel Disease

Crohn's disease and ulcerative colitis are chronic inflammatory diseases of unknown etiology that predominantly affect the intestinal tract (69). A multitude of causes have been proposed including infectious, autoimmune, or toxic events, yet

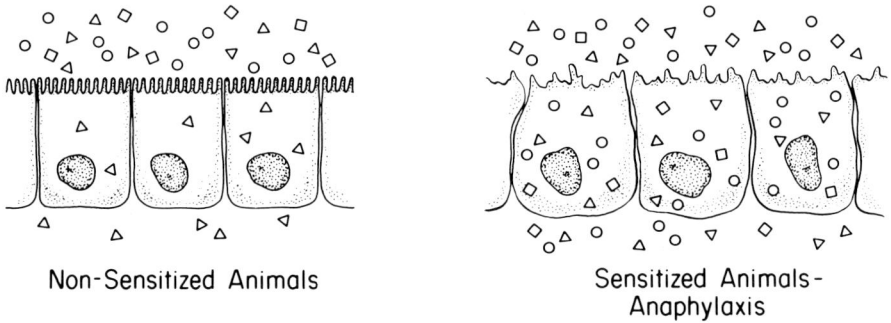

Non-Sensitized Animals   **Sensitized Animals-
                                      Anaphylaxis**

FIG. 2. Under conditions of intestinal anaphylaxis, more bystander antigen is taken up across the intestinal surface than under normal conditions. This enhanced uptake of bystander antigen may contribute to an expanded allergic (immunologic) response to bystander antigen.

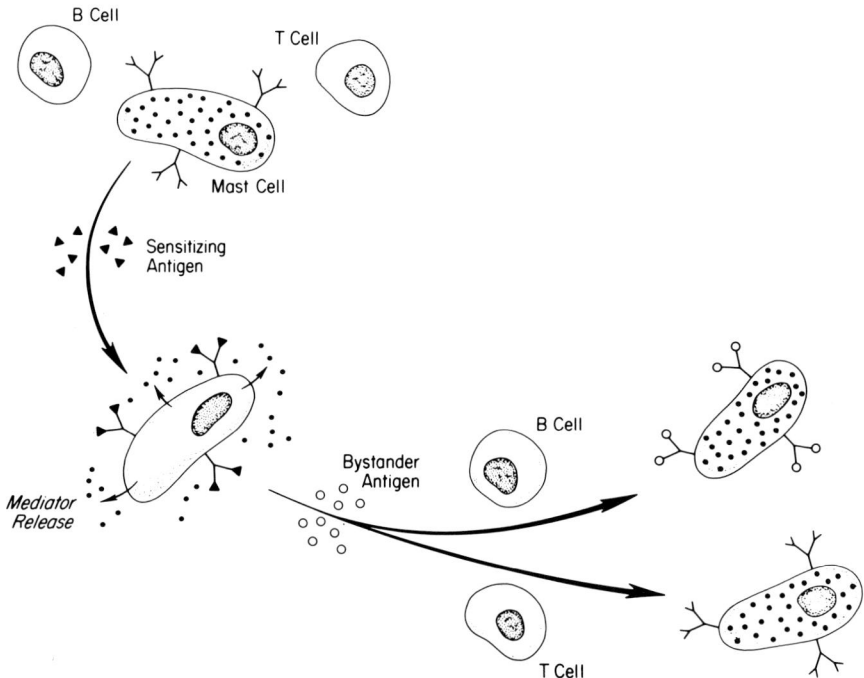

FIG. 3. Broadening of the intestinal anaphylaxis response. When sensitizing antigens stimulate an IgE response and create mast-cell triggering oral challenge, bystander antigens can cross the altered musoca and create additional IgE-mediated mast-cell response. This phenomenon produces a broadening of the IgE–mast-cell response to the antigens.

extensive investigations have failed to elicit a definitive agent. There is, however, substantial evidence to suggest that immunological processes are fundamental to the pathogenesis of inflammatory bowel disease (70). Interestingly, Shorter et al. (71) suggested that the immature mucosal barrier may play a crucial role in the development of this condition. According to their theory, in early life, when there is increased intestinal permeability, excess passage of immunogenic antigens may prime the intestine into a state of hypersensitivity for a particular antigenic moiety. In later life, if the mature intestinal barrier is disrupted (as occurs with infection), chance reexposure of the mucosal immune system to this same antigenic moiety could potentially induce a hypersensitivity reaction and initiate the cell-mediated inflammatory response that is characteristic of inflammatory bowel disease.

Celiac Disease

Celiac disease or gluten enteropathy is an intestinal disease that occurs in certain susceptible individuals who, following the ingestion of cereals (wheat, barley, rye, and possibly oats), develop a malabsorption syndrome associated with intestinal villous atrophy (72). This condition usually presents in infancy, subsequent to the introduction of cereals into the child's diet. However, in some adults, whose gastrointestinal symptoms are mild, celiac disease may be heralded by the appearance of dermatitis herpetiformis, an associated vesicular skin eruption (73). Gluten enteropathy likely results from a hypersensitivity reaction to gliadin, a protein fraction of wheat gluten. The disease has a strong association with the human lymphocyte antigen (HLA) B8, DR3 and DQw2 histocompatibility antigens, suggesting an autoimmune pathogenesis (72). Recently, it has been demonstrated that gliadin has sequence homology to a nonpathogenic gastrointestinal (GI) tract virus, adenovirus 12 (74). In accordance with this finding, Kagnoff proposes that patients with certain HLA markers who are infected with adenovirus 12, at a time of intestinal barrier immaturity, may prime or sensitize the local intestinal immune system to that viral antigen. At a later date, introduction of gliadin to GALT, by virtue of its immunological cross-reactivity with the viral protein, will induce a cell-mediated immune response causing intestinal injury and inflammation (75). Aside from this cellular response, other environmental factors and antibody immune responses also probably contribute to the pathogenesis of celiac disease.

THE GASTROINTESTINAL BARRIER AND HUMAN MILK

As alluded to throughout this discussion, breast milk contains factors that may both passively protect the immature mucosal barrier and actively stimulate its maturation (60,62,65). Among the substances that pass with human milk are lactoferrin, lysozyme, secretory antibody, lymphocytes, and macrophages. Widdowson et al. (76) have demonstrated that the intestinal epithelium proliferates more rapidly in animals fed maternal milk compared with those given formula feeds. Heird and Hansen (77) have shown that brush border enzyme activity (lactase, sucrase, alkaline phosphatase) is enhanced after ingestion of colostrum. Udall et al. (38) have demonstrated a decrease in antigen penetration across the immature mucosal barrier in newborns, following colostrum feedings. Breast milk contains high levels of sIgA. This immunoglobulin is synthesized by mammary plasmacytes derived from the common mucosal immune system (78). In lactating animals, B cells originating from the gut may home to the breast, forming an enteromammary immune system (79). Through this route, breast milk supplies sIgA that is specifically directed against antigens or microorganisms present in the maternal intestine. Once ingested by the neonate, this maternally derived sIgA confers protection of the neonatal intestine against these noxious agents. That breast-feeding protects the infant from food allergy, eczema, or infectious diseases has not yet been convincingly proven (80). Nevertheless, because breast milk may have an important functional role in the maturation of the intestinal mucosal barrier, we advocate breast-feeding of all infants at least until 6 months of age.

In conclusion, the development of a mucosal barrier represents an important adaptation of the gastrointestinal tract to the extrauterine environment. This barrier includes both nonimmune and immune processes, such as the mucous coat, gastric acid, the microvillous membrane, sIgA, and lamina propria immunocytes, which operate independently or in concert to provide maximal protection for the intestinal surface. There is now ample evidence to suggest that the intestinal barrier of the neonate is immature. As a result of this delay in the maturation, newborns are susceptible to pathologic penetration by noxious intraluminal substances. The consequences of this altered defense include susceptibility to infection and the potential for hypersensitivity reactions to ingested antigens. Thus, necrotizing enterocolitis, food allergy, celiac disease, and other diseases may, in part, result from a damaged or immature mucosal barrier. Fortunately, nature (via breast milk) has provided a means of passively protecting and nurturing the intestinal defense system during this period of vulnerability.

ACKNOWLEDGMENTS

Dr. Schreiber is the recipient of a Medical Research Council of Canada Fellowship Award.

REFERENCES

1. Walker WA. Gastrointestinal host defense: importance of gut closure in control of macromolecular transport. *Ciba Found Symp* 1976;70:201–19.
2. Walker WA. Pathophysiology of intestinal uptake and absorption of antigens in food allergy. *Ann Allergy* 1987;59:7–16.
3. Walker WA. Role of the mucosal barrier in antigen handling by the gut. In: Brostoff J, Challacombe SJ, eds. *Food Allergy and Tolerance*. Ballière Tindall 1987;11:209–22.
4. Mestecky J, Russell MW, Jackson S, Brown T. The human IgA system: a reassessment. *Clin Immunol Immunopathol* 1986;40:105–14.

5. Walter WA, Isselbacher KJ. Uptake and transport of macromolecules by the intestine: possible role in clinical disorders. *Gastroenterology* 1974;81:531–50.
6. Challacombe SJ, Tomasi TB. Systemic tolerance and secretory immunity after oral immunization. *J Exp Med* 1980;152:1459–72.
7. Walker WA. Antigen handling by the small intestine. *Clin Gastroenterol* 1986;15:1–20.
8. Tenuvuo J, Lehtonen O, Daltonen A, et al. Antimicrobial factors in whole saliva of human infants. *Infect Immunol* 1986;54:49–53.
9. Cook GC. Infective gastroenteritis and its relationship to reduced gastric acidity. *Scand J Gastroenterol* 1985;S111:17–23.
10. Kraft SC, Rothberg RM, Knauer CM, et al. Gastric acid output and circulating antibovine serum albumin in adults. *Clin Exp Immunol* 1967;2:321–30.
11. Hyman PE, Clarke DD, Everett SL, et al. Gastric acid secretory function in preterm infants. *J Pediatr* 1985;106:467–71.
12. Snyder JS, Walker WA. Structure and function of intestinal mucin: developmental aspects. *Int Arch Allergy Appl Immunol* 1987;82:351–6.
13. Specian RD, Neutra MR. Mechanism of rapid mucous secretion in goblet cells stimulated by acetylcholine. *J Cell Biol* 1980;85:626–40.
14. Lake AM, Bloch KJ, Sinclair KJ, et al. Anaphylactic release of goblet cell mucous. *Immunology* 1980;39:173–8.
15. Walker WA, Able SN, Wu M, et al. Intestinal uptake of macromolecules. V. Comparison of the *in vitro* uptake by rat small intestine of antigen antibody complexes prepared in antibody or antigen excess. *J Immunol* 1976;117:1028–32.
16. Elliot K, O'Connor M, Whelan J, eds. Adhesion and microorganism pathogenicity. *Ciba Found Symp* 1981;80:1–346.
17. Shub MD, Pang KY, Swann DA, et al. Age related chemical changes in rat small intestinal mucous glycoprotein. *J Biochem* 1985;215:405.
18. Stern MS, Pang KY, Walker WA. Food proteins and gut mucosal barrier. II. Differential interaction of cow's milk proteins with the mucous coat and the surface membrane of adult and immature rat jejunum. *Pediatr Res* 1984;18:1252–7.
19. Bresson JL, Pang KY, Walker WA. Microvillous membrane differentiation: quantitative difference in cholera toxin binding to the intestinal surface of newborn and adult rabbits. *Pediatr Res* 1984;18:984–7.
20. Tomasi TB, Grey WM. Structure and function of immunoglobulin A. *Prog Allergy* 1972;16:81–213.
21. Mestecky J, McGhee JR. Immunoglobulin A: molecular and cellular interactions involved in IgA biosynthesis and immune response. *Adv Immunol* 1987;40:153–245.
22. Kuhn LC, Kraehenbuhl JP. Role of secretory component, a secreted glycoprotein, in the specific uptake of IgA dimer by epithelial cells. *J Biol Chem* 1979;254:11072–81.
23. Walker WA, Isselbacher KJ. Intestinal antibodies. *N Engl J Med* 1977;297:767–73.
24. Walker WA. Intestinal transport of macromolecules. In: Johnson LR, Christensen J, Grossman ML, Jacobson ED, Schultz SG, eds. *Physiology of the Gastrointestinal Tract*. New York: Raven Press, 1981:1271–89.
25. Allansmith M, McClellan BH, Butterworth M, Maloney JR. The development of immunoglobulin levels in man. *J Pediatr* 1968;72:685–9.
26. Burgio GR, Lanzavecchia A, Pievani A, et al. Ontogeny of secretory immunity: levels of secretory IgA and natural antibodies in saliva. *Pediatr Res* 1980;14:1111–4.
27. Cunningham-Rundels C, Brandeis WE, Good RA, Day NK. Bovine antigens and the formation of circulating immune complexes in selective immunoglobulin A deficiency. *J Clin Invest* 1979;64:272–9.
28. Bach GL, Pillay VKG, Kark RM. Immunoglobulin (IgA) deficiency in systemic lupus erythematosis. *Acta Rheum Scand* 1971;17:63–71.
29. Ammann AJ, Hong R. Selective IgA deficiency: presentation of 30 cases and a review of the literature. *Medicine* (Baltimore) 1971;50:223–36.
30. Craig SW, Cebra JJ: Peyer's patches; an enriched source of precursors for IgA producing immunocytes in the rabbit. *J Exp Med* 1971;134:188–200.
31. Owen RL, Jones AI. Epithelial cell specialization within human Peyer's patches in the human small intestine. *Gut* 1965;6:225–33.
32. Owen RL. Sequential uptake of horseradish peroxidase by lymphoid follicle epithelium of Peyer's

patches in the neonatal unobstructed mouse intestine; an ultrastructural study. *Gastroenterology* 1977;72:440–51.

33. Wolf JL, Rubin DH, Finberg R, et al. Intestinal M cells: a pathway for entry of reovirus into the host. *Science* (Wash DC) 1981;212:471–2.

34. Bienenstock J, McDermott M, Befus D. A common mucosal immune system. In: Ogra P, Dayton D, eds. *Immunology of the Breast Milk*. New York: Raven Press, 1979;91–104.

35. Perkkis M, Savilahti E. Time of appearance of immunoglobulin containing cells in the mucosa of the neonatal intestine. *Pediatr Res* 1980;14:953–5.

36. Selnar JC, Merril DA, Claman HN. Salivary immunoglobulin and albumin development during the newborn period. *J Pediatr* 1968;72:685–9.

37. Spencer J, Macdonald TT, Finnn T, et al. The development of the gut associated lymphoid tissue in the terminal ileum of fetal human intestine. *Clin Exp Immunol* 1986;64:536–43.

38. Udall JN, Pang K, Fritze L, et al. Development of the gastrointestinal barrier. The effect of age on intestinal permeability to macromolecules. *Pediatr Res* 1981;15:241–4.

39. Chandra RK. Development of gastrointestinal tract cellular immunity during the perinatal period. In: *Textbook of Gastroenterology and Nutrition in Infancy*. New York: Raven Press, 1981;219–39.

40. Nossal GJV. The basic components of the immune system. *N Engl J Med* 1987;316:1320–5.

41. Elson CO, Heck JA, Strober W. T cell regulation of murine IgA synthesis. *J Exp Med* 1979;149: 632–43.

42. Kawanishi H, Strober W. Regulatory T cells murine Peyer's patches directing IgA specific isotope switching. *N Y Acad Sci* 1983;409:243–57.

43. Kiyono H, McGhee JR, Mosteller LM, et al. Murine Peyer's patch T cell clones: characterization of antigen specific helper T cells for immunoglobulin A responses. *J Exp Med* 1982;156:1115–30.

44. Richman LK, Graeff AS, Yarchoan R, Strober W. Simultaneous induction of antigen specific IgA helper T cells and IgG suppressor T cells in the murine Peyer's patch after protein feeding. *J Immunol* 1981;126:2079.

45. Challacombe SJ, Tomasi TB. Systemic tolerance and secretory immunity after oral immunization. *J Exp Med* 1980;153:1459–72.

46. Green DR, Gold J, St. Martin S, et al. Microenvironmental immunoregulation: possible role of contrasuppressor cells in maintaining immune tissues. *Proc Natl Acad Sci USA* 1982;79:889–92.

47. Jackson GDF, Lensitre Coelho I, Vaerman JP, et al. Rapid disappearance from serum of intravenously injected rat myeloma IgA and its secretion in to bile. *Eur J Immunol* 1978;8:123–26.

48. Manning RJ, Walker PG, Carter L, et al. Studies on the origins of biliary immunoglobulins in rats. *Gastroenterology* 1984;87:173–9.

49. Sztul ES, Howell KE, Palade GE. Biogenesis of polymeric IgA receptor in rat hepatocytes I. Localization of its intracellular forms by cell fractionation studies. *J Cell Biol* 1985;100:1255–61.

50. Stochert RJ, Kressner MS, Collins JC, et al. IgA interaction with the asialoglycoprotein receptor. *Proc Natl Acad Sci USA* 1982;79:6229–31.

51. Delacroix DL, Hodgson HJF, McPherson A, et al. Selective transport of polymeric immunoglobulin A in bile. *J Clin Invest* 1982;70:230–41.

52. Altorfer J, Hardesty SJ, Scott JH, et al. Specific antibody synthesis and biliary secretion by the rat liver after intestinal immunization with cholera toxin. *Gastroenterology* 1987;93:539–49.

53. Walter WA, Wu MM, Isselbacher KJ, Block KJ. Intestinal uptake of macromolecules. IV. The effect of pancreatic duct ligation on the breakdown of antigen and antibody complexes on the intestinal surface. *Gastroenterology* 1975;69:1223–9.

54. Lake AM, Block KJ, Sinclair KJ, Walker WA. Anaphylactic release of intestinal goblet cell mucous. *Immunology* 1979;39:173–8.

55. Walker WA. Role of the mucosal barrier in toxin/microbial attachment to the gastrointestinal tract. *Ciba Found Symp* 1985;112:34–47.

56. Brown EG, Sweet AY: Neonatal necrotizing enterocolitis. *Pediatr Clin North Am* 1982;29:1149–70.

57. Kliegman RM, Fanaroff AA. Necrotizing enterocolitis. *N Engl J Med* 1984;310:1093–103.

58. Santulli TV, Schullinger JN, Heird WC, et al. Acute necrotizing enterocolitis in infancy: a review of 64 cases. *Pediatrics* 1975;55:376–87.

59. Lake AM, Walker WA. Neonatal necrotizing enterocolitis: a disease of altered host defense. *Clin Gastroenterol* 1977;6:463–80.

60. Hanson L, Ahlstedt S. Andersson B, et al. Protective factors in milk and the development of the immune system. *Pediatrics* 1985;75:172–5.

61. Mizrahi A, Barlow O, Berdon W, et al. Necrotizing enterocolitis in premature infants. *J Pediatr* 1965;66:697–706.
62. Welsh JK, May JT. Anti-infective properties of breast milk. *J Pediatr* 1979;94:1–9.
63. Barlow B, Santulli TV, Heird WC, et al. An experimental study of acute neonatal enterocolitis— the importance of breast milk. *J Pediatr Surg* 1974;9:587–95.
64. Pitt J, Barlow B, Heird WC, et al. Protection against experimental necrotizing enterocolitis by maternal milk. I. Role of milk leukocytes. *Pediatr Res* 1977;11:906–9.
65. Udall JN, Pang KY, Scrimshaw NS, Walker WA. The effect of early nutrition on intestinal maturation. *Pediatr Res* 1979;13:409.
66. Eibl MM, Wolf HM, Furnkranz H, Rosenkranz A. Prevention of necrotizing enterocolitis in low birth-weight infants by IgA-IgG feeding. *N Engl J Med* 1988;319:1–7.
67. Hanson DG. Ontogeny of orally induced tolerance to soluble proteins in mice. I. Priming and tolerance in newborns. *J Immunol* 1981;127:1516–24.
68. Strobel S, Ferguson A. Immune responses to fed protein antigens in mice. 3. Systemic tolerance or priming is related to age which antigen is first encountered. *Pediatr Res* 1984;18:588–94.
69. Kirsner JB, Shorter RG. Recent developments in "nonspecific" inflammatory bowel disease. *N Engl J Med* 1982;306:775–837.
70. MacDermitt RP, Stenson WF. Alterations of the immune system in ulcerative colitis and Crohn's disease. *Adv Immunol* 1988;42:285–328.
71. Shorter RG, Huizenga KA, Spencer RJ. A working hypothesis for the etiology and pathogenesis of nonspecific inflammatory bowel disease. *Am J Dig Dis* 1972;17:1024–32.
72. Auricchio S, Greco L, Troncone R. Gluten sensitive enteropathy in childhood. *Pediatr Clin North Am* 1988;35:157–87.
73. Kalis JB, Malkinson FD. Dermatitis herpetiformis. *JAMA* 1983;250:217–21.
74. Kagnoff MF, Austin RK, Hubert JJ, et al. Possible role for human adenovirus in the pathogenesis of celiac disease. *J Exp Med* 1984;160:1544–57.
75. Kagnoff MF. Coeliac disease: genetic, immunological and environmental factors in disease pathogenesis. *Scand J Gastroenterol* 1984;114:45–54.
76. Widdowson EM, Colombo VE, Artavams CA. Changes in the organs of pigs in response to feeding for the first 24 h after birth. II. The digestive tract. *Biol Neonate* 1976;28:272–4.
77. Heird WC, Hansen IH. Effect of colostrum on growth of intestinal mucosa. *Pediatr Res* 1977;11:406A.
78. Bienenstock J. The local immune response. *Am J Vet Res* 1975;36:488–91.
79. Kleinman RE, Walker WA. The enteromammary immune system: an important new concept in breast milk host defense. *Dig Dis Sci* 1979;24:876.
80. Kramer M. Does breast feeding help protect against atopic disease? Biology, methodology, and a golden jubilee of controversy. *J Pediatr* 1988;112:181–90.

Food Intolerance in Infancy: Allergology, Immunology, and Gastroenterology, edited by Robert N. Hamburger. Carnation Nutrition Education Series, Vol. 1. The Carnation Co., Los Angeles/Raven Press, Ltd., New York © 1989.

Atopic and Nonatopic Intolerance to Foods

Robert J. Dockhorn

University of Missouri School of Medicine, Kansas City, MO 64108

A dictionary definition of intolerance is the inability to endure. Therefore, one might say that the intolerance to food is the inability of an individual to endure a specific food. The term, food intolerance, refers to a wide variety of disorders. Food intolerance can be divided into two groups, the first being reactions involved with immunologically mediated sensitivity, and the second being those reactions that show no evidence of an immunologic phenomenon.

There are at least four types of immunologic reactions that may be involved in the process of immunologic intolerance to foods (1). Type I allergic reactions, or atopic reactions, are dependent upon immunoglobulin E (IgE) antibodies. The reaction, which is initiated by an allergen reacting with tissue-fixed mast cells or basophils, passively sensitized by the IgE antibody produced elsewhere, results from the release of pharmacologically active substances, such as vasoactive amines.

Type II reactions are known as cytotoxic reactions. They are initiated by an antibody other than IgE antibody reacting with either an antigenic component on a cell or tissue surface or an antigen or hapten that has become immediately associated with these cell surfaces. Complement is usually but not always necessary to effect the cellular damage.

Type III reactions, known as immune complex reactions, are initiated when an antigen reacts in the tissue spaces with potentially precipitating antibody, forming microprecipitates in and around the small vessels, causing damage to the tissues. Another mechanism in connection with Type III reactions is excess antigen reacting in the bloodstream with potentially precipitating antibody forming soluble circulating complexes, which are deposited in blood vessel walls or in the basement membrane, causing local inflammation.

Type IV reactions, also known as delayed or cell-mediated reactions, essentially are initiated by the reaction of specifically modified lymphocytes containing substances capable of responding specifically to allergens deposited at a local site.

Atopic or IgE-mediated food hypersensitivity is characterized by a variety of symptoms including anaphylaxis, angioedema, urticaria, asthma, atopic eczema, allergic rhinitis, gastrointestinal upset, headache, and allergic tension fatigue syndrome. The diagnosis of atopic IgE-mediated food hypersensitivity is established by

59

careful history, physical examination, and proper skin test or radioallergosorbent test (RAST) to demonstrate the presence of antigen-specific IgE antibody (2).

Type II food hypersensitivity reactions involve tissue-fixed antigens, in which the tissue is really an innocent bystander that becomes involved in an immune reaction when complement is activated on the tissue cell surface. Cytotoxic antibodies with pathogenic potential bind to the surface of cells by means of antigen-specific configurations on the fragment antigen-binding (Fab) portion of the immunoglobulin molecules. These cytolytic antibodies generally belong to the IgG class. The antigen may be an intrinsic component of the cell, or it may be an antigen or hapten that has become intimately associated with the cell (3).

The coating of circulating blood cells by cytolytic antibodies renders them more susceptible to intra- and extravascular destruction. One particular food, the Mexican fava bean, seems to have predilection for this type of reaction with red blood cells deficient in glucose-6-phosphate dehydrogenase. The red cell involved in this reaction is lysed (4).

Type III food hypersensitivity reactions involve circulating food antigens and circulating IgG antibodies. Usually these IgG antibodies are precipitating antibodies that can form toxic immune complexes. Toxic complexes are formed by antigen and precipitating antibodies in the zone of moderate antigen excess. Immune complexes formed in tissue spaces precipitate around small blood vessels, fixing complement, and producing a local inflammatory response (5).

A typical Type III food reaction can be demonstrtaed in patients with Heiner's syndrome who develop precipitating antibodies to milk protein. This antigen antibody reactivity causes gastrointestinal bleeding, as well as a pulmonary inflammatory reaction (6).

Type IV food hypersensitivity reactions involve food antigen and sensitized circulating lymphocytes. The food antigen causes the sensitized lymphocyte to release lymphokines. The lymphokine substances have recently been shown to possess a variety of biologic activities that are thought to be the *in vitro* correlates of cell-mediated immunity (7). Type IV food hypersensitivity reactions may occur locally in the gastrointestinal tract leading to villous atrophy. This can then result in malabsorption (8).

Nonimmunologic intolerance to foods may occur through a number of pathways including anaphylactoid reactions, poisoning, metabolic disturbances, and psychogenic causes. Anaphylactoid reactions mimicking true anaphylaxis can result from histamine intoxication after ingestion of food containing large quantities of histamine. This occurs after eating poisoned fish of the tuna or mackerel family and mahi-mahi. Histamine poisoning may also follow the ingestion of Swiss cheese. This problem is more frequently recognized in patients treated with isoniazid because they are particularly sensitive to histamine.

Poisoning by other noxious substances may occur causing adverse reaction to food. These poisons are frequently seen after ingestion of toxic mushrooms. Ingestion of poisonous plants like foxglove, which contains digitalis, or groundsel, which contains alkaloids, or poisonous pufferfish, may lead to serious disease states. Many other foods such as green potatoes, insufficiently cooked beans, and rhubarb leaves may cause illness. Some commonly eaten foods may also result in toxicity if excessive quantities are consumed.

Poisoning from food contaminated by infectious agents or their products may occur. Mycotoxins found in some foods can cause liver disease. Some algal toxins result in neurotoxicity following the ingestion of fish such as grouper, snapper, or barracuda which have been contaminated. Certain food-borne diseases may arise from contamination of food with toxic metals including arsenic, cobalt, mercury, and selenium. Also, vasoactive amines such as tyramine, tryptamine, and serotonin can be food contaminants.

Metabolic disturbances such as inborn errors of metabolism, fat intolerance, and carbohydrate intolerance also manifest themselves as food intolerances (9).

A common example of a metabolic derangement leading to food-induced disease is the gastrointestinal disorder associated with intolerance to lactose in milk. This disorder is secondary to the deficiency of the lactase enzyme. Intolerance to other carbohydrates is far less common. Celiac disease is caused by intolerance of glutens and gliadins found in wheat that leads to the classic gastrointestinal and systemic manifestations seen in the disorder (10).

The diagnosis of intolerance to food requires a thorough and detailed history, not only of the patient's symptoms but of the patient's past dietary habits. This is then followed by a careful physical examination after which appropriate tests may be ordered. If the food intolerance appears to be an atopic disease, then appropriate allergy skin tests and appropriate laboratory tests to demonstrate the presence of antigen-specific IgE antibody would be in order. If, however, the food intolerance is not of the IgE type, then appropriate laboratory tests to determine what type of antigen antibody reaction or cell-mediated reaction is occurring.

Once the diagnosis has been established and the offending food has been identified, then the treatment of choice for intolerance to foods, whether it be atopic or nonatopic, is to avoid the suspected food.

In 1978, Bock et al. (11) described the manifestations of sensitivity reactions to foods. They described two groups of reactions, one being reaginic and the other nonreaginic. The reaginic group of manifestations consisted of those seen in the typical IgE food reactions, such as anaphylaxis, abdominal pain, vomiting, diarrhea, angioedema, rash, urticaria, allergic dermatitis, rhinitis, and asthma. In the nonreaginic group the manifestations consisted of: enteropathies leading to vomiting, diarrhea, occult bleeding, protein-losing enteropathies, and malabsorption, as well as urticaria, allergic dermatitis, pneumonitis, and hemosiderosis. Their description of reaginic food sensitivity has an onset at all ages. The duration of the illness can either be transient or permanent. Allergy skin tests to foods are positive. Mucosal reactions demonstrate erythema, edema, and mucous production. On the other hand, food sensitivities of the nonreaginic variety have their onset in infancy or childhood. The duration is usually transient except for those who have gluten sensitivity. Allergy skin tests to foods are negative. However, serum antibodies to foods, particularly of the IgG class, are elevated. Mucosal surfaces show villous atrophy, with cellular infiltration. Their findings showed that the majority of the patients they studied had positive histories to cow's milk; less than half of those patients had positive allergy skin tests to milk and less than one-third had positive double-blind challenge reactions to milk. However, peanut and egg showed a lower positive history but a statistically higher reaction in those with a positive history to allergy skin tests as well as to double-blind food challenges.

Bock et al.'s findings demonstrated that 100% of the patients reacting to allergy skin tests to food antigens had the onset of their symptoms within 2 hr after ingestion of the food. This correlates excellently with the immediate onset symptomatology in IgE-mediated food reactions.

Sampson and McCaskill (12) reported on 160 patients with atopic eczema who had food sensitivities to egg, peanut, milk, fish, soy, and wheat. Of that group, 35% had positive food challenges, 86% had positive skin tests to food antigens, and the onset of their symptoms occurred within 2 hr after ingestion of the food. These findings, once again, demonstrate that IgE food sensitivities are skin test positive but may well not show positive reactions to double-blind food challenges.

A study done by Atkins et al. (13) evaluating patients with food allergies found that the common food offenders were shrimp, peanut, and egg. Once again, food challenge was approximately 40% reliable as a diagnostic tool, whereas skin testing had 90% reliability with the onset of the symptoms coming within 30 min. A study by Bernstein et al. (14) in adult patients with histories of food allergies to tomatoes, milk, chocolate, and shrimp showed only a 28% correlation with food challenges, 31% correlation with skin tests, and a highly variable onset of symptoms after ingestion of the food. It would appear in this group of patients that other immunologic phenomena are occurring besides IgE-mediated food sensitivity.

During 1986, I had the opportunity to study a group of infants and children who had symptoms of food allergy. There were 50 patients ranging in age from 3 months to 10 years. There were 27 males and 23 females. Their symptoms consisted of runny nose, frequent infections, wheezing, cough, ear infections, rash, gastrointestinal problems, and headache. Their total serum IgE levels, for the most part, were quite low. Evaluating IgE antibodies to foods demonstrated low level reactivity to milk, wheat, corn, and eggs. However, when IgG antibodies were measured to specific foods, a large number of these patients had high levels of antibody to egg, milk, wheat, and a lesser number to corn (15).

This information reinforces the observations that immunologic intolerance to foods involves other mechanisms besides IgE. No matter what the underlying cause of the food intolerance is, the basic modality for therapy is strict elimination diet. Pharmacologic agents have been utilized in Type I IgE food hypersensitivity for relief of the symptoms, and these agents include corticosteroid, antihistamines, and cromolyn sodium. However, to actually prevent the reaction from occurring, the suspected food must be removed from the diet.

In summary, if the ingestion of the food happens to trigger an allergic reaction, then the reaction may be immediate or delayed but of IgE mediation or a reaginic type reaction. However, if the allergic reaction is of the delayed type, then the hypersensitivity reaction can be Type II, III, or IV. On the other hand, with the nonimmunologically related reactions, the trigger can cause immediate or delayed reactions caused by toxic, idiosyncratic, or metabolic intolerance.

ACKNOWLEDGMENTS

This work was partially supported by grants from the Carnation Company.

REFERENCES

1. Coombs RRA, Gell PGH. Classification of allergic reactions responsible for clinical hypersensitivity and disease. In: RRA Coombs, PGH Gell, eds. *Clinical Aspects of Immunology*, 2nd ed. Philadelphia: FA Davis, 1968, p. 575.
2. Orange RP, Austen KF. In: B Amos, ed. *Progress in Immunology*. New York: Academic Press, 1971, p. 173.
3. Knogshavn PAL, Hawkins D, Schuster J. The biology of the immune response. In: SO Freedman, P Gold, eds. *Clinical Immunology*, 2nd ed. New York: Harper and Row, 1976, p. 48.
4. Dockhorn RJ. Laboratory tests for food hypersensitivity. In: JC Breneman, ed. *Handbook of Food Allergies*. New York: Marcel Dekker, Inc., 1987, p. 172.
5. Biondi RM. Damage by toxic complexes. In: F Speer, RJ Dockhorn, eds. *Allergy and Immunology in Children*. Springfield, IL: Charles C Thomas, 1973.
6. Heiner DC, Sears JW, Kniker WT. Multiple precipitins to cow's milk in chronic respiratory disease. *Am J Dis Child* 1962;103:40–60.
7. Bellanti JA, Rocklin RE. Cell-mediated reaction. In: JA Bellanti, ed. *Immunology II*. Philadelphia: WB Saunders, 1978, p. 233.
8. Ferguson A, MacDonald TT. Effects of local delayed hypersensitivity on the small intestine. In: *Ciba Foundation Symposium No. 46*, North Holland, New York: Elsevier, 1977, pp. 305–27.
9. Lifshitz F. Food intolerance. In: LT Chairamonte, AT Schneider, F Lifshitz, eds. *Food Allergy*. New York: Marcel Dekker, Inc., 1988, pp. 3–11.
10. Kniker WT, Rodriguez LM. Non-IgE-mediated and delayed adverse reactions to foods or additives. In: JC Breneman, ed. *Handbook of Food Allergies*. New York: Marcel Dekker, Inc., 1987, p. 132.
11. Bock SA, Lew WY, Remigio LK, May CD. Studies of hypersensitivity reactions to foods in infants and children. *J Allergy Clin Immunol*, 1978;62:327–34.
12. Sampson HA, McCaskill CM. Food hypersensitivity in atopic dermatitis: evaluation of 113 patients. *J Pediatr* 1985;107:669–75.
13. Atkins FM, Steinberg SS, Metcalfe DD. Evaluation of immediate adverse reactions to foods in adult patients. II. A detailed analysis of reaction patterns during oral food challenge. *J Allergy Clin Immunol* 1985;75:356–63.
14. Bernstein M, Day JH, Walsh A. Double-blind food challenges in the diagnosis of food sensitivity in the adult. *J Allergy Clin Immunol* 1982;70:205–10.
15. Dockhorn RJ. Clinical studies of food allergy in infants and children. *Ann Allergy* 1987;59:137–40.

Food Intolerance in Infancy: Allergology, Immunology, and Gastroenterology, edited by Robert N. Hamburger. Carnation Nutrition Education Series, Vol. 1. The Carnation Co., Los Angeles/Raven Press, Ltd., New York © 1989.

General Discussion for Section I

Kjell Aas, Robert J. Dockhorn, Robert N. Hamburger, Steven B. Machtinger, Buford Lee Nichols, Jr., and W. Allan Walker

Dr. Nichols: I would like to ask Professor Aas a question just for fun. He mentioned immunoacrobatics. His paper is full of definitions, and I would like him to define immunoacrobatics.

Dr. Aas: I see a resemblance between the acrobatic sequences in a circus and all the different combinations of beautiful methods that you have in immunology and protein chemistry today. You can do amazing work with the available techniques in combination. It is like exercises between two acrobats in immunology and protein chemistry. Advances and progress made in protein chemistry propagate progress in immunology, and immunology propagates progress in protein chemistry. I would like to add that to me, immunology is a branch of protein chemistry.

Dr. Nichols: Immunology is protein chemistry. Well, certainly immunology is the hallmark of the new biology and recombinant deoxyribonucleic acid (DNA) depends upon immunological mechanisms for protein identification and characterization. I would like to ask Dr. Dockhorn a practical question. In his presentation, he stated that it's very important to take a good history when you are evaluating a patient for food intolerance. What percent of the histories taken very carefully do in fact prove to be clinically relevant to your management of the case?

Dr. Dockhorn: At our level of science and knowledge today as far as food allergies are concerned, I think it's terribly important that the histories be taken in a very detailed manner because the diagnosis of the food allergic or intolerant state is probably made 85 to 90% by history. What you're doing with the tests, whether they be skin tests or laboratory tests, is just trying to add proof to your diagnosis that you've already made after you did the careful history and the physical exam.

Dr. Nichols: To follow up on that, you said that you had to do adequate laboratory evaluation. What constitutes adequate laboratory evaluation when perhaps it only confirms your clinical impression?

Dr. Dockhorn: At the present state of the art, that is an excellent question, because most of the practicing physicians in the United States have only limited access to laboratory evaluations for food sensitivity, and therefore it is a limiting factor. If we look at statistics, probably 80 to 85% of physicians use skin tests to verify immunoglobulin E (IgE)-mediated sensitivity and use no other laboratory tests to help them to make the diagnosis of food intolerance.

Dr. MacPherson: Jeff MacPherson from San Diego, California. I would be happy to hear about the possibility of an obviously small number of women who might possess or have flawed breast milk; breast milk, if you will, that will not induce gut maturation.

Dr. Walker: I can only theorize on this question because I am not aware of anyone who has systematically analyzed growth factors in breast milk of a large enough sample of women to determine this. It is certainly conceivable that there are deficiencies in any one of a number of factors that are present in breast milk which could influence or act to influence the neonate's gut maturation. The problem is that we haven't begun to define the effect on gut maturation or the actual absence of such factors. We are still trying to define the extent to which these factors in breast milk may have a cause/effect relationship with gut development.

Dr. Kahn: My name is Andre Kahn from Belgium. We heard that for some patients with clinical evidence of allergy or atopy that tests can be negative and challenge tests can be negative as well. So, I would like to have your comments on what should we think about laboratory tests being negative, and what should we think about challenge tests being negative? Are these necessary to correctly define an allergy, or do you mean that perhaps the clinical history may not be sufficient to define an allergic situation?

Dr. Dockhorn: If I may paraphrase the question, what if a patient comes to your office and has a history that you suspect is related to food intolerance, and there are negative skin tests, there are negative food challenges, and there are negative laboratory tests? If so, then is your diagnosis correct by the history alone? I still think that today, despite the fact that we do not have all of the necessary tools and all the laboratory tests, and we don't know all of the situations involved in food intolerances and, as Dr. Aas says, we really don't have the adequate tools and the right antigenic material we need to work with, if a patient comes to your office with a strong history of food intolerance, the diagnosis can be made and the treatment can be recommended to simply avoid that food. I don't think you have to have positive laboratory tests and skin tests before you place a patient on an elimination diet.

Dr. Nichols: But would you agree, Dr. Dockhorn, that it's more difficult with the non-IgE-mediated immune reactions to document the benefit of elimination diet?

Dr. Dockhorn: Absolutely. I agree wholeheartedly. It certainly would be nice if we had the all-inclusive, all-telling test for all of these conditions so that we wouldn't have to depend so heavily on our clinical acumen. But I do believe that we still have to be thinking physicians and thinking patients, and it does require time on an elimination diet as well as compliance, which is not only a problem with medications but with diets.

Dr. Fish: Lloyd Fish, Minneapolis, Minnesota. Is there a significant difference in terms of maturation of the gut in the infants that have selective IgA deficiency or those infants that have a secretory piece missing or a J chain missing?

Dr. Walker: Dr. Fish, I don't know that there has ever been a well-documented case of secretory component deficiency. There was an article in the *New England Journal of Medicine* that allegedly demonstrated this, but the authors subsequently retracted their observation. There have been a few cases of IgA-deficient nursing mothers, that is, the child nursing from an IgA-deficient mother.

Dr. Fish: And an IgA-deficient infant?

Dr. Walker: Adequate prospective studies have not been performed since all infants have a transient decrease in IgA. Thus, it would be necessary to follow these patients sequentially until they do or do not ultimately produce secretory IgA. I don't think that this has ever been done, and therefore we can't answer this question. From the maternal side, that is, IgA-deficient mothers who are nursing, there are no studies that have shown a difference in maturation of either the intestinal epithelium or the other intestinal lymphoid elements.

Dr. Dolovich: Jerry Dolovich, Hamilton, Canada. I would like to ask the panel to examine the question of non-IgE food reactions a little more critically. My specific question is, can you give a single example where it is proven that a non-IgE immunological mechanism is responsible for food intolerance or, in Dr. Hamburger's broader sense, food allergy? In other words, quite apart from the hypothetical possibilities, can we say there is an example where it's been proven?

Dr. Nichols: I would like to comment that there is one line of investigation coming out of Glasgow which is fascinating in this regard. These are experiments done by Dr. D. M. V. Parrott and Dr. Allan Mowat. They found that by careful genetic manipulation of purebred mice and transplanting across immunotolerant genes that they can produce hypertrophy or atrophy of the villus or the crypt associated with infiltration or absence of interepithelial lymphocytes. That is proof that the immune system does influence intestine morphology. Does that answer your question?

Dr. Dolovich: No, I'm talking about disease, examples of non-IgE immunologically mediated disease. Now, we understand the immune complex damage that happens elsewhere, particularly the kidney, but are there examples in the gastrointestinal tract?

Dr. Hamburger: Are you excluding Heiner's disease, Heiner's syndrome, the IgG-mediated bleeding from the gastrointestinal tract? I mean, that is about as dramatic and sometimes lethal a disease as you can want and it's certainly IgG-mediated.

Dr. Aas: First of all, I think the question is very appropriate. The answers will be diffuse because we are not speaking about IgE antibodies and reactions to food. The question may be precise, but we do not have any method to prove that there are connections between antigens in the food and other sorts of immune reactions in the body, except for a few exceptions. It has, for example, been shown and adequately controlled that some nickel substances in food may provoke contact allergic Type 4 reactions in the skin. We need to go much deeper into just that question and hold it open as a challenge to ourselves.

Dr. Prenner: Dr. Bruce Prenner, San Diego, California. Is there any rationale or justification for physicians of any type, whether they be pediatricians or specialists, to order immune complex assays, IgG-4 and so forth, in the real world? In our area in Southern California it seems to be a popular type of test, and in view of the question, I would like to hear the panel's answer since the cost of these tests is much higher than most of the things the physicians who practice allergy ordinarily do. I would like to know if these tests are justifiable.

Dr. Machtinger: I'll give you my opinion. Certainly there are a number of tests looking at immune complex disease or gastrointestinal (GI) disease and the presence of immune complexes in the blood. Brostoff has done studies on that; and Frick and Kaufman have also published. Where I am in California, there are practitioners who order immune complex tests, but I don't use them in my practice, and I see at this time no reason to do it.

Dr. Nichols: It's very common in pregnancy, by the way.

Dr. Walker-Smith: I want to come back to the question that was posed before. There is a clear example—there are several examples—but there is one very clear example of non-IgE-mediated immunological reaction in the gut, and that is cow's milk-sensitive enteropathy in infancy. This is when there is clear morphological evidence of an almost flat mucosa becoming normal under milk elimination diet, recurring with milk challenge, and with a rise in intraepithelial lymphocytes, etc. I'll be talking about this tomorrow. Granted there isn't absolutely overwhelming evidence, but I think there is strong evidence that this is cell-mediated immunity. Then you could also look at cow's milk colitis. I think that there is good evidence of non-reaginic reactions in the gut in infancy.

Dr. Ziegler: I would like to reply to Dr. Dolovich's question regarding the same thing, the non-IgE-mediated gastrointestinal reactions. I think the most common example that was mentioned already is the occult bleeding in the gastrointestinal tract in infants. About half of the iron-deficient infants have a high precipitating titer of the IgG and to a lesser extent IgM antibodies, and also the example of Dr. Walker-Smith regarding the protein-losing enteropathies. There are also a few scattered reports about gastroduodenitis as well as certain patients with colitis. These are selected patients of course, not all of them. I think the most impressive example is the pulmonary disease or Heiner's syndrome where the confirmation by X-ray as well as by precipitating antibodies is very impressive.

Dr. Nichols: Dr. Buts has some comment to make along this line. He showed that iron deficiency reduces secretory component in the gut.

Dr. Buts: If secretory IgA in breast milk has a protective role against food antigens, are there clinical observations about the reactivity of milk in the woman while deficient in IgA?

Dr. Nichols: Dr. Walker, do you know of any studies in women deficient of IgE or IgA?

Dr. Walker: No, I don't know of any such studies.

Dr. Dockhorn: I would like to make a comment on Dr. Prenner's question about IgG food studies and immune complex food studies. The practicing physician in the United States today has a mind-set against the study of IgG food antibodies and immune complexes. As Dr. Aas said, if the antigens that we are using are no good, how can the laboratory tests be effective? It doesn't necessarily mean that immune complexes are not a part of a disease state. We get things somewhat confused. If it doesn't fit into a category where a specific laboratory test will tell us what is going on, then that disease doesn't occur. I don't believe that is true. I do believe however, that the commercialization of food immune-complex studies as well as food IgG studies has no place in the general practice in our offices, but that doesn't necessarily mean that later on, as we develop better antigens and better techniques, that it isn't going to be a whole lot better than the allergy skin test for specific conditions. So let's not get a mind-set and "throw the baby out with the bathwater." Let's keep looking and keep investigating and be advocates for the study of food allergy rather than advocates against new knowledge in food allergy.

Dr. McGeady: Steven McGeady from Philadelphia, Pennsylvania. If I understood you correctly, Dr. Walker, you equated antigen uptake with up-modulation of Class 2 major histocompatability complex (MHC) antigens in the intestinal epithelium. Can you elaborate on the mechanism of the association between antigen uptake in the Class 2 MHC antigens in the gut?

Dr. Walker: The work I was quoting was principally done by Dr. Paul Bland of Manchester, England. Under conditions of inflammation, such as an inflammatory bowel disease, presumably with release of gamma interferon, there seems to be an increase in the expression of Class 2 antigens. Experimentally, Dr. Bland suggests that the presence of Class 2 MHC antigens, expression on epithelial cells may participate in the uptake and presentation of intestinal antigens. What I was suggesting is that, as we become more knowledgeable in the mechanisms which express Ia antigen on enterocytes and of the extent the epithelial cell is involved in antigen presentation, we might be able to answer some questions about immune suppression as well as helper activity, under conditions of intestinal antigen presentation.

Dr. Nichols: Let me ask you a question, Dr. Walker. Ia is a rat Class 2 antigen. What is the human equivalent and what is the correct terminology when you're talking about human disease?

Dr. Walker: Our work has been principally in the rodent. Therefore, I can only comment on that. I think the work that has been observed, with the exception of studies on inflammatory bowel disease, has been in the rodent.

Dr. Nichols: As I understand the Class 2, it's called the DQ complex, and there is a genetic series within that. If you read the human literature, it will be referring to DQ, but it's the same as Ia in the rodent.

Dr. Sandberg: I want to address this question to Dr. Walker. Would you expand on how you look at intestinal permeability using small molecules or variable sized molecules like PEG versus pinocytosis in your evaluation of this whole process of intestinal function and maturation?

Dr. Walker: We haven't had experience with small molecules, with the exception of work done in an inflammatory bowel model using polyethylene glycol (PEG). I think they are handled entirely differently than proteins. In much of the recent studies of macromolecular molecules researchers have become aware of this fact and are returning to the use of proteins. I don't think we can answer questions related to protein transport with large molecular weight sugars or the use of polyethyleneglycol molecules as evidence of macromolecular transport other than to demonstrate that there is increased permeability. This uptake is a different situation to proteins or protein fragments which are taken up probably through a pinocytosis process.

Dr. Nichols: Do you agree with Claude Morin's observation that D-xylose absorption is altered by the feeding of specific antigens to sensitive individuals?

Dr. Walker: I think that's probably true because, with any kind of an insult to the intestinal surface, you're going to get increased uptake of large molecules.

Dr. Gryboski: Joyce Gryboski, New Haven, Connecticut. I think everyone knows for years that I have been expounding on milk-induced colitis, and in the past couple of years we have seen some children who have been exclusively breast-fed who have had a bloody colitis not related to any other cause. We still work with stool precipitins because I can't find high IgEs and I can't find positive radioallergo-sorbent test (RASTs) in these babies. No matter what has been said about precipitins, I think we are only looking at the tip of the iceberg. If you have nothing else to use to make a diagnosis, and we don't seem to have it, precipitins are still helpful. We have had a couple of breast-fed babies with positive milk and soy and have restricted the mother's diet, which has been terribly difficult, and those babies have stopped bleeding within 24 hr. So I think that is cause and effect. As for the immunoglobulins involved in that kind of reaction, I'm not sure, but I think the precipitins most likely are IgA precipitins. But then you have the baby who, when accidentally fed milk when he has been on a careful milk-restricted diet, blows out his belly, goes into shock, and sloughs blood, mucus, and colonic-epithelium. I think that has got to be caused by an IgE reaction.

Dr. Nichols: Do you agree with that, Dr. Hamburger?

Dr. Hamburger: Oh, absolutely, that's authoritative.

Dr. Ancona: Bob Ancona form Baltimore, Maryland. I would like to ask this question of the whole panel, particularly Dr. Walker. We certainly know the nutritional content of breast milk changes with time and also with gestation, but has anyone looked at any of the immunological components of breast milk when delivery is premature? Are the contents of IgA or lymphocytes changed in the colostrum, for example, day 1 versus day 3 either in human or animal models?

Dr. Walker: We have stated many years ago that IgA levels in breast milk are a mirror image of the decreased levels in neonatal intestinal secretions and have suggested a cause/effect association. I don't know that anyone has systematically looked at breast milk from mothers delivering preterm infants, and it's an area that needs to be studied.

Dr. Nichols: Furthermore, it's necessary to comment that most people are looking at total immunoglobulin fractions and they are not looking at functional antigen-specific antibodies. It's very difficult to trace functionality as well as the total immunoglobulin concentration.

Question: This is actually a follow-up question on Dr. Dolovich's, and it has to do with the question of proof for non-IgE-mediated mechanisms. As immunology becomes more sophisticated, it becomes possible to track interleukins and various cell subsets without ever getting down to the fundamental question of proving that any of them is involved in the actual mechanism of disease. Transfer experiments have been around for the last 30 years or so, and it should have been possible, either in animal models or in humans. I reviewed the immune complex question for the American Academy of Allergy to put together a position statement, and I concluded that it lacks proof at the level of Koch's postulates. The same with thymus-derived cells (T cells), bone-marrow-derived cells (B cells), and the various other hypotheses such as the interleukins, now up to 6 to 8, play any part in disease. Thus, there is no proof that they are there to do damage. So, after this long introduction, are there transfer experiments to show that if you transfer sensitized T cells, you do get the bowel defects or that you can recreate some of the diseases in an animal model system?

Dr. Machtinger: There aren't any transfer studies of that sort. I agree that before you start looking for immune complexes and other immune changes in an organism, you had better make sure that there is pathology there.

Dr. Hamburger: I'm struck by the different levels of statements one makes when talking about science and scientific proof as against what we need as clinicians. I want to remind everybody that when we're talking about lack of proof for fulfilling Koch's postulates, it's asking a bit much of us as clinicians. I would urge you to continue to treat your patients in the best clinical manner until the data that Dr. Dockhorn asked us to get are in.

Food Intolerance in Infancy: Allergology, Immunology, and Gastroenterology, edited by Robert N. Hamburger. Carnation Nutrition Education Series, Vol. 1. The Carnation Co., Los Angeles/Raven Press, Ltd., New York © 1989.

Introduction to Section II

Laurence Finberg

Department of Pediatrics, State University of New York, Health Sciences Center at Brooklyn, Brooklyn, New York 11203

Pediatrics in all likelihood had its origins because of the special problems of infant feeding. At the end of the 19th century, when it became apparent that it was possible to feed human infants something other than human milk, namely the milk of animals, a great need arose to make this practice safe and nutritious. The earliest concerns had to be hygienic and therefore dealt primarily with the then emerging science of microbiology. Decades later, with more knowledge and greater safety from contamination, the focus turned to the specific nutritional content of the milk. Biochemistry and physiology then became the scientific foci, and to a very large extent solutions to the problems were then found. Certainly we now have appropriate safe infant formulas which provide nutrients in appropriate proportions for the vast majority of term infants.

It now follows reasonably, as the science of immunology rapidly develops and our understanding of immunologic problems unfolds, that the next focus for evaluation of infant feeding should be from the perspective of this exciting and exploding science. The words allergy and intolerance may be used to express problems and perceived problems with precise definitions, but more commonly, they are used very imprecisely. We need to address that specificity.

The clinical significance of food allergy, particularly that related to cow's milk, has long been a controversy in pediatrics. My initial training and my subsequent experience have allowed me to align myself with those who think that both cow's milk allergy and cow's milk intolerance are uncommon events with allergy in fact being rare. I speak now not of simple pasteurized cow's milk but that which has been through the evaporation process or those modifications employed by the infant formula industry. I have been able to practice pediatrics essentially without ever giving consideration to these phenomena with two exceptions, each rather rare or at least uncommon.

The first of these is true cow's milk enteropathy, sometimes associated with generalized vascular reactions. These patients can be desperately ill and they require elimination of lactoglobulin from their diet as a lifesaving measure. Even in a teaching hospital these are rare patients.

The second group for which I have seen some clinical evidence is that of lactose intolerance. One variety, the genetically determined, total absence of lactase, is very rare in infancy and even the acquired variety causing clinically significant change is uncommon.

Our task at this meeting is to illuminate as much as possible what is known about immunologic problems associated with infant feeding. We need just to see if there are solutions to the problems already at hand; perhaps most important, we need to define those problems for which we now have the scientific basis for resolution. Having identified myself as a skeptic, I now propose to introduce a session on the techniques for diagnosing food allergy, keeping an open mind as we all evaluate the evidence.

Food Intolerance in Infancy: Allergology, Immunology, and Gastroenterology, edited by Robert N. Hamburger. Carnation Nutrition Education Series, Vol. 1. The Carnation Co., Los Angeles/Raven Press, Ltd., New York © 1989.

In Vivo Diagnosis of Food Allergy

Sami L. Bahna

Department of Allergy and Immunology, The Cleveland Clinic Foundation, Cleveland, Ohio 44195–5305

The diagnosis of food allergy is predominantly clinical. Information on the offending food(s) may be obtained from the medical history, a food/symptom diary, trials of elimination diets, and skin testing. To verify the role of suspected foods, each should be subjected to well-controlled oral challenge testing.

Skin testing is probably the most commonly utilized diagnostic procedure in food allergy. Its reliability, however, is generally suboptimal and varies from one food to another. It has an overall positive predictive accuracy of 48% and a negative predictive accuracy of 74%.

Elimination-challenge testing is the most definitive procedure for verification of the role of suspected foods. Placebo-controlled blind challenges are ideal, yet have limitations; disguising an adequate quantity of food or choosing an appropriate placebo may be difficult. The challenge method also may be very different from the method of natural exposure. The test should be done under medical supervision to document the occurrence of reaction and to treat any potentially severe ones.

In evaluating patients suspected of having food allergy, information on the offending food may be pursued in several ways (1). Medical history, food/symptom diary, trials of elimination diets, and skin testing are widely used (Table 1). Certain *in vitro* tests may also be used and are addressed in *this volume*. To verify the role of a certain food in inducing a particular symptom, appropriate challenge tests should be conducted.

The underlying hypersensitivity mechanism, however, may be difficult to document, although it may be guessed by the nature of symptoms and time of onset following exposure to food. A positive immediate-type skin test or an increased serum level of specific immunoglobulin E (IgE) antibodies supports an IgE-mediated reaction. More than one immunologic mechanism, however, may be involved in the same patient, particularly when there are multiple manifestations (2).

MEDICAL HISTORY

A thorough history may provide valuable information to support or exclude food allergy. Occasionally the medical history may be so obvious as to settle the diagno-

TABLE 1. In vivo *diagnostic procedures of food allergy*

1. Medical history
   a. Relation of symptoms to food intake
   b. Specific foods suspected
   c. Association with other factors
2. Food/symptom diary
   a. Regular daily recording
   b. Recording whenever symptoms appear
3. Trials of elimination diets
   a. Conventional elimination diets (e.g., Rowe's)
   b. Individualized diets devoid of certain foods
   c. Elemental diet
   d. Hypoallergenic formula for infants
4. Skin testing
   a. Epicutaneous (scratch; puncture; prick)
   b. Intracutaneous
5. Challenge testing
   a. Oral
   b. Inhalation

sis without the need for further tests. This would be the case in patients whose symptoms are objective and well defined (e.g., urticaria, angioedema, or wheezing), have occurred intermittently, and on multiple occasions have appeared shortly after exposure to a particular food. The history may reveal the involvement of other factors in addition to food (e.g., physical exercise, emotional events, or premenstrual time).

FOOD/SYMPTOM DIARY

A regular tabular recording by date and time of all foods eaten and the appearance or exacerbation of symtpoms may assist in suspecting the offending foods. The food/symptom diary is most effective when the symptoms are well defined, occur intermittently, last for a short time, and appear shortly after exposure to a food that is not eaten on a daily basis. The recording should encompass a few recurrences of symptoms.

The diary is of little help if the recording is incomplete, if the offending food is incorporated in frequently eaten dishes, or in cases of delayed-onset reactions. The patient may not be aware of a "hidden" food allergen in a commercially prepared food, either because it is not listed on the label or is listed under a name unfamiliar to the public (e.g., whey, casein, calcium caseinate, ovalbumin, ovomucoid, or ovomucin).

In addition to foods, other events may need to be recorded, such as places visited, social activities, emotional events, menses, and physical exercise. Any such factors may contribute to the patient's symptoms or potentiate the effect of food allergens.

If symptoms occur very infrequently, compliance in recording is usually poor. In these cases, recording may be done only whenever symptoms occur and should include a sequential recording of foods eaten and events happening during the preceding 12 to 24 hr.

DIAGNOSTIC ELIMINATION DIETS

Certain elimination diets may be tried in patients whose symptoms are frequent or persistent and whose medical history suggests food allergy without pointing to any particular food. Some conventional diets are devised to be devoid of certain group(s) of commonly allergenic foods. Rowe Elimination Diets Number 1, 2, 3, and 4 are widely known examples (3,4). Elemental formula (Tolerex or Standard Vivonex by Norwich Eaton Pharmaceuticals, or Vivasorb by Phrimer A/S) is a strict elimination diet. The protein in this formula consists of synthesized amino acids (5,6). These elimination diets have some advantages and several disadvantages (7). In infants, a hypoallergenic formula may be given, e.g., casein hydrolysate (Nutramigen by Mead Johnson Nutritional Division) or the recently available whey hydrolysate (Good Start H.A. by Carnation).

Selection of the initial elimination diet may vary from one patient to another. If no improvement in symptoms is noted within 2 to 4 weeks, other elimination diets may be tried. Once improvement occurs, the eliminated foods are reintroduced one at a time to identify the offending ones.

SKIN TESTING

In evaluating patients for food allergy, physicians have shown divergent attitudes towards the usefulness of skin testing. At one extreme are those who do not use food extracts for skin testing, and at the other extreme are those who diagnose food allergy by skin testing alone. At present, skin testing is probably the most commonly used procedure in evaluation of food allergy. Reports on its reliability, however, have shown inconsistent results (8–12).

The allergen extract is usually applied epicutaneously (i.e., by scratch, prick, or puncture techniques). Commercial food extracts for epicutaneous testing are mostly provided in a concentration of 1:20 or 1:10 wt/vol (50% glycerinated). Fresh food, however, may be superior to the commercial extracts (13–15). If the test is negative to the foods suspected from the history, intracutaneous testing may be performed by injecting 0.02 ml of aqueous extract, usually 1:1,000 wt/vol. Performing epicutaneous testing first minimizes the risk of systemic or large local reactions that might result from intradermal administration of an allergen to which the patient is highly sensitive.

The test sites are inspected after 15 to 20 min for the size of the wheal-and-flare response, which reflects an IgE-mediated reaction. A score from 0 to 4+ is given as compared with the response to a diluent and to histamine (2). Most allergists consider a reaction of 2+ or greater as positive, but not necessarily clinically relevant.

The role of each food provoking such a reaction should be verified by elimination-challenge test.

We studied 49 allergy patients, mostly children, whose histories were highly suggestive of food allergy (16). They were subjected to scratch testing with commercial food extracts; whenever the reaction score was 1 + or 0 and the food was suspected from the history, intradermal testing was done. Double-blind, placebo-controlled oral challenges were performed with the food that showed a positive skin test (2 + or greater) or were suspected from the history. The results of skin testing and challenge were concordant in 63% of all instances (Table 2). In the positive challenge group, skin testing was positive in 58% of instances, but varied from one food to another, being lowest for tomato (33%) and highest for fish (83%). In the negative challenge group, skin testing was negative in 65% of instances, lowest for fish (50%) and highest for orange (89%). The overall positive predictive accuracy of skin testing was 48%, lowest for crab (33%) and highest for fish (83%). The overall negative predictive accuracy was 74%, lowest for cow's milk (44%) and highest for egg white (89%). The presenting symptoms in our series were asthma and/or rhinitis in 76%, atopic dermatitis in 47%, urticaria/angioedema in 47%, gastrointestinal symptoms in 27%, and systemic anaphylaxis in 12%. Nevertheless, the results previously reported on atopic dermatitis patients were not much different (17).

A discordance between the results of skin testing and challenge testing might be caused by any of several factors, such as technical errors, non-IgE-mediated reactions, the specific reagins being more localized in the shock organ, or the presence of subclinical hypersensitivity (2).

The suboptimal reliability of skin testing with the currently available food extracts should not deter its use as a screening test, particularly since none of the currently available *in vitro* tests has optimal reliability (1). In a series of 102 adults who had a history of idiopathic anaphylaxis, skin testing with food extracts assisted in identifying the cause in 7 subjects (18).

A high concordance rate between positive skin-test reaction and challenge testing has been noted in studies that used purified allergen extracts, such as codfish (9) and peanut (19). Purification and standardization of food allergy extracts are complex processes, but may be forthcoming (20).

TABLE 2. *Concordance between the results of skin testing and double-blind oral food challenge*

Group	N	Overall	Lowest	Highest
			Concordance, %	
All challenges	107	62.6	53.3 (milk)	75.0 (fish)
Positive challenge group	38	57.9	33.3 (tomato)	83.3 (fish)
Negative challenge group	69	65.2	50.0 (fish)	88.9 (orange)

ELIMINATION CHALLENGE TEST

To verify the role of foods suspected (by history, diary, trials of elimination diets, skin testing, or *in vitro* tests), the patient should first avoid all these foods, and then be subjected to oral challenge with each separately. The challenge must be avoided, however, if the food being considered may have been the cause of a life-threatening reaction in the past.

The first phase of the test aims at documenting definite improvement in symptoms following a trial of dietary elimination. All suspected foods should be simultaneously and completely avoided for 1 to 2 weeks. If the symptoms do not improve substantially, either that food is not the offender or additional offending factors were not controlled. If the symptoms definitely improve, the patient should be subjected to oral challenge tests while taking no or minimal symptomatic medications and having no intercurrent illness.

The second phase of the test aims at documenting recurrence of symptoms following exposure to the offending food. Generally, the challenge test should be done under supervision and in a place where facilities exist for the management of any possible severe reaction. We, as well as others (21,22), have witnessed severe reactions, including systemic anaphylaxis, from oral challenge tests in some patients who had had no such reactions before.

The initial challenge dose of food should depend on the anticipated severity of symptoms and on the quantities of the food the patient had been accustomed to eating while symptomatic. Increasing quantities may be administered every 30 min, as long as no reaction appears, until a cumulative quantity is reached that is equivalent to what the patient usually used to eat. On another visit, a challenge with an appropriate placebo should be carried out in the same way as with the suspected food. In addition to documenting all clinical symptoms and signs, the physician should record, whenever applicable, any changes in relevant laboratory findings. In a clinic setting, if no reaction occurs during the challenge procedure (usually 3 to 4 hr), the patient is sent home with instructions to maintain the elimination diet and to report any symptoms. If no symptoms occur by the next day, more of that food may be eaten at home unless the physician prefers not to disclose the nature of the challenge tests until all the challenges are completed.

In infants and young children, where reactions are mostly objective, the challenge may be conducted in an open manner. In older children and adults, however, the test should be conducted in a blind manner, usually single-blind and occasionally double-blind. Difficulties may be encountered in providing a placebo that matches the suspected food in consistency, color, odor, taste, and quantity. Because of this problem, the physician may choose to use open challenge testing first, then verify by a blind test only those foods that cause a reaction. This approach would save much time because a negative result occurs in approximately two-thirds of blind challenge tests (11,12,23,24). A common method of hiding the test food is providing it in a freeze-dried powder in opaque capsules. It can be also disguised in a hypoallergenic formula, an elemental formula, or in another appropriately selected food.

In our series of 107 double-blind oral challenges in patients highly suspected to be food-sensitive, a clinical reaction was noted in 36% (12). The reproduced symptoms were mostly similar to the presenting symptoms. In a few instances, additional symptoms were noted, including systemic anaphylaxis in one. With few exceptions, all positive reactions appeared while the patient was being observed in the clinic. In a few instances the reaction occurred at home within 24 hr after challenge.

Although oral challenge is the most definitive test for identification of the offending food, it has some limitations. It relies on the appearance of clinical symptoms and might miss a subclinical reaction (25,26). It is conducted under controlled conditions that might be different from the usual circumstances of exposure in certain patients, such as food preparation, combination with other foods, association with other contributory factors, or route of exposure. Certain food hypersensitivity reactions, mostly respiratory, are precipitated by inhalation rather than ingestion (1,2). Verification of these reactions requires specially designed bronchial inhalation challenge tests (27).

ACKNOWLEDGMENT

The author thanks Ms. Helen Thams for her assistance in preparation of the manuscript.

REFERENCES

1. Bahna SL. Diagnostic tests for food allergy. *Clin Rev Allergy* 1988;6.
2. Bahna SL. The dilemma of pathogenesis and diagnosis of food allergy. *Immunol Allergy Clin North Am* 1987;7:299–312.
3. Rowe HA. *Food Allergy: Its Manifestations and Control and Elimination Diet. A Compendium.* Springfield, IL.: Charles C Thomas, 1972;43–54.
4. Anderson JA, Sogn DD, eds. Adverse reactions to foods. American Academy of Allergy and Immunology Committee on Adverse Reactions to Foods, and National Institute of Allergy and Infectious Diseases. *NIH Publication* No. 84–242, 1984.
5. Dockhorn RJ, Smith TC. Use of a chemically defined hypoallergenic diet (Vivonex) in the management of patients with suspected food allergy/intolerance. *Ann Allergy* 1981;47:264–6.
6. Hill DJ, Lynch BC. Elemental diet in the management of severe eczema in childhood. *Clin Allergy* 1982;12:313–5.
7. Bahna SL. Critique of various dietary regimens in the management of food allergy. *Ann Allergy* 1986;57:48–52.
8. May CD. Objective clinical and laboratory studies of immediate hypersensitivity reactions to foods in asthmatic children. *J Allergy Clin Immunol* 1976;58:500–15.
9. Aas K. The diagnosis of hypersensitivity to ingested foods. Reliability of skin prick testing and the radioallergosorbent test with different materials. *Clin Allergy* 1978;8:39–50.
10. Bernstein M, Day JH, Welsh A. Double-blind food challenge in the diagnosis of food sensitivity in the adult. *J Allergy Clin Immunol* 1982;70:205–10.
11. Atkins FM, Steinberg S, Metcalfe DD. Evaluation of immediate adverse reactions to foods in adult patients. I. Correlation of demographic, laboratory, and prick skin test data with response to controlled oral food challenge. *J Allergy Clin Immunol* 1985;75:348–55.
12. Bahna SL, Gandhi MD. Reliability of skin testing and RAST in food allergy diagnosis. In: Chandra RK, ed. *Food Allergy.* St. John's, Newfoundland, Canada, Nutrition Research Foundation, 1987;139–47.

13. Hannuksela M, Lahti A. Immediate reactions to fruits and vegetables. *Contact Dermatitis* 1977;3:79–84.
14. Kauppiner K, Kousa M, Reunala T. Aromatic plants—A cause of severe attacks from angio-edema and urticaria. *Contact Dermatitis* 1980;6:251–4.
15. Pauli G, Bessor JC, Dietemann-Mollard A, et al. Celery sensitivity: Clinical and immunological correlations with pollen allergy. *Clin Allergy* 1985;15:273–9.
16. Bahna SL, Gandhi MD. Reliability of skin testing in food allergy diagnosis. *N Engl Reg Allergy Proc* 1986;7:256.
17. Sampson HA, Albergo R. Comparison of results of skin tests, RAST and double-blind, placebo-controlled food challenges in children with atopic dermatitis. *J Allergy Clin Immunol* 1984;74:26–33.
18. Stricker WE, Anorve-Lopez E, Reed CE. Food skin testing in patients with idiopathic anaphylaxis. *J Allergy Clin Immunol* 1986;77:516–9.
19. Sach MI, Jones RT, Yunginger JW. Isolation and partial characterization of a major peanut allergen. *J Allergy Clin Immunol* 1981;67:27–34.
20. Lemanske RF, Taylor SL. Standardized extracts, foods. *Clin Rev Allergy* 1987;5:23–36.
21. Goldman AS, Anderson DW Jr., Sellers W, et al. Milk allergy. I. Oral challenge with milk and isolated milk proteins in allergic children. *Pediatrics* 1963;32:425–43.
22. Walker-Smith JA. Gastrointestinal allergy. *Practitioner* 1978;220:562–73.
23. May CD, Bock SA. A modern clinical approach to food hypersensitivity. *Allergy* 1978;33:166–88.
24. Simpson SI, Somerfield SD, Wilson JD, et al. A double-blind study for the diagnosis of cows' milk allergy. *NZ Med J* 1980;92:457–9.
25. Vitoria JC, Aranjeulo ME, Rodriguez-Soriano J. Jejunal biopsy in cow's milk protein intolerance. *Lancet* 1978;1:722–3.
26. Wilson N, Silverman M. Diagnosis of food sensitivity in childhood asthma. *JR Soc Med* [Suppl 5] 1985;78:11–6.
27. Lybarger JA, Gallagher JS, Pulver DW, et al. Occupational asthma induced by inhalation and ingestion of garlic. *J Allergy Clin Immunol* 1982;69:448–54.

Food Intolerance in Infancy: Allergology, Immunology, and Gastroenterology, edited by Robert N. Hamburger. Carnation Nutrition Education Series, Vol. 1. The Carnation Co., Los Angeles/Raven Press, Ltd., New York © 1989.

The Use of the Allergy Immunology Laboratory in Food Allergy

Richard D. O'Connor

Division of Asthma, Allergy and Clinical Immunology, Sharp Rees-Stealy Medical Group, San Diego, California 92101

The laboratory diagnosis of food allergy is a complex subject. It began in the late 1960s when an assay to detect *in vitro*-specific immunoglobulin E (IgE) antibodies was developed (1) and there have been numerous papers published since that time. There are several investigators in attendance who have done excellent research studies over the past 20 years and it really is quite an acknowledgment of the importance of this symposium that so many of them are here. In order to reduce the enormous volume of data to a manageable size I have been very selective.

In keeping with Dr. Finberg's skepticism of food allergy (a skeptic being defined in Greek philosophy as one who must be convinced), I'm going to try to convince you that the topic is important and deserves our attention. For example, Dr. John Yunginger and colleagues (2) recently detailed seven deaths from food-allergic responses that they had accumulated over a 16-month period. In California, I personally am aware of two deaths within the last 6 months from food allergy. Systemic anaphylactic reactions to foods do occur and can be dangerous.

In 1981 the International Union of Immunological Societies formed a working group in conjunction with the Immunology Division of the World Health Organization. This group reviewed a variety of immunological assays including an assessment of the use of IgE-specific *in vitro* assays, such as paper radioimmunosorbent test (PRIST) and radioallergosorbent test (RAST). Their conclusion was that IgE-specific assays are very useful in the evaluation of food allergies (3). This is, however, not a universal opinion. In current textbooks and articles one finds statements such as: "Tests based on IgE antibody RAST used in the diagnosis of immediate hypersensitivity reactions have not been tested carefully in the gastrointestinal syndromes and no firm conclusions can be reached about their validity" (4) or: "The use of RAST for the diagnosis of food allergy is controversial" (5). Faced with these divergent opinions, I developed criteria for critically evaluating published studies.

I have approached my review from two perspectives. First, as the co-director of an allergy immunology laboratory, I am interested in the proper use and evaluation of new laboratory diagnostic assays. Secondly, as a practicing allergist, it is critical to realize that not every laboratory test approved by the Food and Drug Administration (FDA) may be clinically valuable.

First, I will review with you three themes: how to evaluate a laboratory test, the effect disease prevalence has on laboratory tests, and the importance of performing double-blind food challenges in clinical studies of food allergy.

EVALUATION OF A LABORATORY TEST

There is an article that appeared in *Pediatric Infectious Diseases* by Drs. Radetsky and Todd (6) entitled "Criteria for the Evaluation of New Diagnostic Tests" and I recommend it highly. The criteria that I have utilized in reviewing the utility of laboratory tests are summarized in that article.

There are four issues that must be considered in evaluating a laboratory assay: sensitivity, specificity, predictive value of a positive test, and the predictive value of a negative test. These terms are defined in Table 1.

A new diagnostic test is usually compared to a standard test (commonly referred to as the gold standard). The positive and negative results for both the new test and the gold standard are displayed in Table 2. Referring to Table 2, sensitivity, specificity, and the predictive values of a positive and negative test can be calculated. The hypothetical results of such a comparison are given below.

The number of positives that are obtained with the new test that concurred with the standard test, divided by the total number of positives obtained with the standard test, determines sensitivity. Referring to Table 2:

$$\text{Sensitivity} = A/A + B = 45/45 + 5 = 45/50 \times 100 = 90\%.$$

A test that is 90% sensitive, is positive in 90% of patients with the disease.

Specificity is defined as the percentage of negative tests in patients without the disease.

$$\text{Specificity} = D/C + D = 47/3 + 47 = 47/50 \times 100 = 94\%.$$

It is appropriately negative in nondiseased patients 94% of the time.

TABLE 1. *Evaluation of diagnostic tests*

Sensitivity:
Percentage of positive tests in patients with the disease
Specificity:
Percentage of negative tests in patients without the disease
Predictive value of a positive test:
Percentage of diseased patients among those with a positive test
Predictive value of a negative test:
Percentage of healthy patients among those with a negative test

---

TABLE 2. *The positive and negative results for the new diagnostic test compared to the gold standard*

| | | New test | | Total |
		Positive	Negative	
Gold	Positive	45 (A)	5 (B)	50
standard	Negative	3 (C)	47 (D)	50
test	Total :	48	52	100

In conjunction with sensitivity and specificity, there are two additional useful values. The predictive value of a positive test is the percentage of diseased patients among all those with a positive test. The predictive value of a negative test is the percentage of healthy patients among all those with a negative test.

Pred. value pos. test $= A/A + C = 45/45 + 3 = 45/48 \times 100 = 94\%$.
Pred. value neg. test $= D/B + D = 47/5 + 47 = 47/52 \times 100 = 90\%$.

EFFECT OF DISEASE PREVALENCE ON LABORATORY TESTS

In addition to these principles, there is an another point that must be borne in mind. The prevalence of a disease has an important influence on the value of a positive test (7).

It is necessary not only to consider the sensitivity and specificity of a test, but also to use it in the correct population of patients. Table 3 illustrates the effect of disease prevalence on the positive and negative predictive value of an assay that is 95% sensitive and 95% specific. If you randomly examine a population in whom the disease prevalence is only 0.1%, the positive predictive value of that assay would be approximately 2%. If you have selected a population in whom the disease is 50% prevalent, the value of a positive assay now becomes 95%. It becomes apparent that you must refine criteria for which patients you are actually going to order this assay.

TABLE 3. *Effect of disease prevalence*

| Sensitivity and specificity $= 95\%$ | |
Disease prevalence, %	Positive predictive value, %
0.1	2
1.0	16
2.0	28
5.0	50
50.0	95

This then is the second major point I wanted to drive home with regard to the use of the laboratory. That is, it is important to define the population of patients in whom you plan to order a particular test. You cannot randomly use laboratory tests to evaluate patients who have vague symptoms. You have to focus on well-defined, well-characterized syndromes in which the test is likely to be of real value.

IMPORTANCE OF FOOD CHALLENGES

Throughout the 1970s it became apparent that one of the things required in clinical research in allergic disease, especially in food allergy, was to develop objective standards that better characterize patients.

Dr. Charles May (8) and colleagues performed double-blind food challenges in 41 children who had a convincing history for an adverse clinical response subsequent to ingestion of milk. Placebo challenges were also performed. Eleven positive challenges were observed in these 41 patients (27%). Similar results were obtained by Bernstein et al. (9) in adults with a positive clinical history. Bernstein et al. performed 46 challenges in adults who had convincing histories for adverse responses to foods. Twenty-eight percent (13 of 46) of his patients had a positive response to a double-blind challenge. The importance of challenges is further strengthened by the results of aspirin challenges at Scripps Clinic where approximately 30% of patients with convincing histories had negative challenges (Dr. Ronald Simon, *personal communication*).

With these three issues in mind, namely, the evaluation of a laboratory test, the effect of disease prevalence on laboratory tests, and the use of double-blind food challenges, we can approach the literature with the point of view: ''Can this article give us information about sensitivity, specificity, and the predictive value of a test, based on data confirmed by double-blind food challenges in susceptible populations?''

The majority of studies reported in the literature prior to the development of double-blind food challenges correlated RAST with either clinical history or open challenges. I have confined my review to those studies reporting challenge data.

Dr. Bahna (10,11) recently reported data from studies that he had performed over several years. In his study, 61 patients who had a history of an adverse response to food were included. The symptoms about which these patients complained were respiratory in 42, dermatologic in 40, gastrointestinal in 15, and systemic anaphylaxis that occurred in 6 patients. Many patients had combined dermatologic and respiratory complaints. Dr. Bahna conducted double-blind food challenges and performed RASTs for 11 selected foods. Both children and adults were included. It may be useful in future studies to study children and adults separately because the prevalence of food allergy may be different in these two populations and may affect the value of a positive test as shown earlier. Overall, the RAST was concordant in 58% of the patients (Table 4); that is, the RAST was positive and a double-blind challenge with the same food antigen was positive in 58% of the cases. However, the

TABLE 4. *Radioallergosorbent*
and double-blind challenge

Both positive	
range 33 to 100%	58%
Both negative	
range 0 to 71%	47%

range for individual foods went from a low of 33% to a high of 100% with different food antigens. The RAST and the double-blind challenges were both negative in 47% of the patients; the range varied from 0 to 71%. The data specifically for milk and egg from Dr. Bahna's paper are shown in Table 5. In the RAST column, the assay for milk was 56% sensitive and 67% specific, the positive predictive value was 71% and the negative predictive value was 50%. The RAST data are comparable to the results of skin testing. Other food antigens varied even more and the overall results (Table 6) are also shown.

What is clear from these studies is that the RAST assay can be utilized in conjunction with double-blind food challenges in a clinical investigational protocol. One of the problems that may occur in this type of study is defining which subjects should be included; that is, should all patients with any history of an adverse reaction to food be included? What are the advantages of a more refined definition of the patient population?

With definition of the disease group being studied as atopic dermatitis, additional useful information is obtained. Dr. Hugh Sampson and colleagues (12,13) began a series of studies published in 1984 in 40 children with atopic dermatitis. The diagnosis of atopic dermatitis was established according to the accepted dermatological criteria of Hanifin (14). Sampson and colleagues conducted 155 double-blind, placebo-controlled challenges in these children. Nine challenges were deferred because life-threatening anaphylaxis had occurred. Thirty-three of the 155 double-

TABLE 5. *Assessment of reliability for skin test and radioallergosorbent test compared*
to double-blind food challenge for milk and egg

	Milk, %		Egg, %	
	ST[a]	RAST	ST	RAST
Sensitivity	44	56	67	33
Specificity	67	67	80	40
Positive predictive accuracy	67	71	50	14
Negative predictive accuracy	44	50	89	67

[a]ST, skin test; RAST, radioallergosorbent test.

TABLE 6. *Assessment of reliability for skin test and radioallergosorbent test compared to double-blind food challenge for all food antigens*

	Overall results, %	
	ST[a]	RAST
Sensitivity	58	58
Specificity	65	33
Positive predictive accuracy	48	44
Negative predictive accuracy	74	67

[a]ST, skin test; RAST, radioallergosorbent test.

blind challenges (21%) were positive: 94% of the reactions were cutaneous, 42% involved gastrointestinal responses, whereas ocular or nasal responses occurred in 27% of the positive challenges and 18% involved respiratory complaints. All of these reactions, it is important to note, occurred in less than 20 min after the double-blind food challenge.

Looking at the value of a RAST versus double-blind food challenges, I have listed sensitivity, specificity, positive predictive value, and the negative predictive value for various antigens (Table 7). The data for cow's milk: sensitivity is 60%, specificity 77%, and the negative predictive value is very good at 93%. However, the positive predictive value is not very helpful at 27%. You will observe better results with egg and especially peanut, in which the RAST was very sensitive; that is, 100% of the patients with the disease were appropriately identified by the assay. However, it wasn't very specific because it only excluded 58% of the healthy population. However, the negative predictive value was excellent in this study: a negative peanut RAST was 100% predictive for the absence of disease caused by the ingestion of peanuts. When we look at well-defined populations, such as children with atopic dermatitis, the true value of a RAST appears not so much in the value of a positive test but in the value of a negative test. Eighty-two percent for egg, 100% for peanut, 93% for milk, 95% for wheat, 94% for soy, and 94% for fish. The other values for specificity, sensitivity, and the value of a positive test do not yet meet current acceptable laboratory standards.

TABLE 7. *Laboratory evaluation of radioallergosorbent test versus food challenge*

	Milk	Wheat	Egg	Soy	Peanut	Fish
Sensitivity, %	60	75	80	67	100	67
Specificity, %	77	64	64	64	58	81
Positive predictive value, %	27	20	57	18	44	33
Negative predictive value, %	93	95	82	94	100	94

The third study that I will review was performed by Dr. Hill and his group in Australia (15). The data are based on a patient population of children suspected to be allergic to milk by clinical history. This is somewhat similar to Dr. Bahna's study because clinical history is utilized rather than a specific disease. It was the history of an adverse response with the ingestion of milk rather than a disease itself. In Dr. Hill's study *(this volume)*, milk was withheld from the diet for 6 to 12 weeks. Children were then hospitalized and milk challenges were done either in a single-blinded fashion or in open challenges. This was not a double-blind study. The children were however, followed prospectively in the hospital. One reason to discuss this study is because of the time course of the responses to challenge. He was able to divide the patients into three groups based upon their response to challenge (Table 8). In Group 1 there were 27 children whose responses were cutaneous and the responses all occurred in less than 45 min after ingestion of the food. In Group 2 there were 53 children. Their responses were gastrointestinal. They began to vomit or experienced diarrhea. Forty-eight of these 53 patients had their reactions occur between 45 min and 20 hr. In Group 3 there were 20 patients. These were children who had a combination of complaints. Seventeen patients experienced symptoms more than 24 hr after ingestion of the offending antigen whereas 3 patients experienced symptoms at 8, 12, or 16 hr.

The RAST data for Dr. Hill's study are seen in Table 9. Eighteen RASTs were positive among the 26 positive challenges (69%) in Group 1. There were 19 of 52 positive RASTs (37%) in Group 2, and 4 of 19 in Group 3 patients (21%). RAST was positive infrequently in those patients who reacted more than a day after challenge.

I have confined my presentation to studies of IgE-mediated reactions because that's where the greatest amount of reproducible and reliable information exists. If we look at other immunological mechanisms, whether they be humoral, cellular, or complement-mediated, very little or no data of an adequate nature exist in conjunction with blinded food challenges. The studies of Dr. Hill and his group observing the time and the type of reactions allow us to begin to explore possible alternative mechanisms for these sorts of responses. It may be important to include placebo challenges in future studies, especially in those responses occurring several hours after challenge.

TABLE 8. *Response to challenge*

Group	N	Predominant response
1	27	Angioedema, urticaria all < 45 min
2	53	Vomiting, diarrhea
		48 Patients between 45 min and 20 hr
3	20	Diarrhea, eczema, cough/wheeze
		17 Patients after 24 hr

TABLE 9. *Milk-specific antibodies*

	Groups		
	1	2	3
RAST	18/26	19/52	4/19[a]

[a]Positive only in patients with cutaneous reactions.

The data in Table 10 are from a survey that was carried out by the Centers for Disease Control. The Centers mailed negative and positive sera to a variety of laboratories around the country that agreed to participate in a "proficiency survey." That is an important consideration because the information is only from those laboratories that agreed to participate! Secondly, the survey was performed blinded. The laboratories didn't know what was in the serum samples that they received. At least one negative standard was reported as being positive by 10% of the participating laboratories; 17% reported a positive IgE for wheat in the negative standard. Looking at positive standards, 7% of the laboratories reported that the positive standard was negative for milk but none of them missed it for wheat. We have known for years that wheat is a very difficult antigen to use both *in vivo* and *in vitro* because of its cross-reactions with grass pollen. However, I think it is sobering to realize that 1 of 10 laboratories could have given you a positive result for milk when it really was negative and 7% of the laboratories would have reported a negative result, when in fact the serum sample was known to be positive. So another aspect of food allergy *in vitro* diagnosis which we have to take into consideration is to be sure that we are using laboratories that know what they are doing. Unfortunately a lot of in-office laboratories (as well as commercial laboratories) are performing allergy assays just because kits are readily available. Most of them do not have sufficient background, experience, or skill to warrant being involved in the field of laboratory immunology and allergy.

It is customary to conclude a talk on the laboratory diagnosis of food allergy by

TABLE 10. *Proficiency survey—radioimmunosorbent test for Centers for Disease Control*

Negative sera standard	
Positive milk	10%
Positive wheat	17%
Positive sera standard	
Negative milk	7%
Negative wheat	0%

pointing out that the RAST is valuable only in patients with certain types of disorders. For example, patients with atopic dermatitis often cannot be skin tested because of their disease. In these patients RAST is of inestimable value.

RAST is of critical use in the study of patients with anaphylaxis in whom there is danger of performing any type of challenge, including skin testing. In the interpretation of RAST, as with all laboratory tests, caution is required and correlation with history is critical. RAST is one component of your allergy evaluation but you cannot base recommendations on the RAST value alone, especially in a person who was truly life-threateningly allergic to a food. At the present time we are on safe ground in saying that RAST has an excellent negative predictive value, particularly in atopic dermatitis.

We now need to design and perform well-controlled studies in a variety of other food allergy-related disorders: asthma is the next prime one. Ocular and nasal responses should also be a consideration. The gastrointestinal syndromes are an important area for us to take a look at as well as syndromes such as migraine headaches. These disorders, with the development and use of proper clinical trials, can now be evaluated in a selective and objective way.

The other point to be made about the value of RAST and food allergies is that positive results vary by antigen and they vary by country. In Norway and Sweden, where fish allergy is an extremely important problem, investigators have been able to identify specific offending antigens that cause most allergic reactions. We have not yet developed sufficient biochemical knowledge of the antigenic determinants of other foods.

In this paper, the words *in vitro*-specific IgE and RAST have been used interchangeably, but there are several other assays currently available from a variety of commercial sources. Most of the literature and certainly the three studies which have been presented in this paper utilized the Pharmacia RAST. This is not to promote Pharmacia, it is to point out that results may be very different unless careful studies are performed with any other *in vitro* assay. When our laboratory has performed comparative evaluations of different kits and assays, there have been enormous differences in results with certain serums, even though overall the majority of the tests may be acceptably comparable by FDA regulatory standards.

What we have seen in the last 20 years is the development of a model which we can apply to a wide variety of other situations. Clinical researchers now need to use prospective double-blind placebo-controlled challenge studies. These studies should be designed to examine relatively homogenous populations with specific diseases or syndromes that are well-characterized and well-defined in advance. These studies will allow us to determine accurately how useful RAST can be in the clinical practice of food allergy.

I want to stress that a new test must be evaluated in relationship to what is the current standard. We are adopting the attitude that the standard test, known as the gold standard for the diagnosis of food allergy, is a response that occurs during the double-blind placebo-controlled food antigen challenge. In 1989, to accept anything less than that is inadequate.

ACKNOWLEDGMENTS

I thank Dr. Robert N. Hamburger for his collaboration and encouragement. This work was partially supported by grants from the Carnation Company, Mead Johnson & Company, the Elizabeth and Carroll Boutell Fund, and the U.C.S.D. Pediatric Immunology and Allergy Foundation. The assistance of Janice R. Turner, Linda Galbreath, and Maria Ware is very much appreciated. Clinical laboratory work was performed in the Advanced Allergy Management, Inc. laboratory, La Jolla, CA 92037.

REFERENCES

1. Wide L, Bennich H, Johansson, SGO. Diagnosis of allergy by an in vitro test for allergen antibodies. *Lancet* 1967;2:1105.
2. Yunginger J, et al. Fatal food-induced anaphylaxis. *JAMA* 1988;260:1450–2.
3. The use and abuse of immunologic tests. *Clin Immunol Newsletter* 1981;2:178–88.
4. Powell GK. Gastrointestinal manifestations of food allergy. In: Chiaramonte LT, Schneider AT, Lifshitz F, eds. *Food Allergy*. New York: Marcel Dekker, 1988.
5. Hawryiko E, Murali MR. Immunologic tests for food allergy. In: Chiaramonte LT, Schneider AT, Lifshitz F, eds. *Food Allergy*. New York: Marcel Dekker, 1988.
6. Radetsky M, Todd JK. Criteria for the evaluation of new diagnostic tests. *Pediatr Infect Dis* 1984;3:461–6.
7. Cebul RD, Beck JR. Applications in ambulatory screening and preadmission testing of adults. *Ann Intern Med* 1987;106:403–13.
8. May CD, Remigio L, Bock SA. Usefulness of measurement of antibodies in serum in diagnosis of sensitivity to cow milk and soy proteins in early childhood. *Allergy* 1980;35:301–10.
9. Bernstein MB, Day JH, Welsh A. Double-blind food challenge in the diagnosis of food sensitivity in the adult. *J Allergy Clin Immunol* 1982;70:205–10.
10. Bahna SL, Gandhi MD. Reliability of skin testing and RAST in food allergy diagnosis. In: *Food Allergy*, Chandra RK, ed. St. John's, Newfoundland, Canada, Nutrition Research Foundation, 1987:139–47.
11. Bahna SL. The dilemma of pathogenesis and diagnosis of food allergy. *Immunol Allergy Clin North Am* 1987;7:299–312.
12. Sampson HA, Albergo R. Comparison of results of skin tests, RAST, and double-blind, placebo-controlled food challenges in children with atopic dermatitis. *J Allergy Clin Immunol* 1984;74:26–33.
13. Sampson HA. IgE-mediated food intolerance. *J Allergy Clin Immunol* 1988;81:495–504.
14. Hanifin JM, Lobitz WC. New concepts of atopic dermatitis. *Arch Dermatol* 1977;113:663.
15. Hill DJ, Firer MS, Shelton MJ, Hosking CS. Manifestations of milk allergy in infancy: clinical and immunologic findings. *J Pediatr* 1986;109:270–6.
16. Przybyszewski VA, Taylor RN. Allergen-specific immunoglobulin E performance evaluation results. USPHS Centers for Disease Control, Atlanta, 1983.

Food Intolerance in Infancy: Allergology,
Immunology, and Gastroenterology, edited by
Robert N. Hamburger. Carnation Nutrition
Education Series, Vol. 1. The Carnation Co., Los
Angeles/Raven Press, Ltd., New York © 1989.

Predictive Value of Blood Immunoglobulin E in Childhood Allergy

Jean Bousquet and François-Bernard Michel

Clinique des Maladies Respiratoires, Centre Hospitalier Universitaire,
34059 Montpellier, France

Allergic diseases are important causes of morbidity throughout the world. The majority of estimates of allergy prevalence indicate a percent range between 20 and 35%, and the prevalence rates of the 10 leading pathologic conditions in the United States show that allergies rank second in order, after dental problems, and are among the most costly health problems (1). The severity of allergic diseases should not be underestimated because (a) asthma deaths may be increasing in numbers (2) and (b) a large number of school and working days are lost in direct relationship to them (1). Moreover, the incidence of atopic disorders appears to increase steadily (3,4), perhaps owing to environmental cofactors such as pollution (5,6). Although many of the proposed preventive measures were inconclusive, it is important to try to prevent atopic disorders by means of food and aeroallergen avoidance (7–9) as well as by reducing air pollution in the infant's environment. Because the risk of developing allergy seems to be greater in early infancy than later in life (8,9), their implementation should begin immediately after birth, before the expression of the allergic phenotype. Preventive measures should be strict and applied for a long period of time, so that they may appear difficult to follow in the whole population, and for these reasons, only the "high-allergic risk newborn" (10) should be a candidate for prevention methods.

The expression of the allergic phenotype is caused by the combination of genotypic and environmental factors, and in the genetically susceptible individual minute amounts of allergens will lead to an immunoglobulin E (IgE)-mediated immune response, whereas the normal individual will not respond to the same immunologic stimulus (11). It appears that genetically predisposed newborns have a greater IgE production than others so that the prediction of allergy is mainly based upon the atopic family history and the titration of IgE in cord blood.

GENETIC FACTORS

The hereditability of allergic diseases has been confirmed by carefully conducted genetic studies (11,12). Many studies in different countries have shown that be-

TABLE 1. *Risk of developing atopy based on family history of allergy*[a]

Family history	Risk, %
Both parents atopic	40–60
Both parents atopic with the same manifestation	50–80
One parent atopic	20–40
One sibling atopic	25–35
Neither parent nor sibling atopic	5–15

[a]From Bousquet and Kjellman, ref. 17, with permission.

tween one-half and three-quarters of patients with allergies have a positive family history of allergic diseases. Moreover, there is a trend toward a genetic predisposition to end-organ hereditability (13–15). Genetic factors are more important in determining allergy in early life because the allergic phenotype is expressed soon after the interaction between the immune system and allergens; in adults, allergen-independent environmental factors are more prevalent. However, adults encountering allergens to which they were not previously exposed can easily mount an IgE-mediated allergy as shown in natives of Papua New Guinea exposed to house dust mites (16). A newborn's approximate risk of developing allergy based on the family history of allergic disease is listed in Table 1 (17). However, the risk in infants to develop atopic diseases is 23% when both parents are allergic, 13% if only one parent presents atopic symptoms, and 5% when there is no allergy in the family (18). These data indicate that the efficiency of a family history as a screening method for the prediction of allergy is poor (19).

The correlation between human lymphocyte antigen (HLA) and allergy is well established, and the relative risk of allergy in individuals who possess an HLA phenotype might in the future provide useful predictive information. At present, it is known that the relative risk for a patient sensitive to ragweed with HLA-Dw2 to be sensitized to ragweed antigen Ra5 is as high as the risk for a patient with HLA-B27 who presents with Reiter's syndrome (20). Other genetic markers might be used. A possible link between blood groups or α_1-antitrypsin phenotypes and allergy was suggested, but the data have been conflicting (for review see ref. 21). More recently, adenosine deaminase phenotypes have been proposed to predict wheezing in infancy and childhood asthma, but this study has to be confirmed (22).

MATERNAL-FETAL FACTORS

Prematurity and low weight birth do not affect the development of allergy (10). Drugs administered during pregnancy may have some immunoregulatory activities. Progesterone was shown to cause a significant increase ($p<0.001$) in total serum IgE levels (10,23), but it is not known whether its use may result in an increase in allergic disorders in infancy. It has been recently observed that β-blocking drugs taken by the pregnant mother increase the levels of cord blood IgE (Björkstén, *unpublished observations*). Maternal tobacco smoking during pregnancy was found to increase cord serum IgE, especially in nonatopic families (24).

Fetal sensitization may occur *in utero* (10,25) and it has been recommended that potential high-risk mothers should avoid or minimize the intake of highly allergenic food during the last 2 or 3 months of pregnancy (9). However, a prospective well-controlled study did not confirm the relevance of diet during late pregnancy (26,27).

CORD BLOOD MARKERS

Cord blood markers are of great importance in the determination of allergic risk in newborns, but markers must fulfill some criteria: (a) Markers must be of fetal origin; (b) a very small sample quantity should be required for titration; (c) titration should not be influenced by nonspecific factors that may be unknown in cord blood; (d) titration should be simple and results rapidly obtained; (e) cord blood must be collected carefully, perferably by direct puncture of the cord vein to avoid contamination from maternal blood (an alternative may be to draw blood during the first few days of life) (28); and (f) a very sensitive and specific technique should be used, because most markers in cord blood are present in very small quantities.

Cord Serum Immunoglobulin

Several criteria make cord blood IgE a good candidate for the prediction of atopy: (a) the fetus is able to synthesize IgE after the 11th week of gestation (29), and IgE were found to be present in cord blood after the 37th week of gestation (10); (b) IgE is thought not to cross the placenta (30); (c) there is an established correlation between IgE and allergy; and (d) it has been observed that infants with high IgE levels were prone to develop allergic diseases in later life (31).

The IgE concentrations in cord blood are normally very low and may be undetectable in a majority of newborns if sensitive methods are not used. The measurement of cord serum IgE is one of the valuable cord blood markers, but only few IgE techniques are able to discriminate very small levels of IgE antibodies. Moreover, some laboratories are not confident enough with the IgE tests to accurately measure such low levels. It is therefore of paramount importance to test the reproductivity of IgE titration in serums containing less than 1 KU/L of IgE (Fig. 1). The contamination of cord blood by maternal blood has to be accurately characterized because IgE levels are much greater in adults, especially if they are atopic. Fälth-Magnusson and Kjellman (26) observed that cord blood samples are contaminated in 3% but others have found a much greater incidence of contamination (32,33). Contamination may be found by titrating cord IgA levels and IgE may be subsequently measured on a capillary sample.

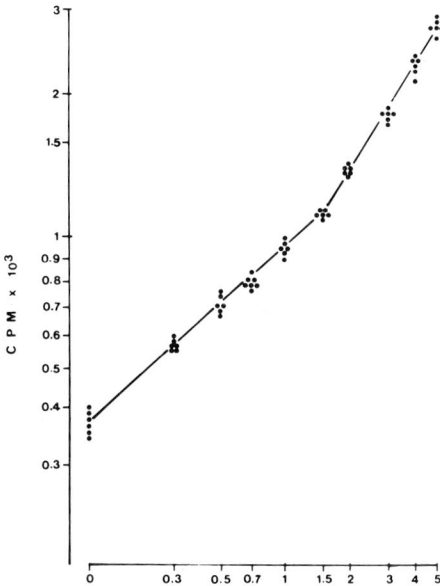

FIG. 1. Evaluation of the accuracy of the Phadebas® paper radioimmunosorbent test to discriminate very low levels of total immunoglobulin E (IgE). (From Michel et al., ref. 67, with permission.)

Cord serum IgE levels range from 0 to 10 KU/L with paper radioimmunosorbent test (PRIST) (Pharmacia Diagnostics, Uppsala, Sweden), the Enzygnost (Behring Laboratories, West Germany), and PACIA (Technicon Instruments Corp., Tarrytown, N.Y.) tests (10,18,34–41). Other techniques were not yet shown to accurately test these low levels, and proper control studies have to be performed before these methods are used. Higher concentrations are found in black infants than in white infants (42) and in those whose mothers are infested by helminths (43). Other factors increasing cord blood IgE are maternal progesterone administration during pregnancy (Fig. 2) (10,23), maternal smoking (24), and β-blockers administered to pregnant mothers. The first study examining the predictive capacity of elevated cord blood IgE was reported in 1976; 21% of 33 infants with atopic disease that developed before 2 years of age had high cord blood IgE (34). Several studies using the PRIST and one using the PACIA technique have confirmed and extended these findings (Fig. 3; Table 2 (10,18,23,28,34–37,44–50)), with one possible exception (49). The cord blood IgE determination provides more predictive information than does the family history (10,45,48) but it does not predict the severity of symptoms of atopic diseases although 94% of children with severe long-lasting symptoms of atopic diseases were identified by an elevated cord blood IgE level. In the same study of over 1,600 children followed for more than 6 years, it was calculated that the sensitivity of cord blood IgE was 40% and the specificity was over 90% (18).

In Scandinavia, infants with elevated cord blood IgE have a double atopic risk when born in May than in November owing to the early pollen exposure (50). It was

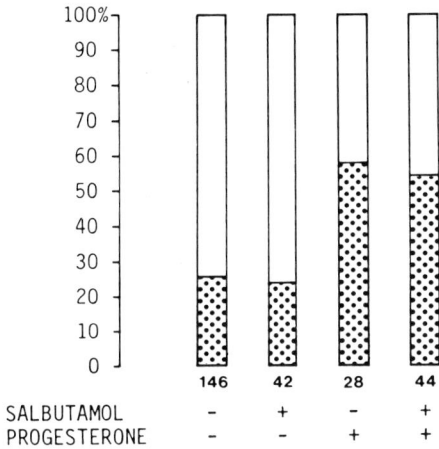

FIG. 2. Influence of salbutamol and progesterone on the levels of cord blood immunoglobulin E (IgE). (From Bousquet and Michel, ref. 21, with permission.)

also observed that infants with elevated cord blood IgE are at greater risk when fed cow's milk (37,47,48). It is interesting to note that these environmental influences were not obvious in newborns with low cord blood IgE levels.

Cost-benefit studies were recommended for the evaluation of the entire prediction-prevention program. Assuming that prevention (breast-feeding and aeroal-

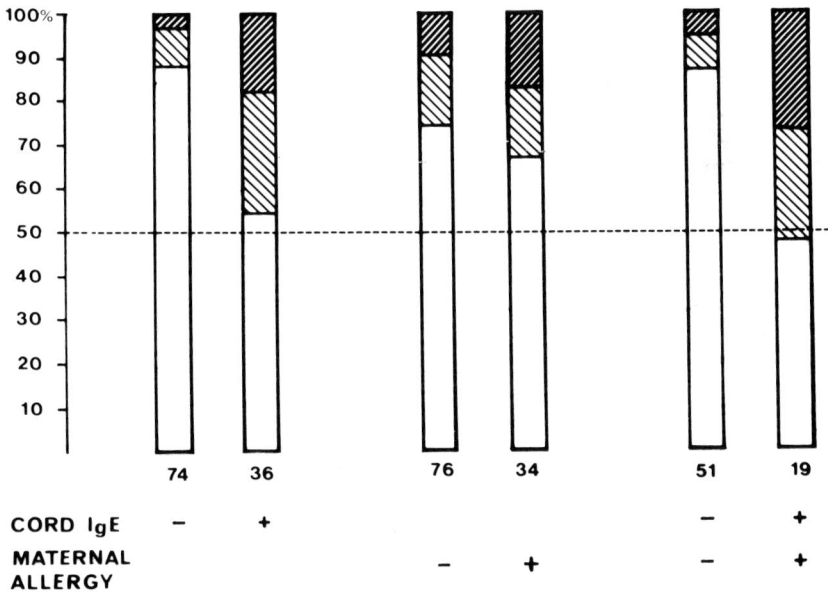

FIG. 3. Predictive capacity of family atopic history and cord blood immunoglobulin E (IgE) in children of 36 months of age. (From Bousquet et al., ref. 23, with permission.)

TABLE 2. *Predictive value of cord blood immunoglobulin E*

	Dannaeus et al. (34)	Croner et al. (18)	Bousquet et al. (23)	Businco et al. (37)	Kjellman and Croner (48)	Chandra et al. (46)	Magnusson (45)
No. subjects followed	53	1,701	281	102	1,651	226	190
Selection							
on atopic families		No	Yes	Yes	No	No	No
on breast-feeding		No	No	Yes	No	Yes	No
Duration of survey	18 months	18 months	36 months	24 months	7 years	24 months	18 months
Cord blood IgE							
Method	PRIST[a]	PRIST	PRIST	PRIST	PRIST	PRIST	PACIA
Cutoff point (KU/L)	1	0.9	1	0.5	0.9	0.7	1.2
Atopy (%)							
Low IgE	0	5	11	21	13	3–12[b]	19
High IgE	50	70	61	52	82	35–81[b]	72
No family atopy		12	16				
Family atopy		43	45		40		
Family atopy + high IgE		78	74		86		

[a]PRIST, paper radioimmunosorbent test.
[b]First value: breast-fed infants; second value: cow's milk-fed infants.

lergen avoidance) was effective, Hjalthe et al. (51) studied the relative costs of preventive measures and treatments of the diseases and compared three different screening methods followed by preventive measures with that of the absence of prediction and prevention: (a) IgE screening of all newborn babies; (b) IgE screening solely of those with a positive family history; (c) prediction only based on family history; and (d) no prediction and no prevention.

The results of this study support the potential value of IgE screening studies in newborns. However, the prevention of allergy by breast-feeding is far from being effective.

Cord Blood Lymphocytes

The peripheral blood of infants of atopic parents showed thymus-derived cells (T cells) that were significantly decreased in number ($p<0.05$) (52). In bottle-fed infants, there was an inverse correlation between lymphopenia and eosinophilia (53). Bottle-fed infants who had a low T-cell count developed significantly higher IgE levels before 9 months of age (54), suggesting that T-cell counts may be of particular value in the prediction of allergy. In a prospective study, Chandra and Baker (55) showed that before 1 month of age, T cells were quantitatively and functionally different in normal and subsequently atopic infants. Those who developed atopic dermatitis had a reduced number of CD8+ cells and an elevated T4/T8 ratio. Moreover, functional suppressor activity was lower than normal.

Other Cells in Cord Blood

Eosinophils easily enumerated in cord blood have been found to be elevated significantly ($p<0.02$) in blood collected from newborns from allergic families (56). Similarly, platelet counts were low in cord blood of infants with a family history of atopy (Magnusson and De Weck, *manuscript in preparation*). Because of the simplicity of determination, eosinophils or platelets might become an important parameter if their predictive value can be established.

Other Markers

Other markers will undoubtedly be found in the future and will increase our ability to predict the onset of allergic disease. Phosphodiesterase is a marker that seems to be promising in predicting atopy (57,58), but a long-term follow-up study is required.

POSTNATAL PARAMETERS

The sex of the neonate is of relevance, because in infancy, boys develop atopic disease more often than do girls. Cord serum IgE concentrations were more often el-

TABLE 3. *Predictive capacity of parameters at birth for the subsequent development of allergy in infancy and childhood*

Parameter	Predictive capacity	Feasibility
Elevated cord serum IgE	Very strong	Good
Positive family history of allergy	Strong	Very good
Sex of newborn (boy)	Strong	Very good
Month of birth	Intermediate	Very good
Aeroallergen eviction	Intermediate	Difficult
Breast-feeding	Possible	Possible
Eviction of air pollution and passive smoking	Possible	Difficult
Cord blood eosinophils	Unknown	Good
Cord blood lymphocyte subsets	Unknown	Poor
Conditions of pregnancy	Unknown	
Others	To be confirmed	

evated in boys than in girls (18,28,40). Early allergen contacts and events may also influence the development of allergic disorders in genetically predisposed newborns. Aeroallergen exposure during the first months of life increases allergy onset. Pollens (59–62), animals (59,63), and even house dust mites (53,63) were shown to be implicated in an increased incidence of allergy. Food allergens are also important, but at present, it is not yet known whether breast-feeding (62,64,65) or delayed solid feeding (62,66) will prevent or delay allergy onset.

CANDIDATES FOR PREVENTION

Although it may be desirable to try to prevent allergy in all newborns, it is reasonable to select candidates for prevention and to define a strategy for prevention. At present there are two factors that have been shown to be predictive: family history of atopy and cord serum IgE (17) (Table 3). When both parents are atopic, preventive measures for the infant are recommended. On the other hand, infants of nonatopic parents and those who have no siblings with allergies do not need preventive measures. All others should be studied more carefully. At present, the most important parameter is cord-blood IgE concentration. The family allergy score described above may be helpful in selecting candidates for allergy prevention and IgE determinations in cord blood. When the total cord serum IgE is elevated, then preventive measures should be implemented.

REFERENCES

1. Young P. Asthma and allergies: an optimistic future. Washington, DC: United States Government Printing Office, 1980: US Department of Health and Human Service, Public Health Service, NIH Publication No. 30:388.
2. Sheffer AL, Buist AS. Report of the asthma mortality task force. *J Allergy Clin Immunol* 1987;80:361–514.

3. Eaton KK. The incidence of allergy—has it changed? *Clin Allergy* 1982;12:107–10.
4. Taylor B, Wadsworth J, Wadsworth M, Peckham C. Changes in the reported prevalence of childhood eczema since the 1939–1943 war. *Lancet* 1984;i:1255–7.
5. Muranaka M, Suzuki S, Koizumi K, et al. Adjuvant activity of diesel exhaust particulates for the production of IgE antibody in mice. *J Allergy Clin Immunol* 1986;77:616–23.
6. Ishizaki T, Koizumi K, Ikemori R, Ishiyama Y, Kuhibiki E. Studies of prevalence of Japanese cedar pollinosis among the residents in a densely cultivated area. *Ann Allergy* 1987;58:265–70.
7. Kjellman N-IM. Prediction and prevention of atopic allergy. *Allergy* 1982;67:463–70.
8. Soothill JF. Prevention of food allergy. In: Brostoff J, Challacombe SJ, eds. *Clinics in Immunology and Allergy,* vol. 2, no. 1. London: WB Saunders Co. Ltd, 1982;243–55.
9. Hamburger RN, Heller S, Melon MH, O'Connor RD, Seiger RS. Current status of the clinical and immunologic consequences of a prototype allergic disease prevention program. *Ann Allergy* 1983;51:281–90.
10. Michel FB, Bousquet J, Greillier P, et al. Comparison of cord blood immunoglobulin E concentrations and maternal allergy for the prediction of atopic disease in infancy. *J Allergy Clin Immunol* 1980;65:422–30.
11. Marsh DG, Meyers DA, Bias W. The epidemiology and genetics of atopic allergy. *N Engl J Med* 1981;305:1551–9.
12. De Weck AL. HLA and allergy. *Monogr Allergy* 1977;11:3–19.
13. Gerrard JW, Vickers P, Gerrard CD. The familial incidence of allergic disease. *Ann Allergy* 1976;36:10–159.
14. Kjellman N-IM. Atopic disease in seven-year-old children. *Acta Paediatr Scand* 1977;66:465–73.
15. Sibbald B, Horn MED, Brain EA, Greeg I. Genetic factors in childhood asthma. *Thorax* 1980;35:671–4.
16. Turner KJ. Changing prevalence of asthma in developing countries. In: Michel FB, Bousquet J, Godard P, eds. *Highlights in Asthmology.* Munich: Springer Verlag, 1987;37–44.
17. Bousquet J, Kjellman N-IM. Predictive value of tests in childhood allergy. *J Allergy Clin Immunol* 1986;78:1019–22.
18. Croner S, Kjellman N-IM, Eriksson B, Roth A. IgE screening in 1701 newborn infants and the development of atopic disease during infancy. *Arch Dis Child* 1982;57:364–8.
19. Kjellman N-IM, Croner S, Fälth-Magnusson K, Odleram H, Björsktén B. Prediction of allergy in infancy. *Ann Allergy, (in press).*
20. Marsh DG, Hsu SH, Roebber M, et al. HLA-Dw2: a genetic marker for human immune response to short ragweed pollen allergen Ra5. I. Response resulting primarily from natural antigenic exposure. *J Exp Med* 1982;155:1439–48.
21. Bousquet J, Michel FB. Prediction of allergic risk in infants. In: Businco L, ed. *Advances in Pediatric Allergy.* Amsterdam: Excerpta Medica, 1983;55–68.
22. Ronchetti R, Lucarini N, Lucarelli P, et al. A genetic basis for the heterogeneity of asthma syndrome in pediatric ages: adenosine deaminase phenotypes. *J Allergy Clin Immunol* 1984;74:81–5.
23. Bousquet J, Menardo JL, Viala JL, Michel FB. Predictive value of cord serum IgE determination in the development of "early-onset" atopy. *Ann Allergy* 1983;51:291–5.
24. Magnusson CGM. Maternal smoking influences cord serum IgE and IgD levels, and increases the risk for infant allergy. *J Allergy Clin Immunol* 1986;78:898–904.
25. Kaufman HS. Allergy in the newborn: skin test reactions confirmed by the Prausnitz-Küstner test at birth. *Clin Allergy* 1971;1:363–7.
26. Fälth-Magnusson K, Kjellman N-IM. Development of atopic diseases in babies whose mothers were on exclusion diets during pregnancy. *J Allergy Clin Immunol* 1987;80:868–75.
27. Lilja G, Dannaeus A, Fälth-Magnusson K, et al. Immune response of the atopic woman and fetus: effects of high- and low-dose food intake during late pregnancy. *Clin Allergy* 1988;18:131–41.
28. Casimir G, Verleylev D, Duchâteau J. Concentrations sériques en IgE: prédiction des manifestations atopiques. Avantages de l'allaitement maternel. *Rev Med Brux* 1983;4:323–6.
29. Miller DL, Hirvonin T, Gitlin D. Synthesis of IgE by the human conceptus. *J Allergy Clin Immunol*1973;52:182–8.
30. Bazaral M, Orgel HA, Hamburger RN. IgE levels in normal infants and mothers and an inheritance hypothesis. *J Immunol* 1971;107:794–801.
31. Orgel HA, Hamburger RN, Bazaral M, et al. Development of IgE and allergy in infancy. *J Allergy Clin Immunol* 1975;56:296-307.
32. Zeiger RS, Heller S, Mellon M, O'Connor RD, Hamburger RN. Effectiveness of dietary manipulations in the prevention of food allergy in infants. *J Allergy Clin Immunol* 1986;78:224–38.

33. O'Connor RD, Zeiger RS, Mellon MH, Heller S, Hamburger RN. The occurrence of elevated cord sera IgE levels due to maternal admixture. *NER Allergy Proc* 1984;5:149.
34. Dannaeus A, Johansson SGO, Foucard T. Clinical and immunological aspects of food allergy. II. Development of allergic symptoms and humoral immune response in infants of atopic mothers during the first 24 months of life. *Acta Paediatr Scand* 1978;67:497–504.
35. Dutau C, Enjaume C, Rochiccioli P. Valeurs normales des IgE sériques totales chez l'enfant de la naissance à 16 ans. *Arch Fr Pediatr* 1979;36:795–804.
36. Basuyau JP, Mallet E, Lenormand JJ, et al. IgE sériques chez les nourissons normaux et intolérants aux protéines du lait de vache. *Nouv Presse Med* 1977;9:591–3.
37. Businco L, Marchetti F, Pellegrini G, Perlini R. Predictive value of cord blood IgE levels in "at risk" newborn babies and influence of type of feeding. *Clin Allergy* 1983;13:503-8.
38. Ringel KP, Dati F, Buchholtz F. IgE-Normalwerte bei kindern. *Laboratoriumblätter* 1982;32: 26–8.
39. Kjellman N-IM, Johansson SGO, Roth A. Serum IgE levels in healthy children quantified by a sandwich technique (PRIST). *Clin Allergy* 1976;6:51–9.
40. Magnusson CGM, Masson PL. Immunoglobulin E assayed after pepsin digestion by an automated highly sensitive particle counting immunoassay. Application to human cord blood. *J Allergy Clin Immunol* 1985;75:513–24.
41. Kjellman N-IM, Johansson SGO. IgE and allergy in newborns and infants with a family history of atopic disease. *Acta Paediatr Scand* 1976;65:601–7.
42. Thomas J, Abrishami MA, Cheref MN, Walters CS. Neonatal IgE values in the black populations. *Ann Allergy* 1979;43:144–5.
43. Weil GJ, Hussain R, Kumaraswami V, et al. Prenatal allergic sensitization to helminth antigens in the offspring of parasite-infected mothers. *J Clin Invest* 1983;71:1124–9.
44. Casimir G, Duchâteau J. Neonatal serum IgE concentration as predictor of atopy. *Lancet* 1983; 1:413.
45. Magnusson CGM. Cord serum IgE in relation to family history and as a predictor of atopic disease in early infancy. *Allergy* 1988;241–51.
46. Chandra RK, Puri S, Cheema PS. Predictive value of cord blood IgE in the development of atopic disease and role of breast feeding in its prevention. *Clin Allergy* 1985;15:517–22.
47. Van den Plas Y, Sacre L. Influences of neonatal serum IgE concentrations, family history and diet on the incidence of cow's milk allergy. *Eur J Pediatr* 1986;145:493–5.
48. Kjellman N-IM, Croner S. Cord blood IgE determination for allergy prediction—a follow-up to seven years of age in 1,651 children. *Ann Allergy* 1984;53:167–71.
49. Weliky N, Lee WY, Meyers BS, Heiner DC. A prospective study of cord blood and amniotic fluid immunoglobulins in 48 infants at risk for allergy and 29 controls. *J Allergy Clin Immunol* 1981;67:104.
50. Croner S, Kjellman N-IM. Predictors of atopic disease: cord IgE and month of birth. *Allergy* 1986;41:68–70.
51. Hjalthe K, Croner S, Kjellman N-IM. Cost-effectiveness of neonatal IgE-screening for atopic allergy before seven years of age. *Allergy* 1987;42:97–103.
52. Juto P. Elevated serum immunoglobulin E in T-cell deficient infants fed cow's milk. *J Allergy Clin Immunol* 1980;66:402–7.
53. Juto P, Strannegard O. T lymphocytes and blood eosinophils in early infancy in relation to heredity for allergy and type of feeding. *J Allergy Clin Immunol* 1979;64:38–42.
54. Björkstén B, Juto P. Allergy and cell-mediated immunity in infants. In: Businco L, ed. *Advances in Pediatric Allergy*. Amsterdam: Excerpta Medica, 1983;19–28.
55. Chandra RK, Baker M. Numerical and functional deficiency of suppressor T cells precedes development of atopic eczema. *Lancet* 1983;2:1393.
56. Dry L, Leynadier F, Asuaf N, et al. Cord blood eosinophilia and family history of atopic disease. In: Oehling A, ed. *Advances in Allergy and Applied Immunology*. Oxford: Pergamon Press, 1980;779.
57. Heskel N, Chan SC, Stevens SR, Hanifin JM. Leukocyte cAMP-phosphodiesterase as a marker for atopy in neonates. *Clin Res* 1983;31:573.
58. Grewe SR, Chan SC, Hanifin JM. Elevated leukocyte cyclic AMP-phosphodiesterase in atopic disease: a possible mechanism for cAMP-agonist hyporesponsiveness. *J Allergy Clin Immunol* 1982;70:452–8.
59. Björkstén B, Suoniemi I. Early allergen contacts, adjuvant factors and subsequent allergy. In: Kerr

JW, Ganderton MA, *Proceeding of the XI International Congress of Allergology and Clinical Immunology*. London: Macmillan Press Ltd, 1983;145–8.

60. Kemp AS. Relationship between the time of birth and the development of immediate hypersensitivity to grass-pollen antigens. *Med J Aust* 1979;1:263–6.
61. Morrison-Smith J, Springett VH. Atopic disease and month of birth. *Clin Allergy* 1979;9:153–62.
62. Zeiger R. Development and prevention of allergic diseases in childhood. In: Middleton E Jr, Ellis EF, Reed CE, Adkinson NF Jr, Yunginger JW, eds. *Allergy, Principles and Practice*, 3rd ed. 1988;930–68.
63. Soothill JF, Stokes CR, Turner MW, et al. Predisposing factors and the development of reaginic allergy in infancy. *Clin Allergy* 1976;6:305–14.
64. Björkstén B. Does breast feeding prevent the development of allergy? *Immunol Today* 1983;4: 215–8.
65. Kramer MS. Does breast feeding help protect against allergic disease? Biology, methodology, and a golden jubilee of controversy. *J Pediatr* 1988;112:181–90.
66. Fergusson DM, Horwood LJ, Beautrais AL, Shannon FT, Taylor B. Eczema and infant diet. *Clin Allergy* 1981;11:325–32.
67. Michel FB, Bousquet J, Coulomb Y, Robinet-Levy M. Prediction of the "high-allergic-risk" newborn. In: Johansson SGO, ed. *Diagnosis and treatment of IgE-mediated diseases*. Amsterdam: Excerpta Medica, 1981;35–47.

Food Intolerance in Infancy: Allergology, Immunology, and Gastroenterology, edited by Robert N. Hamburger. Carnation Nutrition Education Series, Vol. 1. The Carnation Co., Los Angeles/Raven Press, Ltd., New York © 1989.

Epidemiology of Food Allergy: With Emphasis on the Influence of Maternal Dietary Restrictions During Pregnancy and Lactation on Allergy in Infancy

N-I.M. Kjellman, G. Hattevig, K. Fälth-Magnusson, and B. Björkstén

Department of Pediatrics, University Hospital and Faculty of Health Sciences, S-581 85 Linköping, Sweden

Adverse reactions to foods are seen in approximately 25% of infants and young children (1,2). Usually such reactions are transient but occasionally they continue into adult life (2,3). Immunoglobulin E (IgE)-mediated, immediate (but not delayed) food-allergic reactions are often the first sign of an atopic constitution (4). Genetic factors are of great importance for the development of immediate type food allergy and apparently also for other types of food reactions (1,5). Recurrent food-allergic reactions were seen by the parents of 58% of children with a bilateral family history of atopic disease as compared with 29% of children with a unilateral history, and only 12% of children with no family history of atopic disease (Table 1).

There have been many attempts to clarify the incidence, prevalence, and natural history of food allergy but still there is a wide range of results (2,3). Some studies focus on infants at high risk for the development of food allergy and atopic disease and other studies are made on samples from the general population. The age of the study group is of great importance (2). There is no symptom which is specific for food allergy. The varying criteria used to establish a diagnosis of food allergy may explain some of the differences but there may also be other reasons, such as genetic and socioeconomic differences between populations. Furthermore, there are differences in traditions as to, for example, at what age a food is introduced into the diet, and this may explain regional differences. What the infant eats during the first few days of life appears especially important (6). Delayed introduction of allergenic foods reduces the immune response to them (7). Differences between various foods in allergenicity and in resistance to, for example, enzymatic degradation, are other factors of importance for the development of sensitization.

History is often unreliable especially regarding food allergy, as it may be based on mistake or even on a series of mistakes. For scientific purposes, it is difficult to

TABLE 1. *The 10 most common causes of repeated food reactions (mechanism not elucidated) in 144 children followed prospectively from birth to 4½ years of age*[a]

Citrus fruits	17%
Strawberries	14%
Chocolate	8%
Egg	8%
Tomato	8%
Fish	6%
Nuts	6%
Rose hip	5%
Milk	4%
Carrots	3%

[a]From Kjellman, ref. 5, with permission and follow-up.

rely on retrospective information as many people tend to forget all previous symptoms and signs of disease—especially teenagers. The allergy may have disappeared a long time ago but the family still fears to reintroduce the food into a child's diet.

Repeated eliminations and subsequent provocations, preferably done double-blind, are often needed for a diagnosis of food allergy (2,8). The skin prick test (SPT) and radioallergosorbent test (RAST) may help to identify relevant foods for elimination and provocation. The tests seem to be particularly valuable in the diagnosis of food allergy in infants (9). They may also be used for the prediction of development of allergy to a particular food (10) or of other allergies (11). SPT and RAST results must, however, always be carefully evaluated and related to clinical history as positive tests may be present for several years after a previously food-allergic child has developed clinical tolerance (12). There are also many false-negative tests caused by poor extracts or the use of too weak allergen concentrations. Unfortunately, standardized extracts are not available. Furthermore, subjects with delayed-type symptoms usually show negative SPT and RAST results.

This paper aims at summarizing present knowledge regarding factors of importance for sensitization to food and development of food allergy. We have chosen to lay emphasis on the influence of maternal food intake during pregnancy and/or lactation on the development of symptoms and signs of allergy during childhood. Data from some not yet published studies are included.

INTERACTION BETWEEN MOTHER AND FETUS/INFANT

Sensitization *in utero* is probably rare but IgE antibodies against milk and/or egg have been demonstrated in cord blood and by skin tests in newborn infants (summarized in ref. 13). Allergens are readily transmitted through the placenta which would explain the occurrence or sensitization. Another possible but not proven mechanism for sensitization would be transplacental passage of IgG antibodies directed towards antibodies to foods (or other antigens), so-called anti-idiotypic antibodies. This mechanism has been demonstrated in transfer of immunity to polio virus from mother to baby (14). Such antibodies would act as the antigen itself, and stimulate the production of antibodies of various classes.

The immunological interaction between a mother and her fetus/infant is complex (13). The placenta permits transfer of antibodies and allergens but also of cells and various mediators, for example, for modulation of immune responses and for cell maturation. The fact that sensitization occurs only rarely during pregnancy but more frequently during lactation may partly be explained by the immune suppression imposed on the fetus during pregnancy to avoid graft-versus-host reactions. It is also possible that allergen, when presented through the placenta, is accompanied by antibodies in an ideal balance for the induction of tolerance. After birth, the suppression ends as the infant has to build up its own immune defense system to be able to survive, and, therefore, IgE antibodies to foods, for example, are more readily produced.

Breast milk contains antibodies mainly of the IgA class, directed towards infectious agents, foods, etc. (15). Gut maturation factors and factors of importance for the induction of the immune system of the infant are also present (13). Breast milk, however, also contains allergenic material from the maternal diet (e.g., proteins from cow's milk, egg, and fish). Sensitization during the period of exclusive breast-feeding is common. Therefore, breast milk is not hypoallergenic. Any allergy-protective capacity is therefore more likely caused by effects on the infant's immune system and/or simply caused by the protection from gastrointestinal or respiratory infections.

We have been looking for IgE antibodies to food allergens of fetal origin using a sensitive RAST technique. Several hundred cord serums of allergy-risk infants (identified either by a bilateral family history of atopic disease and/or by a high cord blood IgE concentration) in several studies (among them refs. 1,11, and 16) have been analyzed with no positive finding. Always when a positive RAST towards inhalants or a food was found, the same antibodies were also present in maternal serum samples in a much higher concentration, indicating contamination of the sample with maternal blood (16).

INFLUENCE OF MATERNAL FOOD INTAKE DURING PREGNANCY

Dietary restrictions (avoidance of egg, cow's milk, beef, etc.) during pregnancy and lactation have been recommended in high allergy-risk pregnancies (13). Many studies have included these recommendations with no attempt to identify which period, pregnancy, or lactation, if any of them, was important for the development of atopic disease and food allergy during infancy.

In a cooperative prospective study, the effect of four dose levels of maternal intake of highly allergenic foods (egg and cow's milk) during pregnancy has been analyzed in Sweden. Mothers-to-be, expecting high allergy-risk infants, were randomized to four groups during midpregnancy for intake of either no, low, normal, or high amounts of these nutrients from week 28 to delivery. Compliance to the diet was checked by personal statements and analyses of levels of food antibodies in the serum of the IgG, IgA, IgM, and IgE isotypes during pregnancy and in the infant.

In one part of the study (16), 180 infants completed a follow-up to 18 months of age (out of 212 mothers entered). Mothers-to-be were randomized either to complete avoidance of egg and cow's milk or to normal food intake. Despite support from a dietitian, 22 mothers could not accept the diet or had problems in having a nutritionally adequate diet, caused by the taste of the supplement offered. Another seven mothers in the control group were so interested in keeping a diet that they avoided egg and milk and therefore could not be accepted for the calculations. These 29 were, however, subject to follow-up as all the other families. The dropouts, owing to noncompliance or moving away from our region, were thus reduced to three.

In the other part of the study, mothers were randomized either to a low intake of cow's milk and egg (no visible amounts) or a high intake (1 liter of milk and one egg a day) during late pregnancy (Lilja et al., *manuscript in preparation*).

From delivery, mothers in all four groups were instructed to take normal food. All infants were fed according to the recommendations of the Swedish Pediatric Allergy Association including late introduction of milk and egg with a casein hydrolysate (Nutramigen®) as supplement to breast milk (13). Food antibody concentrations were determined also in colostrum and in the infants at birth (cord blood) as well as at 6 and 18 months of age.

Food antibodies in maternal serum were highly influenced by maternal intake (17). They decreased significantly more with no intake of milk and egg than with a low intake of these foods and increased significantly with a high intake of milk and egg. On the other hand, neonatal food-antibody concentrations seemed virtually uninfluenced by maternal food intake and the concentrations were usually higher than in the corresponding maternal serums at delivery.

High concentrations of food-specific IgG, IgA, or IgM antibodies in maternal serum or in cord blood did not seem to protect against the development of atopic disease during infancy (18) in contrast to what has been suggested by others (9,19).

Similarly, food-antibody concentrations in colostral samples were lower than the corresponding serum concentrations and no significant difference was found between breast milks of mothers who during pregnancy had been on an elimination diet and those who had been in the control group (Fälth-Magnusson et al., *manuscript in preparation*).

More importantly, none of more than 200 risk infants had IgE antibodies to cow's milk or egg in cord blood. Sixteen percent of the infants in the first part of the study showed sensitization to egg during the 1st year despite the intention not to deliberately give them egg before 12 months of age (except via breast milk). There was no significant difference in egg sensitization between the two diet groups (with no intake or normal maternal intake during pregnancy). Eight percent of the infants had proven egg allergy and no significant group difference was found in this respect.

Partial or complete tolerance was reached by 12 of 16 egg-allergic children by 3½ years of age.

In all but 3 of the 35 children with a positive SPT towards egg before 18 months of age this was accompanied or followed by symptoms of atopic disease. A positive egg SPT was found significantly more often at 6 months of age in a subgroup of children completely breast-fed to 3 months of age (16%) as compared to a group fed breast milk supplemented with Nutramigen® from an early age (4%; $p<0.01$). The type of maternal food intake during pregnancy did not seem to influence the development of atopic disease (mostly atopic dermatitis) to 18 months (study completed by blinded evaluation, ref. 16) nor to 3½ years of age (questionnaires only; *manuscript in preparation*) when 35% of children in both groups had prevalent atopic disease.

From the second part of the study (which was done in Stockholm and Uppsala), preliminary results from the follow-up at 18 months of age indicate no protective effect from high maternal food intake during pregnancy (Lilja et al., *manuscript in preparation*). The development of atopic disease and food allergy during infancy was quite similar in the group with a high maternal intake of milk and egg during pregnancy (23%) and in the group where mothers had avoided all visible egg and milk during pregnancy (19%).

INFLUENCE OF MATERNAL FOOD INTAKE DURING LACTATION

The importance of maternal food intake during lactation has been investigated in another prospective, randomized study in 115 allergy-risk infants (Hattevig et al., *manuscript in preparation*). After normal food intake during pregnancy, one group of nursing mothers took normal amounts of cow's milk, egg, and fish during the first 3 months of lactation, whereas the experimental group avoided these nutrients completely with the help of a dietitian.

At 3 and 6 months of age, infants of mothers who were on elimination diets showed significantly less atopic dermatitis than the control group. At 9 months, the experimental group showed less severe eczema. At 12 and 18 months there was still a difference in favor of the elimination diet but the difference was no longer statistically significant. Food sensitization as judged from SPT did not show any significant differences at 9 months. At 3 months, but not at 6 months, presence of IgE antibodies in serum was significantly less common in infants of mothers on diet. Thus, maternal allergen avoidance seems to delay, but not prevent, appearance of infant allergy. This study confirms results from Chandra's group (20), where significantly less atopic disease occurred in breast-fed allergy-risk infants as compared to bottle-fed risk babies but only so in the subgroup where the mothers had been on a diet during lactation (and during pregnancy). Food allergen present in most normal breast milk samples may explain the lack of allergy protection from breast-feeding reported in many studies (21–24).

FOOD SENSITIZATION IN RELATION TO FOOD INTAKE

From previous studies (11) we know that sensitization (IgE antibody production) to common foods is a normal phenomenon during infancy. Using sensitive RAST assay, 22% of girls followed from birth developed IgE antibodies in low concentrations (but well above background). As also pointed out by others (21,25) many children got their IgE antibodies to foods before the relevant food had been given to the child deliberately, thus indicating sensitization via the breast milk. The IgE antibodies decreased and disappeared in almost all children before school age (26). High concentrations (RAST class 1 or more) were in this study almost exclusively found in children with current or subsequently developing atopic disease.

Late introduction of a food appears to reduce the immune response. This was indicated by a study in which the frequency of infants producing IgE antibodies to cow's milk decreased when milk was introduced after, as compared to before, 6 months of age (25). Also the IgG antibody response to introduction of cow's milk is reduced significantly with late introduction of milk (23). Most importantly, allergic symptoms occur less often when cow's milk is introduced after, as compared to before, 6 months of age (24).

In a nonselected population 1 to 2% of infants have IgE-mediated cow's milk allergy (27) and 3 to 4% have egg allergy (11). How common sensitization and symptomatic allergy are toward, for example, soy and peanuts in the population seems to be relatively unknown but Halpern et al. (24) found approximately 0.5% soy allergy in a large population offered soy as a substitute for cow's milk. Soy-specific IgE was found by RAST in 6 of 165 infants investigated for atopic symptoms out of 1,701 infants followed from birth (1). Peanut allergy is common in the United States (3) but also in Swedish children with atopic disease a high prevalence of peanut sensitization was recently reported (28).

In schoolchildren, most reactions to foods result from the ingestion of birch pollen-associated foods such as hazelnuts, raw apples, pears, raw carrots, etc. The symptoms are usually limited to the oral cavity but generalized symptoms may occur. Birch-associated food reactions are found in approximately 50% of children investigated for birch pollen allergy (29). An increasing number of birch-associated food reactions are reported (and confirmed in, e.g., SPT) with increasing birch SPT wheal sizes or RAST class.

For food-specific skin tests the prick-prick method is recommended as it is simple and reproducible (29). This is done by first pricking a lancet into, for example, a hazelnut and then into the skin of the subject. We have evaluated the effect of oral hyposensitization with enterocoated tablets containing megadoses of birch pollen extract on the birch-associated food allergies (Björkstén et al., *manuscript in preparation*). SPT wheals to hazelnut decreased significantly and in parallel to the birch pollen SPT during active, but not during placebo, therapy. A trend toward a decreased SPT was seen with apple. At the same time, the patients reported less symptoms when eating the food in question.

THE NATURAL HISTORY

The normal way of treating food allergy is to eliminate the food completely for a given period of time and then to reintroduce it. The period of elimination is decided according to the type of food and type and severity of symptoms (3). At reintroduction, it is often found that the food is tolerated, partially or totally. The favorable prognosis of food allergy has been described by Esteban (30) who found that 50% of subjects lost their symptoms after approximately 4 to 5 years. Fish allergies tended to endure longer than allergy to cow's milk. Similarly, Bock (31) demonstrated that allergy to nuts and peanuts tended to be present during a longer period than, for example, egg allergy.

The following factors have been shown to indicate a less favorable prognosis of a food allergy (32): start of symptoms during lactation, sensitization to several allergens, a family history of food allergy, symptoms from organs other than the gastrointestinal tract. Cord blood IgE concentrations seem to influence the risk for egg sensitization but not the prognosis of egg allergy (33).

A decreasing SPT wheal or reduced RAST score were indications of favorable prognosis (34). Positive SPT may, however, be found years after the development of clinical tolerance to the food (31).

Early sensitization to foods as indicated by a positive RAST (class 1 or more) or a positive SPT to egg (diameter 3 mm or more) during infancy was found to predict later sensitization toward inhalant allergens better than the total IgE concentration during infancy, including the cord blood IgE (26).

CONCLUSIONS

1. Food sensitization occurs rarely antenatally but often during lactation. Minute amounts of food allergen are present in normal breast milk and these low amounts appear ideal for the sensitization process. This must be kept in mind when discussing early feeding in babies at high risk for allergy development, also when it comes to choice of infant formula.
2. Production of low concentrations of IgE antibodies is a normal phenomenon when the infant first meets a food allergen but high concentrations of such antibodies in a healthy child predict subsequent development of atopic disease.
3. Allergy to egg, peanuts, cow's milk, wheat, soy, and fish is common during infancy, especially when there is a bilateral family history of atopic disease or a high neonatal IgE concentration.
4. Subjects at high risk for food-allergic symptoms can be identified and prevention started already during the neonatal period. Thus, preventive measures could be instituted already neonatally. It is, however, important that any manipulation with maternal food intake during lactation or major change from normal infant feeding should be supported and supervised by a dietitian in order to avoid suboptimal nutrition, calcium deficiency, etc.

5. Elimination of highly allergenic foods from the maternal diet during lactation may delay the onset of atopic eczema and reduce the intensity of symptoms during infancy but diet during pregnancy does not influence the development of atopic disease or food allergy.

6. Late introduction of a highly allergenic food may reduce the IgE and the IgG antibody responses and the frequency of overt symptoms of allergy to that particular food.

7. In regions where birch pollen is common, birch-associated food allergies predominate in schoolchildren. Oral birch-pollen hyposensitization may reduce symptoms and immunological parameters of these birch-associated food allergies.

8. In most cases the prognosis of food allergy is favorable and tolerance, partial or complete, is reached within months or years. However, subjects with immediate-type food allergies should be regarded as at risk for subsequently developing respiratory allergies including asthma and therefore preventive measures should be taken.

9. When used sequentially, SPT are of definite value for the follow-up of certain food allergies. If no good extract is available, fresh foods and the prick-prick test method may be used to get more reliable results. However, long-term elimination should never be done solely on the basis of a positive SPT—provocation tests are almost always necessary.

10. Until generally accepted diagnostic criteria and standardized food allergen extracts are available, comparisons over time and between various parts of the world are difficult.

ACKNOWLEDGMENTS

Financial support by the Swedish Medical Research Council (grant 7510), the Medical Research Fund of the County of Östergötland, King Gustaf Vth 80-Year-Anniversary Fund, the First of May Flower Annual Campaign for Children's Health, Konsul Th Berg Foundation, Riksförbundet mot Astma-Allergi, and the Expressen Perinatal Research Fund is gratefully acknowledged.

REFERENCES

1. Croner S, Kjellman N-IM, Eriksson B, Roth A. IgE screening in 1701 newborn infants and the development of atopic disease during infancy. *Arch Dis Child* 1982;57:364–8.
2. Kajosaari M. Food allergy in Finnish children aged one to six years. *Acta Paediatr Scand* 1982;71:815–9.
3. Anderson JA, Sogn DD, eds. Adverse reactions to foods. *AAAI and NIAID Report,* NIH Publication No. 84-242, 1984.
4. van Asperen PP, Kemp AS, Mellis CM. A prospective study of the clinical manifestations of atopic disease in infancy. *Acta Paediatr Scand* 1984;73:80–5.
5. Kjellman N-IM. Development and prediction of atopic allergy in childhood. In: H Boström,

N Ljungstedt, eds. *Skandia International Symposia: Theoretical and Clinical Aspects of Allergic Disease*. Stockholm: Almqvist & Wicksell. Stockholm 1983;57–73.

6. Stinzing G, Zetterström R. Cow's milk allergy, incidence and pathogenetic role of early exposure to cow's milk formula. *Acta Paediatr Scand* 1979;68:383–7.

7. Eastham EJ, Lichauco T, Grady MI, Walker AW. Antigenicity of infant formulas: Role of immature intestine on protein permeability. *J Pediatr* 1978;93:561–4.

8. Sampson HA. Role of immediate food hypersensitivity in the pathogenesis of atopic dermatitis. *J Allergy Clin Immunol* 1983;71:473–80.

9. Hamburger RN. Diagnosis of food allergies and intolerances in the study of prophylaxis and control groups in infants. *Ann Allergy* 1984;53:673–7.

10. Dannaeus A, Johansson SGO, Foucard T. Clinical and immunological aspects of food allergy in childhood. II. Development of allergic symptoms and humural immune response to foods in infants of atopic mothers during the first 24 months of life. *Acta Paediatr Scand* 1978;67:497–504.

11. Hattevig G, Kjellman B, Johansson SGO, Björkstén B. Clinical symptoms and IgE responses to common food proteins in atopic and healthy children. *Clin Allergy* 1984;14:551–9.

12. Kjellman N-IM. Food allergy—treatment and prevention. *Ann Allergy* 1987;59:168–74.

13. Björkstén B, Kjellman N-IM. Perinatal factors influencing the development of allergy. *Clin Rev Allergy* 1987;5:339–47.

14. Mellander L, Carlsson B, Hansson L-Å. Secretory IgA and IgM antibodies to E. coli 0 and poliovirus type I antigens occur in amniotic fluid, meconium and saliva from newborns. A neonatal immune response without antigenic exposure: a result of anti-idiotypic induction? *Clin Exp Immunol* 1986;63:555–61.

15. Hansson LÅ, Ahlstedt S, Andersson B, et al. The immune response of the mammary gland and its significance for the neonate. *Ann Allergy* 1984;53:576–82.

16. Fälth-Magnusson K, Kjellman N-IM. Development of atopic disease in babies whose mothers were on exclusion diet during pregnancy—a randomized study. *J Allergy Clin Immunol* 1987;80:868–75.

17. Lilja G, Dannaeus A, Fälth-Magnusson K, Graff-Lonnevig V, Johansson SGO, Kjellman N-IM, Öhman H. Immune response of the atopic woman and fetus: effects of high- and low-dose food allergen intake during late pregnancy. *Clin Allergy* 1988;18:131–42.

18. Fälth-Magnusson K, Kjellman N-IM, Magnusson KE. Antibodies IgG, IgA and IgM to food antigens during the first 18 months of life in relation to feeding and atopic disease. *J Allergy Clin Immunol (in press)*.

19. Casimir G, Gossart B, Vis HL, Duchâteau J. Antibody against betalactoglobulin (IgG) and cow's milk allergy. *J Allergy Clin Immunol* 1985;75:206.

20. Chandra RK, Puri S, Suraiya C, Cheema PS. Influence of maternal food antigen avoidance during pregnancy and lactation on incidence of atopic eczema in infants. *Clin Allergy* 1986;16:563–9.

21. Cant A, Marsden RA, Kilshaw PJ. Egg and cow's milk hypersensitivity in exclusively breast fed infants with eczema, and detection of egg protein in breast milk. *Br Med J* 1985;291:932–5.

22. van Asperen PP, Kemp AS, Mellis CM. Relationship of diet in the development of atopy in infancy. *Clin Allergy* 1984;14:525–32.

23. Kjellman N-IM, Johansson SGO. Soy versus cow's milk in infants with a biparental history of atopic disease: development of atopic disease and immunoglobulins from birth to four years of age. *Clin Allergy* 1979;9:347–58.

24. Halpern SR, Sellars WA, Johnson RB, Anderson DW, Saperstein S, Reisch JS. Development of childhood allergy in infants fed breast, soy or cow's milk. *J Allergy Clin Immunol* 1973;51:139–51.

25. Hamburger RN, Heller S, Mellon MH, O'Connor RD, Zeiger RS. Current status of the clinical and immunological consequences of a prototype allergic disease prevention program. *Ann Allergy* 1983;51:281–90.

26. Hattevig G, Kjellman B, Björkstén B. Clinical symptoms and IgE responses to common food proteins and inhalants in the first seven years of life. *Clin Allergy* 1987;17:571–8.

27. Jakobsson I, Lindberg T. A prospective study of cow's milk protein intolerance in Swedish infants. *Acta Paediatr Scand* 1979;68:853–9.

28. Sigurs N, Hildebrand H, Hultkvist K, et al. Atopy in childhood identified by Phadebas RAST, serum IgE, skin test and Phadiatop™. *Allergy* 1988; 43 (Suppl. 7):8.

29. Dreborg S, Foucard T. Allergy to apple, carrot and potato in children with birch pollen allergy. *Allergy* 1983;38:167–72.

30. Esteban MM, Pascual C, Madero R, Diaz Pena JM, Ojeda JA. Natural history of immediate food

allergy in children. In: L. Businco, F. Ruggieri, eds. *Proceedings of the first Latin Food Allergy Workshop*. Rome, Italy: Fisons SpA. 1985;27–30.
31. Bock SA. The natural history of food sensitivity. *J Allergy Clin Immunol* 1982;69:173–7.
32. Ford PK, Taylor B. Natural history of egg hypersensitivity. *Arch Dis Child* 1982;57:649–52.
33. Kjellman N-IM, Björkstén B, Hattvig G, Fälth-Magnusson K. Natural history of food allergy. *Ann Allergy (in press)*.
34. Businco L, Benincori N, Cantani A. Epidemiology, incidence and clinical aspect of food allergy. *Ann Allergy* 1984;53:615–22.

Food Intolerance in Infancy: Allergology,
Immunology, and Gastroenterology, edited by
Robert N. Hamburger. Carnation Nutrition
Education Series, Vol. 1. The Carnation Co., Los
Angeles/Raven Press, Ltd., New York © 1989.

General Discussion for Section II

Sami L. Bahna, Jean Bousquet, Laurence Finberg,
Max Kjellman, and Richard D. O'Connor

Dr. Bahna: Dr. Kjellman, you mentioned that maternal antibodies to food proteins in the breast milk did not protect the breast-fed baby from food allergy. Were these antibodies of the immunoglobulin G (IgG) class or of the IgA class?

Dr. Kjellman: We looked at all three classes, and even maternal IgA antibodies toward egg did not protect the infant from being sensitized to egg.

Dr. Bahna: This, I think, would be contrary to another study which showed that in breast-fed infants who developed allergy to foods in the maternal diet, the breast milk of their mothers was lacking IgA antibodies to those foods.

Dr. Kjellman: Yes, I am aware of that work but I cannot account for the difference in findings.

Dr. Schmidt: Dr. Bahna, you alluded to the fact that double-blind control studies and food challenges are the gold standard for making a diagnosis of food allergy. One of the problems that I have in doing double-blind control studies is that we have quantitative as well as qualitative changes in patients while doing these studies. In other words, a patient may be able to tolerate a small amount of milk at one time but can't take a large amount without having an allergic reaction. Do you take that into consideration when you're doing double-blind control studies? The second point I want to make is that we have become aware of the fact that late-phase reactions are extremely important in allergic reactions in the respiratory tract, and I'm sure they probably play a role in food allergy as well. Do you take that into account and do you observe patients over several hours when doing double-blind control challenges in your patients? In addition, I want to ask our European colleagues about oral cromolyn in the prevention of food allergies since there is a lot of controversy about this in the literature; and we don't have it here in the United States. Would you make a comment about your experience?

Dr. Bahna: Regarding the first question, the quantitative effect of the challenge dose. It is true that one person differs from another, depending on the degree of sensitivity. But even in the same individual, the offending dose of food may vary from time to time. I think we are not completely aware of the cumulative effect of all the different factors involved in each person or at different times, whether these are extrinsic factors or intrinsic factors. I used to think that the gold standard in food allergy is the challenge test, but I don't think it is very pure gold! We have been aware from our own experience as well as of other investigators that challenge in itself is not always the whole answer. In addition to the dose, the route of exposure may be a factor, such as inhalation, particularly of fried or hot foods. When a person eats a meal and is sitting in front of a dish of food for half an hour, is that equivalent to the freeze-dried foods in capsules that we have him swallow? I don't think this is comparable. How much are we not accounting for the role food inhalation plays? It's difficult to check in a satisfactory manner, to say nothing of the artificial setting that we challenge the person in. The blind oral challenge test is an artificial replica that is often different from the natural exposure. Regarding the second question, the late-onset reactions, I personally observe my patients for at least 3 hr, usually 4 hr, and sometimes longer. Still, I realize that some patients may get reactions later, after they've left for home. At least these are not the immediate- or anaphylactic-type reactions. Unfortunately, not all of them can be objectively documented, especially when they are subjective.

Dr. Bousquet: May I answer your question concerning oral cromoglycate in prevention of food allergy? I don't think that oral cromoglycate would prevent food allergy. It may prevent symptoms when food allergy has developed, but I know that Dr. Atherton found that cromolyn was absolutely ineffective. We have some different experience, but I think cromolyn is effective in a rather small number of children. Yet when it is effective, it is extremely valuable.

Dr. Kjellman: May I add to this that we made a study in the laboratory setting where we gave cromolyn before a provocation test with cow's milk and could increase the amount of cow's milk given before symptoms occurred by a factor of 10, and at the same time prevent the changes in the gut absorption which we mirrored by giving polyethylene glycol ingestion. So it seems theoretically to work well, but from a practical point of view very few patients benefit from it, other than the occasional possibility of eating together with other people.

Dr. Collins-Williams: Collins-Williams, Toronto, Canada. Dr. Kjellman, I know when you were saying that restricting the diet in pregnancy is of no value, you were talking about food allergy in general. However, I've seen well over 200 children who have had violent anaphylactic reactions to peanut on the first known contact after birth. The only explanation I can see is that they were sensitized *in utero* and therefore there might be a value in restricting highly allergenic foods in a susceptible population.

Dr. Kjellman: I would like to see proof that these infants were really already sensitized when newborn, because once they are born they are exposed—highly exposed—to foods in the household dust, with the breast milk and so on (as we have just heard), and it takes no more than 10 days to build up a reaction. At least IgE response and sensitization could be as rapid as that. How old were these children when they had their reactions?

Dr. Collins-Williams: Oh, they varied considerably, but some of them were quite small. There are a lot of children who get peanut butter very early in life. I agree it's possible that they were sensitized after birth, but I just wanted to know your opinion.

Dr. Kjellman: As already indicated, we have been looking for intrauterine sensitization in several hundreds of high-risk infants, some infants with very high total IgE, and we haven't been able to prove it in a single case, even though we looked for it with an extremely sensitive, refined radioallergosorbent test (RAST) technique. So if it occurs, it must be very, very rare.

Dr. McGeady: Steve McGeady of Philadelphia, Pennsylvania. I have two questions. The first is to Dr. Bousquet. I was surprised to see your conclusions on the double-antibody radioimmunoassay, that it's ineffective in detecting cord blood IgE since that test has been widely used, for example, for detection of *in vitro* production of IgE. Do you have any explanation for that?

Dr. Bousquet: Well, it was not the test used by Gleich and Yunginger. It was a European test. In our study, the double-antibody radioimmunoassay was proved non-effective, but I have no experience with other tests. It is the only possible explanation I can give you.

Dr. McGeady: The illustration which you presented looked almost like the mirror image of a normal curve. Did you think there might be an interfering protein in that?

Dr. Bousquet: That might be. It's a possibility. We tested for interfering protein with the paper radioimmunosorbent test (PRIST) only.

Dr. McGeady: My other question is to Dr. Bahna. Clinically, we are frequently asked to evaluate children for cow's milk hypersensitivity very early in life, and yet that is an age when we often have a lot of trouble with skin testing. I wonder how you deal with the very young infant, say in the 3 to 5 month of age range who comes in with suspected cow's milk hypersensitivity?

Dr. Bahna: The medical history is important, particularly in this age where such youngsters have not been exposed to numerous foods. I use the history plus either RAST or skin testing. In infants it is usually easier to draw a blood sample for total IgE and specific IgE antibodies to milk as well as other foods that the baby might have consumed. And even if both the history and the RAST or the skin tests are negative, I would give a trial of elimination of one or two suspected foods for 1 to 2 weeks, and then give back the eliminated food and observe for the recurrence of symptoms.

Dr. McGeady: So the gold standard may not be so tarnished after all.

Dr. Bahna: Most of the time it is not, but occasionally it may be "gold plated," as I hear Dr. Hamburger saying.

Dr. Devries: Jeffrey Devries from Detroit, Michigan. Dr. Kjellman, you recommended that mothers who are breast-feeding infants at risk of developing atopic disease should be on an elimination diet. Would you extrapolate that recommendation to the diet of the infants themselves who are at high risk? Is there a particular period within the first year of life during which you would eliminate from their diet certain foods that are more commonly allergenic?

Dr. Kjellman: The general recommendation in Sweden by the Board of Pediatric Allergists is that high-risk infants are fed without egg and fish during the first 12 months and cow's milk is introduced not before 9 months of age. Of course, families shouldn't smoke or have pet animals at home either.

Dr. Devries: Do you also avoid citric acid juices, such as orange juice and grapefruit juice, until a certain age?

Dr. Kjellman: If possible, delay until 12 months of age because the high-risk population had reactions towards citrus fruits in 50% of cases.

Dr. Devries: Is there any clinical evidence that this recommendation would be beneficial for the general population in reducing the incidence of subsequent food allergy?

Dr. Kjellman: There is no real proof of it because it hasn't been separately evaluated, but from the picture I showed, if you assume that you have a late reaction, including an inflammation, then any food giving a reaction should be avoided, otherwise the inflammation paves the way for sensitization.

Dr. Guesry: Guesry, Vevey, Switzerland. My question is for Max Kjellman. You showed a very provocative slide stating breast milk is not hypoallergenic. I think you need to clarify your statement because a few minutes later, you showed the works of Chandra and of Luisa Businco and your own work showing that breast-feeding reduced by about 50% the manifestation of cow's milk allergy. What would you call a hypocholesteremic drug that could reduce the cholesterol in 50% of the at-risk population? Usually it's called a hypocholesteremic drug and everybody would agree. So I wonder why you refuse to call it hypoallergenic breast-feeding when it works in 50%, at least, of the population?

Dr. Kjellman: Breast-feeding is not hypoallergenic because it really contains allergen in a concentration which is known from animal experiments to be ideal for sensitization. Animal experiments by our group have shown that exactly those concentrations present in normal breast milk are ideal to induce reactions; while if you increase the concentration by a factor of 100 to 100,000, then sensitization decreases with the increasing amount of allergen given.

Dr. Guesry: So you mean that in this business you prefer to believe the animal experimentation rather than the clinical evidence?

Dr. Kjellman: No, not at all. I think to combine it because if we take away the most potent allergens from the breast milk by recommending a diet and supervising the diet, then perhaps even breast milk is acceptable as a hypoallergenic formula.

Dr. Guesry: I'm glad to hear you say that.

Dr. Kjellman: It works as a preventive measure because it also contains positive factors which stimulate the production of IgA and gut maturation. So it is worthwhile from that point of view, and it could be even better if we take away the highly allergenic foods from the maternal diet.

Dr. Bahna: I'm glad that Dr. Guesry opened this issue. I would like to point out that there is no evidence that human milk components per se are allergenic. This excludes human milk contaminated by the maternal diet. There is no clinical or experimental evidence that human milk protein can sensitize human beings. In the laboratory, it is easy to sensitize, for example, the rabbit with bovine milk, but not by rabbit milk. I'm not aware of any researcher who was able to sensitize an animal by the breast milk of the same species. If anyone in the audience has such information, it will help us to hear about it.

Dr. Kjellman: I have no such information. But what I thought you would bring up is why on earth were our children, who were fed both breast milk and Nutramigen together, four times less sensitive towards *egg* at 6 months of age compared to breast-fed infants? That is something surprising! This could mean that Jarrett's ideas really are valid. Instead of giving a hypoallergenic formula, we should give either a really nonallergenic food or we should give cow's milk allergens in very high amounts so that we really induce tolerance. Breast milk in this case was not devoid of allergens because the mothers were supposed to eat a normal diet, and we also demonstrated that allergens were present in their breast milk. So that is probably why their babies were sensitized so often.

Dr. Bahna: I agree with that, but sometimes we are asked whether human milk can cause allergy in human babies, and the answer should be, No, we don't have any information that indicates that human breast milk can sensitize human infants.

Dr. Bousquet: Since human milk is contaminated by food antigens in a vast majority of cases, we must say that human milk in the normal condition usually contains food antigens.

Dr. Sandberg: Could some of the panel members review for me some of the differences in the way infants are fed in different areas in Europe, just to compare them to the way we feed in the United States?

Dr. Kjellman: We had a period where mothers didn't give breast so much, but now they are breast-feeding extremely well, perhaps too well I think, because many mothers are still breast-feeding when their children are over 18 months of age. I think that 98% or so leaving the maternity ward are at least partially breast-feeding, and that after 3 months something like 60% are giving breast milk feedings, at least partially.

Dr. Hill: David Hill, Children's Hospital, Melbourne, Australia. I would like to ask Dr. O'Connor a little more about your gold standard used in the United States for food challenges. I am basing my comments on our studies on children with cow's milk allergy. It seems to me that the gold standard that has been used has not really addressed the question in its broadest context. It seems to me that the test is how that gold standard compares with controlled hospital challenges. I note, for instance, the volume of milk delivered by Sampson and Bock is much smaller than the amount of milk we would require to precipitate reactions in our hospitalized study children with milk allergy.

Dr. O'Connor: It's clear that the use of the double-blind food challenge is very important and the need for its use is dependent upon the patient's age. You can hospitalize patients and do double-blind challenges in the hospital and watch them closely. In the adult population, 20 to 30% of those patients are placebo reactors. In the studies reported by Sampson and Bock, their placebo reaction rates were dependent upon age. Thus, the necessity to do a double-blind challenge with a placebo control is age-dependent. As to the challenge quantity, Bock as well as Sampson first did the double-blind challenge, but when the double-blind challenge was negative, they did an open challenge with larger quantities of milk to prove that it was safe to go ahead and ingest milk. In their open studies where they gave the native food, they had no positive reactions to larger quantities after a negative double-blind challenge. You are really asking the question, is it sufficient to hospitalize a child or put him in a clinical research setting where he can be observed prospectively and then do open studies? I'm not aware of any data directly comparing them. I'm not sure if the answer exists from data in the literature. My feeling is that unblinded study without placebo control probably can only be performed reliably in a very young infant, although no data exist at the present time. My plea for doing double-blind challenges was meant to extend to clinical investigators who report research studies because theirs are the only data which probably will be accepted by everybody. If you don't, there are going to be a lot of detractors from your studies.

Ms. Carpenter: Kathleen Carpenter, and I work with the Women, Infants and Children's Program in the Bronx here in New York. We are naturally mandated to promote breast-feeding and some of us seem to be hearing a case being made here against breast-feeding. Our question is this: What actual percentage in the general population of babies show problems with their mother's breast milk?

Dr. Bahna: I don't think we have accurate figures about allergies in exclusively breast-fed infants. There are multiple variables that are not controlled. It is certainly much less than in bottle-fed infants or in infants who receive solid feedings early in life. Regarding the statement you made, that there are some people on this panel who discourage breast-feeding, I think all of us are strong proponents of breast-feeding. But we realize that there are some infants who, no matter what you do for them, are so genetically engineered that minute quantities of food antigens from the maternal diet in the breast milk can sensitize them. Likewise, grandmother's comforting touch with her finger that has some food on it on the tongue of the infant may sensitize him. But all of us still think "breast is best!"

Dr. Kjellman: I would just add that of course we promote breast-feeding as much as we can, especially in various high-risk situations, including situations where there is a high risk of infections, because infections may very well pave the way for sensitization towards food allergens and inhalant allergens.

Dr. Dolovich: Jerry Dolovich, Hamilton, Canada. I would like to make a comment about late responses and then ask a question. Dr. Siegel asked a question about late responses and it evolved that people have not seen late responses in the gut. Yet if one looks at the respiratory tract, one finds it's quite easy to elicit them in the airway where there is a sensitive test of responsiveness in the lower airway at least, whereas it is hard to elicit them in the nasal mucosa, at least in terms of a visible or observable constriction. Yet the inflammatory process is there in the nose and it's there in the lower airway. The point is that with some challenges you get that late response and inflammation in the airway and with some challenges you don't. This is a tremendously important variable, whether it occurs or not (that is, in challenges in the airway), and it's indeed possible that this variable, sometimes present and sometimes not present, occurs in the gut as well, although one might not find it unless follow-up measurements that somehow detect the inflammation were done. I don't know how you would do it, but it's potentially an important variable as to what happens later following ingestion of antigen. My question has to do with this very common reactivity to citrus in young children, and I wonder if anyone has any insight as to what the mechanism is to citrus fruit, the reaction in infants to citrus fruit, and why does it happen? Is it IgE-dependent?

Dr. Kjellman: We know a few cases where an IgE-mediated reaction to citrus fruits has been proven, but the vast majority is not obviously IgE-mediated and we don't really know the mechanism.

Dr. Siegel: Sheldon Siegel from Los Angeles, California. I'm a little bit surprised that nobody has mentioned anything about soybean, soy preparations, and the treatment of allergic children. Dr. Machtinger did mention the studies in 1922 by Grullee and Sanford (1), in which they showed that babies fed cow's milk had seven times the incidence of eczema versus those babies that were breast-fed. As a consequence of that, Dr. Jerome Glazer, whom I trained with, and whom I was with at the time, did some studies with mothers feeding breast milk or soy-based formula, reasoning that soy was less common in our everyday diet than cow's milk and that if the infants did become sensitized there would not be as much of a problem. Unfortunately, his original studies were not controlled well, but from them it's now common practice in the United States for almost all pediatricians and many allergists to take children and put them on soybean milk as more or less of a prophylactic procedure in preventing food allergy. If they can't breast-feed, they put them on soybean. I would like to have Dr. Kjellman comment on that because I gather that is not done commonly in the Scandinavian countries.

Dr. Kjellman: No. We did a study which was in 48 high-risk infants. We gave soy or cow's milk formula once the breast-feeding period came to an end, and we found no significant differences between the groups, and these were really with a very, very high allergy risk. If anything, the soy group had more problems. Furthermore, we found a few really serious soy reactions among those who were exposed to soy from a rather early age, severe gastrointestinal symptoms and a delay in weight gain and so on, and it took several months until they started growing properly. So soy preparations are allergenic. They induce problems at least as often as cow's milk if they are given to high-risk infants at an early age. And we know from studies where we have given soy to cow's milk allergic children, that if we start it when a child has gastrointestinal symptoms, especially from cow's milk, then almost all children will also react adversely to the soy preparation. To us, cow's milk allergy is almost a contraindication to giving soy if the child is in early infancy or has had gastrointestinal symptoms. For preventive purposes, I really prefer a formula which has proven to be preferably nonallergenic.

Dr. Zucker: Preston Zucker, New Jersey. We talk about cow's milk allergy as if we're dealing with a single entity. Yet, we're dealing with cattle of different breeds who are fed different things and treated with different pharmacological agents. Once the milk is extracted from the cow it then may or may not be pasteurized at different standards, have fat extracted to make it into low-fat or skim milk, or, in some cases, be treated with *Lactobacillus*. How can you make scientific conclusions when you are using something which seems so heterogeneous?

Dr. Bahna: You are right, there are different breeds of cattle, they are fed different things, and the content of the milk varies even in the same cow at different times. But that's what we have to live with. It's true also in pollens. At different times of the year, the protein content of the pollens is different. That is the normal variation. Additionally, I would like to comment on an important issue that Dr. Jerry Dolovich raised again: delayed reactions, which is a dilemma in food allergy. I don't think, Dr. Dolovich, that we can make a parallelism between the late reactions from food allergy and the late reactions from inhalant allergy. In inhalant allergy, a person can get an acute attack of asthma or rhinitis from inhaling microgram or picogram quantities of pollen. This is not the case in food allergy. We need grams or up to a pound of food to cause a food reaction in some patients. It is likely that delayed reactions to foods are different from those to pollen. It is easier to study delayed reactions of inhalant allergy. Food is ingested and processed inside the body in various ways, and the final or actual food allergen may be completely different from the native food.

Dr. Dolovich: Whether it's a gram, an ounce, or a pound, the prospect still exists as a possible variable in what happens in the gut; and whether it's a gram, an ounce, or a pound, you just don't know what is happening. I'm not saying you should know and I'm not expressing criticism. I just would suggest to you it's still out there as a possibility, and something is going on that we just don't understand.

Dr. Kjellman: Regarding cow's milk, for instance, as a source of allergens: cow's milk should be treated like other allergens and when producing an extract, it should be pooled. For instance, *Cladosporium* extract is a pool of various cultivated strains which are then controlled with various methods to ensure that the quality is the same in each batch. So this should of course apply to food extracts, too. Food extracts available on the market are very poor, and that is why we very often use fresh food in the natural concentration in which it is eaten. Thus, for a solid food, we make a prick test by pricking through the food with a lancet into the skin of the patient. This has been shown by Tony Foucard, among others, to be the most reproducible way to establish food allergy, by using fresh food, fresh fruits, meats, and so on.

Dr. Singer: Allan Singer, Los Angeles, California. With patients who have severe life-threatening anaphylactic reactions to foods, you've talked about detecting some of these with RAST and with skin testing, and then later we talked about the fact that a certain percentage of patients will outgrow this sensitivity at 18 months, 3 years of age, or later. Since there is sensitization or, in other words, their skin test or RAST may remain positive even though their clinical symptoms disappear, I was wondering how do the people on the panel find out that these patients actually outgrew their sensitivity? At age three, what do they do? Some on the panel have stated that you don't want to challenge a patient if they give a history of anaphylactic sensitivity and have a positive skin test. How at age three do you find out that they have outgrown it unless they accidentally ingest the food?

Dr. O'Connor: Dr. Alan Bock (2) has looked at the natural history of food allergy in children and followed up with the children for several years. In his studies, approximately 70% of children who were allergic in the first 12 months of life could tolerate the food by age 3 to 5 years. There were still 30% who couldn't tolerate the food based upon challenge data. He rechallenged these children several years later. Those children, however, were not the ones who had life-threatening reactions, and I think it's important to distinguish between those two populations.

Dr. Singer: Bock says that he does challenge patients despite a history of life-threatening anaphylaxis.

Dr. O'Connor: I referred to his published data. The natural history of the children he reported was for those who had allergic reactions early in childhood. I'm not aware of any studies looking at the natural history of anaphylactic reactions of a life-threatening nature later in life.

Dr. Hamburger: There is one published study on that subject by Boyanno et al. (3) from Madrid, and they found high total IgE levels or persistence of high specific IgE antibody was the best guideline to those sensitized children who were not going to outgrow their allergy. Those were the ones who continued to have allergic responses to that food though 9 years of age.

Dr. Kjellman: It has been demonstrated that early onset of allergic symptoms, starting during the period while still breast-feeding, is a bad sign for the prognosis. We evaluated the skin prick test results in relation to open provocation tests with egg in our kids from 12 months of age and found that very often the prick test would still be positive. However, prospectively over a period of time there is often a trend towards a plateau or a decrease in the skin test reactivity when the challenge is going to be negative. So the prick test was much more helpful than we had anticipated. There was a significant difference in the skin-prick test reaction at the time of the provocation test between those who were positive and those who were negative in their provocation test response.

Dr. Bahna: We too expect in those patients with anaphylaxis that sensitization will persist longer than with other (nonanaphylactic) manifestations. I have also noticed that some of these patients who get anaphylaxis from ingestion may get urticaria from touching or from inhaling the food. So, this may be another clinical parameter that we can monitor or ask the patient about. As Dr. Kjellman indicated, skin testing or the RAST can also guide us, but I think the final thing will be a very cautious challenge after a prolonged time of avoidance.

Question: I would like to follow up on an earlier question to Dr. Kjellman about European practices as far as introduction of solid foods. How long do you all recommend just breast milk or formula before the introduction of solid foods or cow's milk? Secondly, for the whole panel, when physicians, through the pressure from mothers, their own practice, or whatever, introduce solid foods earlier than the recommended times (in this country 4 to 6 months), what risk are they putting their infants at for allergic problems in the future?

Dr. Kjellman: Starting with the recommendations in Sweden, we have adjusted our recommendations to reasonable possibilities, and recommend that mothers breast-feed for four months at least before giving any additional food, and preferably in the high-risk group wait until 5½ months of age until any solid food is introduced. How much you increase your risk by earlier solid food introduction can be seen from the literature. About a 30% increase was obvious in the Finnish study, for instance, by the introduction of solid foods before six months of age.

Dr. Bousquet: I would like to make a comment on breast-feeding and solid-feeding. Not being a pediatrician, I may have a cold-blooded outlook on that. The literature, in fact, does not give any strong evidence that breast-feeding can significantly protect patients or infants from being subsequently allergic. I am wondering whether we should advise very long periods for breast-feeding, especially of more than 6 months, which is totally impossible in France, for example. Perhaps we should see if avoidance of air pollution may not be more important.

Dr. Kjellman: Cigarette smoking is of course a very big risk factor.

Dr. Heyman: Mel Heyman, San Francisco, California. Objective tests for food allergy or food reactions were discussed, but you ignored the tests of cell-mediated immune reactions, such as the lymphocyte migration inhibition factor or the other tests that you listed. I wonder if you would care to comment on those.

Dr. O'Connor: When I was reviewing the literature, I concentrated on those areas where some corroborating data could be found. There have been a number of very interesting reports looking at lymphocyte proliferation or alternatively the presence of immune complexes or activation products of the complement system. However, in the context of confirming food challenges, very little exists, and I think this is the area that really deserves a lot of attention, especially the study of cell-mediated immune function with late onset reactions of more than 24 hr, or alternatively the clearance of immune complexes. I think that they offer a great deal of hope for the future in terms of interesting research projects. When I recently reviewed the literature, I paid attention to those areas that (a) were common and (b) where there was some evidence to suggest, from double-blind food challenges, they might be of some help to clinicians.

REFERENCES

1. Grulee CG, Sanford HN. The influence of breast and artificial feeding on food antigen infantile eczema. *J Pediatr* 1936;8:223–5.
2. Bock SA. Prospective appraisal of complaints of adverse reactions to foods in children during the first three years of life. *Pediatrics* 1987;79:683–8.
3. Boyano MT, Martin EM, Pascual C, Ojeda JA. Food allergy in children. II. Prognostic factors and long-term development. *An Esp Pediatr* 1987;26:241–5.

Food Intolerance in Infancy: Allergology, Immunology, and Gastroenterology, edited by Robert N. Hamburger. Carnation Nutrition Education Series, Vol. 1. The Carnation Co., Los Angeles/Raven Press, Ltd., New York © 1989.

Introduction to Section III

William C. Heird

College of Physicians and Surgeons of Columbia University, New York, NY 10032

During pediatric training, I was taught that food allergies are extremely rare. However, my clinical activities since seem to refute this early teaching. Being involved primarily in nutritional management of infants and children with gastrointestinal dysfunction, I am impressed by the rather high percentage of these patients who react adversely to ingestion of bovine milk and/or soy protein. In some, vomiting and/or diarrhea with or without intestinal blood loss and/or protein-losing enteropathy in response to ingestion of these proteins is the only manifestation of intestinal dysfunction, but most have a variety of other manifestations of gastrointestinal dysfunction (e.g., enzyme deficiencies, metabolic derangements, secondary malnutrition, surgically correctable congenital or acquired lesions of the gastrointestinal tract). This experience, of course, is not unique. Interestingly, Keating (1), in one of the first reports of the use of parenteral nutrition in treatment of infants with chronic diarrhea, observed that 4 of 15 survivors had what was called lactose intolerance (possibly bovine milk protein sensitivity) and another 2 had lactose deficiency a year after discharge.

The apparent discrepancy between what I was taught during the early stages of pediatric training and what I deal with in my clinical activities today is easily resolved. On the one hand, primary food allergies probably are rare in a general pediatric population. However, in the population requiring nutritional intervention, this is not the case. This latter group most likely includes both the more severe manifestations of primary food allergy encountered in the general pediatric population as well as a number of infants who have become sensitized secondarily as a result of intestinal damage from a variety of other causes.

Whereas children with severe gastrointestinal manifestations of food allergy represent the bulk of the gastroenterologist's experience with food allergies, the nutritionist's experience is not limited to this entity. For example, I receive a number of calls from other pediatricians and from disturbed parents inquiring about the role of food allergies in sleep disorders, colic, and various dermatoses. In this session, we will hear about these clinical manifestations of food allergy as well as the gastrointestinal manifestations. Hopefully, we will also hear more about what constitutes an adequate diagnosis of food allergy in all of these disorders.

The latter, in my opinion, is extremely important. Although it is relatively easy to devise a nutritious diet that excludes foods to which a child may be sensitive, such a diet is not always sufficiently palatable to assure that the pediatric patient will ingest sufficient quantities to support normal growth. The more subtle effects of such diets also must be considered. For example, the child placed on a restrictive diet is being deprived of a number of taste experiences which many believe may be important factors in development of taste and, hence, intake throughout life. The parents of children placed on restrictive diets also require special consideration. They often feel that their child is missing many of the social aspects of a more varied diet and frequently have mixed feelings about just how strictly the diet should be enforced. If their leniency results in increased symptoms, they experience feelings of guilt. If they choose to be more strict, they are concerned that too much emphasis is being placed on food and that this may contribute to development of feeding disorders, both immediately and later in life. To a parent, perhaps the most devastating aspect of having a child placed on a restricted diet is the fact that it is a constant reminder that their child is not normal.

Obviously the nutritional management of children with food allergies has a number of far-reaching manifestations, some of which we are just beginning to talk about and consider. Certainly, restrictive diets should not be imposed without a reasonably clear indication or diagnosis. The presentations comprising the session may not provide all the answers we need or would like to have, but they are a first step in the right direction.

REFERENCE

1. Keating JP. Parenteral nutrition in infants with malabsorption. In: Winters RW, Hasselmeyer EG, eds. *Intravenous Nutrition in High Risk Infants,* New York: John Wiley & Sons, Inc., 1974;117–25.

*Food Intolerance in Infancy: Allergology,
Immunology, and Gastroenterology,* edited by
Robert N. Hamburger. Carnation Nutrition
Education Series, Vol. 1. The Carnation Co., Los
Angeles/Raven Press, Ltd., New York © 1989.

Intestinal Manifestations of Food Allergy

John A. Walker-Smith

*Department of Pediatric Gastroenterology, Queen Elizabeth Hospital for Children,
London, Great Britain*

Gastrointestinal food allergies may be defined as clinical syndromes which are characterized by the onset of gastrointestinal symptoms following food ingestion where the underlying mechanism is an immunologically mediated reaction within the gastrointestinal tract.

PATHOGENESIS

This chapter first reviews what pathology could be anticipated in the intestinal mucosa on the basis of gastrointestinal food allergy.

In animal models, the local effects of allergic reactions of the Gell and Coombs Classifications type I, III, and IV have been investigated in the small intestinal mucosa (1).

Type I or reaginic allergic reaction may be produced in a rat who has been immunized and then challenged with an intravenous dose of antigen (2). The effect of such an immediate allergic reaction is the development within 5 or 10 min of microscopic edema, mucous secretion, and increased blood flow. Histologically, the mucosa may be entirely normal or just show some edema of the lamina propria and small subepithelial blebs.

In a study of intraluminal antigen challenge of actively or passively immunized pigs to produce a type III or immune complex allergic reaction, a massive influx of polymorphs to the mucosa was shown but without morphological damage (3). In a similar model in rabbits, deposition of immune complexes in the gut wall was shown (4).

A variety of type IV, local cell-mediated reactions in the mucosa have been produced in animals including graft-versus-host disease, rejection of transplanted allografts of intestine, and parasite infections in thymus-derived cell (T-cell)-depleted hosts (5–7). These models show that the earliest changes in these cell-mediated reactions are infiltration of lymphocytes into the lamina propria and the epithelium. The crypts lengthen (i.e., become hypertrophied) and crypt cell production rate is increased. Villi are shortened. These changes are mediated by lymphokines secreted

127

by activated T cells. Thus, there is a compelling morphological incidence in these animal studies to suggest that cell-mediated immunity may produce small intestinal enteropathy.

Similar evidence is now available in human fetal small intestinal mucosa by fetal gut organ culture. The efferent limb of the mucosal immune reponse, namely the effect of activated T cells in the lamina propria, can be studied in human fetal small intestinal cultures (8). T cells may be activated *in situ* by pokeweed mitogen or anti-CD3 antibody. This results in crypt hypertrophy and villous atrophy (i.e., the development of a small intestinal enteropathy with features resembling food-sensitive enteropathy). The degree of mucosal lymphocyte activation relates to the age of the fetus from which the tissue is obtained. For example, no effect was demonstrated in a 14-week-old fetal intestine at which time there are few T cells (9). As the age of the fetal gut increases so do the changes increase, being maximal in the oldest fetus studied at 22 weeks. All these changes could be inhibited by cyclosporine A which is known to inhibit cell-mediated reactions. Lymphokines alone were not responsible for the mucosal changes.

So it could be hypothesized in gastrointestinal food allergy, where there is a cell-mediated reaction, that lymphocytes in the small intestinal mucosa lamina propria, which have been sensitized to dietary antigen, interact with food antigens that enter the mucosa from the gut lumen. This leads to activation of T lymphocytes leading to crypt hypertrophy and reduction in villous height.

CLINICAL SPECTRUM

With this pathogenetic background, let us look at the clinicopathological syndromes which are recognized as being caused by food allergy. Broadly, from a clinical viewpoint, the syndromes of gastrointestinal food allergy have been divided into the quick-onset syndromes where symptoms manifest quickly (i.e., within minutes to an hour of food ingestion) and those in which the onset is slow (i.e., taking hours or days after food ingestion). Hill et al. (10), based on challenge studies, recognizes an intermediate group where symptoms occur 45 min to 20 hr after challenge.

QUICK-ONSET SYNDROMES

These are the syndromes where a type I reaction in the small intestinal mucosa is likely to account for the clinical features, although this remains to be established, as there are few studies of small intestinal mucosa after food challenge in these syndromes.

Acute Anaphylaxis

The most dramatic example of a quick-onset syndrome is acute anaphylaxis after oral food ingestion. Anaphylaxis was first described in 1901, by Charles Richet and

Paul Portier on the yacht of Prince Albert of Monaco after ingestion of foreign protein. Only 4 years later in 1905, Schlossman (11) documented similar symptoms of acute shock in infants not after injection but after ingestion of a foreign protein, namely cow's milk. In the same year, Finkelstein (12) described a death caused by cow's milk ingestion leading to acute anaphylaxis. It is now known that anaphylaxis usually results from a generalized immediate immunoglobulin E (IgE)-mediated reaction following the introduction of sufficient antigens into a previously sensitized individual releasing histamine and other biologically active mediators from sensitized mast cells. However, the term, anaphylaxis, must remain a clinical one as reactions with clinical features of anaphylaxis have been described without IgE mediation. This then is the most severe example of quick-onset gastrointestinal food allergy. It has been described following ingestion of cow's milk, wheat, and eggs.

Acute Gastrointestinal Food Allergy

Less dramatic is the acute onset of vomiting with or without diarrhea within an hour of food ingestion (i.e., acute gastrointestinal food allergy). Swelling of lips and tongue, angioedema, and urticaria may accompany these gastrointestinal symptoms. A classic example is the breast-fed infant who reacts in this dramatic way to cow's milk. The amount of cow's milk responsible for this can be extremely small. It has been proven that infants can be sensitized to cow's milk via its presence in maternal breast milk when the mother herself is drinking cow's milk (13). Other foods producing acute onset of vomiting and diarrhea include wheat or gluten and egg.

Typically, levels of food-specific IgE antibodies are elevated and skin prick tests are positive. These tests characteristically became negative when this temporary syndrome disappears. A good example is provided by the egg prick test in a quick-onset egg allergy (14).

SLOW-ONSET REACTIONS

These reactions include those syndromes where there is structural damage to either the small or large intestinal mucosa. It may not be clinically obvious that ingestion of cow's milk products or other foods has caused the gastrointestinal pathology demonstrated.

The first group of these disorders is food-sensitive enteropathy, of which the most classical example is cow's milk-sensitive enteropathy and the second is food-sensitive colitis and cow's milk-sensitive colitis in particular.

Cow's Milk-Sensitive Enteropathy

This may be defined as a temporary disorder of infancy characterized by a variably abnormal small intestinal mucosa while having milk in the diet. This abnormality is reversed by a cow's milk-free diet only to relapse upon challenge (15,16). It only affects children less than 3 years of age as a general rule (Fig.1). One remarkable exception is the case report of a child with celiac disease whose small intestinal mucosa was responsive to cow's milk until at least the age of 7 years (17). This disorder has not however been described in adult life. The small intestinal mucosal biopsy appearances, although not diagnostically specific, have the following characteristics: (a) The lesion is typically patchy (18). (b) It may be similar but it is usually less severe than that found in celiac disease. (c) The mucosa is characteristically thin (16). (d) Intraepithelial lymphocyte count, although usually elevated, is less than that found in celiac disease (19). (e) In the case of cow's milk-sensitive enteropathy, there is typically an accumulation of fat in the epithelium (20). (f) Disaccharidase levels are depressed overall but to a lesser degree than that found in celiac disease. When all these features are taken together in a child with appropriate clinical features, they are highly characteristic, although none of these features are specifically diagnostic and there are indeed many causes of small intestinal mucosal damage in infancy (21).

In clinical practice, the notion of a milk elimination-responsive enteropathy has been introduced, as it is not always possible to use this approach of serial biopsy related to dietary elimination and challenge (15). Thus, when an infant with chronic diarrhea and malnutrition or other gastrointestinal symptoms has a small intestinal biopsy with the appearances described above and responds rapidly to a cow's milk-free diet with relief of symptoms and weight gain, such a child has a milk elimination-responsive enteropathy. It is very likely that such infants in fact have cow's milk-sensitive enteropathy (22,23). The role of gastrointestinal infection causing secondary cow's milk-sensitive enteropathy has been described (23). From this has come the concept of primary cow's milk-sensitive enteropathy occurring apparently *de novo* usually weeks or months after starting cow's milk feeding and secondary

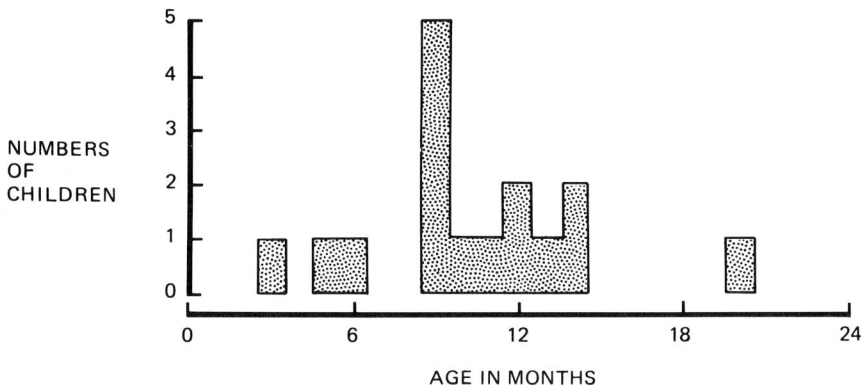

FIG. 1. Ages of 18 children at time of diagnosis of cow's milk-sensitive enteropathy by biopsy.

cow's milk-sensitive enteropathy which may occur as a sequel to gastrointestinal infection.

An hypothesis interrelating acute gastroenteritis and cow's milk-sensitive enteropathy has been proposed (23). The allergenicity of the cow's milk given at the time of the gastrointestinal infection may be of critical importance (24,25).

Management

Treatment involves substituting cow's milk feeds with the commercially available cow's milk protein-free formula feeds. In practice, only protein hydrolysate formulas are recommended as initial treatment. These include casein hydrolysate, Pregestimil and Nutramigen (Bristol-Myers), and the whey hydrolysate, Alfare (Nestlé). In a study comparing Pregestimil and Alfare, there was some advantage for the latter, although the results were not conclusive (26). In the occasional case where this management fails, a comminuted chicken formula can be used. In developing countries where commercially manufactured protein hydrolysates are either not available or are too expensive, a cheap formulation can be made based upon cooked chicken meat. When available, expressed breast milk is very effective treatment (27). Soy formulas are not recommended when there is damage to the small intestinal mucosa as there is a considerable risk of developing in turn soy-sensitive enteropathy (28). A figure of 15% has been reported (29). Likewise, goat's milk is not recommended as there is considerable cross-reactivity with cow's milk protein.

It is important to ensure that both liquid and solid foods are free of cow's milk proteins. Disaccharide intolerance may accompany the protein intolerance, and in such circumstances, disaccharides should also be withdrawn from the diet. In practice, there is little difference between a lactose-free and a milk protein-free diet. The necessity for dietary treatment is always temporary, and reintroduction of a normal diet is normally nearly always possible by the age of 1 to 2 years; this is usually achieved at home, but a history of severe reactions, such as urticaria or anaphylactoid shock, is an absolute indication for reintroduction of a normal diet under very close medical supervision.

Other Food-Sensitive Enteropathies

A number of other food-sensitive enteropathies have been described. Soy protein, gluten, egg, chicken meat, rice, and fish have all been described as causes of food-induced enteropathy in early infancy (30,31).

Other Reactions

There are also a less well-defined group of children with apparent late reactions to cow's milk who do not have structural damage related to cow's milk ingestion. Hill et al. (10) have described these as children who react with gastrointestinal, skin, and respiratory symptoms following cow's milk challenge. Some of these children may also be atopic with elevated IgE antibodies and positive skin-prick tests. In an attempt to clarify the clinical profiles in cow's milk allergy, the clinical features have been analyzed and time to respond in 100 children. In fact, three rather than two clusters of patients were recognized, namely Group 1 (26 patients) who developed symptoms within 45 min of cow's milk ingestion; Group 2 (57 patients) who developed symptoms within 20 hr; and Group 3 (17 patients) who developed symptoms more than 20 hr after challenge. Group 1 had frequent skin reactions and nearly all had positive skin-prick tests to milk. Group 2 had reactions almost confined to the gastrointestinal tract and there was a low incidence of positive skin tests. Group 3 had diarrhea, respiratory symptoms, and eczema. Positive skin tests were found in the eczema patients.

Some children have symptoms with a wide range of other foods. There may be an overlap between quick and late onset reactions. A group of children who react both quickly and slowly with a family history of atopy, peripheral eosinophilia, elevated serum IgE, and RASTs to specific foods have been described by Syme (32) with a remarkable response to oral disodium cromoglycate in some cases.

Such cases need to be clearly distinguished from eosinophilic gastroenteritis, a rare idiopathic disorder characterized by protein-losing enteropathy, peripheral eosinophilia, and iron deficiency anemia secondary to gastrointestinal blood loss. This condition must be distinguished from cow's milk-sensitive enteropathy, although it merges with other disorders such as the allergic gastroenteropathy (33). Some patients appear resistant to elimination diets and require treatment with corticosteroids, thus suggesting different pathogeneses.

Food-Sensitive Colitis

Rubin (34) described rectal loss of fresh blood which responded to cow's milk withdrawal. Gryboski (35) described eight children with cow's milk colitis diagnosed by response to cow's milk elimination. The main clinical features were explosive bloody diarrhea, shock, pallor, and colitis. The diagnosis was based upon evaluation of sigmoidoscopic appearances and rectal biopsy. No pathogens were isolated. The advent of safe colonoscopy and multiple mucosal biopsy even in early infancy has clearly established food-sensitive or allergic colitis as an important case of chronic bloody diarrhea in infancy (36). However, in my own referral practice, chronic inflammatory bowel disease is a more common problem (37,38). Colonoscopically, there is patchy erythema of the mucosa and petechiae and there may be aphthoid ulceration. Histopathologically, edema and infiltration with eosinophils have been reported (36) although others (39) describe a histopathological appearance not dissimilar to ulcerative colitis with an inflammatory infiltrate; however, both changes disappear on a cow's milk free-diet only to reoccur on early challenge. Similar appearances are seen in Crohn's disease, Behçet's disease, amebiasis, and chronic granulomatous disease. Even breast-fed infants whose mothers drink much cow's milk may develop cow's milk colitis (13). β-Lactoglobulin has been demonstrated in the breast milk of lactating mothers although the amounts are very small.

This disorder needs to be distinguished from ulcerative colitis and Crohn's colitis. However ulcerative colitis has been observed to remit in a group of five children when on a milk-free diet, all having both symptomatic and histological relapse after milk was reintroduced (40); such treatment is not curative. It has also been suggested that ulcerative proctitis may at times be caused by local IgE-mediated reaction to cow's milk protein (41). Thus, a response to cow's milk elimination may not accurately discriminate between these disorders and true cow's milk-sensitive colitis. The diagnosis rests upon endoscopy and the histopathology demonstrated by mucosal biopsy and the subsequent clinical course. In food-sensitive colitis, there may be a dense infiltration of eosinophils in the mucosa and the lesion resolves on food elimination *pari passu* with clinical remission.

There is an association with atopy, and serum IgE may be elevated in some cases. Olives et al. (42) have studied the relationship between cow's milk colitis and cow's milk-sensitive enteropathy. Twenty-nine children with cow's milk-sensitive enteropathy were studied. In only 7% was severe colitis observed both endoscopically and histologically, but in 86%, a microscopic colitis was demonstrated. However, it is clear that the large and small intestines are not always affected at the same time and the selectivity of organ damage remains unexplained.

In conclusion, it is now clearly established that a variety of foods, but particularly cow's milk, may be associated with food allergy causing structural and functional damage to the intestinal mucosa both large and small. Such disorders appear to be temporary and are a feature of early childhood.

REFERENCES

1. Ferguson A. Pathogenesis and mechanisms in the gastrointestinal tract. In: *Proceedings of the First Fisons Food Allergy Workshop,* 1980, pp. 28–38. Oxford: Medicine Publishing Foundation.
2. Bloch KJ, Bloch DB, Stearns M, Walker WA. Intestinal uptake of macromolecules. VI Uptake of protein antigen *in vivo* in normal rats and in rats injected with Nippostrongylus brasiliensis or subjected to mild systemic anaphylaxis. *Gastroenterology* 1979;77:1039.
3. Bellamy JEC, Nielsen NO. Immune-mediated emigration of neutrophils into the lumen of the small intestine. *Infect Immunol* 1974;9:615.
4. Accinni L, Brentjens JR, Albini EO, O'Connell DW, Pawlowski IB, Andres GA. Deposition of circulating antigen-antibody complex in the gastrointestinal tract of rabbits with chronic serum sickness. *Am J Dig Dis* 1978;23:1098.
5. MacDonald TT, Ferguson A. Hypersensitivity reactions in the small intestine. 2. Effects of allograft rejection on mucosal architecture and lymphoid cell infiltrate. *Gut* 1976;17:81.
6. MacDonald TT, Ferguson A. Hypersensitivity reactions in the small intestine. 3. The effects of allograft rejection and of graft-versus-host disease on epithelial cell kinetics. *Cell Tissue Kinet* 1977;10:301.
7. Ferguson A, MacDonald TT. Effects of local delayed hypersensitivity on the small intestine. In: *Immunology of the Gut (Ciba Foundation Symposium No. 46).* Amsterdam: Elsevier, North Holland, p. 305.
8. MacDonald TT, Spencer J. Evidence that activated mucosal T-Cells play a role in the pathogenesis of enteropathy in human small intestine. *J Exp Med* 1988;167:1341–9.
9. Spencer J, MacDonald TT, Finn T, Isaacson PE. The development of gut associated lymphoid tissue in the terminal ileum of fetal human intestine. *Clin Exp Immunol* 1986;64:536.
10. Hill DJ, Firer MA, Shelton MJ, Hosking CS. Manifestations of milk allergy in infancy: Clinical and immunologic findings. *J Pediatr* 1986;109:270–6.
11. Schlossman A. Ueber die giftwirkung des artfremden eiweisses in der milch auf den organismus des sauglings. *Arch Kinderheilk D* 1905;42:99–103.

12. Finkelstein H. Kuhmilch als ursache akuter ernahrungstorengen bei sauglingen. *Monatsschr Kinderheilk D* 1905;4:65–72.
13. Lake AM, Whittington BPF, Hamilton JR. Dietary protein induced colitis in breast-fed infants. *J Pediatr* 1982;101:906–10.
14. Ford RPK, Taylor B. Natural history of egg hypersensitivity: immediate and delayed onset clinical patterns. *Arch Dis Child* 1983;58:856–926.
15. Walker-Smith JA, Harrison M, Kilby A, Phillips AD, France NE. Cow's milk sensitive enteropathy. *Arch Dis Child* 1978;53:375–80.
16. Maluenda C, Phillips AD, Briddon A, Walker-Smith JA. Quantitative analysis of small intestinal mucosa in cow's milk sensitive enteropathy. *J Pediatr Gastroenterol Nutr* 1984;3:349–56.
17. Watt J, Lincott JR, Harries JT. Combined cow's milk protein and gluten-induced enteropathy: Common or rare? *Gut* 1983;24:165–70.
18. Manuel PD, Walker-Smith JA, France NE. Patchy enteropathy. *Gut* 1979;20:211.
19. Phillips AD, Rice SJ, France NE, Walker-Smith JA. Small intestinal lymphocyte levels in cow's milk protein intolerance. *Gut* 1979;20:509–12.
20. Variend S, Placzek M, Raafat F, Walker-Smith JA. Small intestinal mucosal fat in childhood enteropathies. *J Clin Pathol* 1984;37:373–7.
21. Walker-Smith JA. *Disease of the Small Intestine in Childhood.* London: Butterworths, 1988.
22. Harrison BM, Kilby A, Walker-Smith JA. Cow's milk protein intolerance: a possible association with gastroenteritis lactose intolerance and IgA deficiency. *Br Med J* 1976;1:1501–4.
23. Walker-Smith JA. Cow's milk intolerance as a cause of postenteritis diarrhoea. *J Pediatr Gastroenterol Nutr* 1982;1:163–75.
24. Manuel PD, Walker-Smith JA. A comparison of three infant feeding formulae for the prevention of delayed recovery after infantile gastroenteritis. *Acta Paediatr Belg* 1981;34:13–20.
25. Walker-Smith JA. Milk intolerance in children. *Clin Allergy* 1986;16:183–90.
26. Walker-Smith JA, Digeon B, Phillips AD. Evaluation of a casein and a whey hydrolysate for treatment of cow's milk sensitive enteropathy. *Eur J Pediatr* 1989 *(in press).*
27. Miller V, Macfarlane PI. Human breast milk in the management of protracted diarrhoea of infancy. In: Walker-Smith JA, McNeish AS, eds. *Diarrhoea and Malnutrition in Childhood,* Chapter 23. London: Butterworths, 1986;225–9.
28. Iyngkaran N, Yadav M, Looi LM. Effect of soy protein on the small bowel mucosa of young infants recovering from acute gastroenteritis. *J Pediatr Gastroenterol Nutr* 1988;7:68–75.
29. Perkkio M, Savilahti E, Kuitunen P. Morphometric and immunohistochemical study of jejunal biopsies from children with intestinal soy allergy. *Eur J Pediatr* 1981;137:63–9.
30. Iyngkaran N, Adidain Z, Meng LL, Yadav M. Egg-protein induced villous atrophy. *J Pediatr Gastroenterol Nutr* 1982;1:29–35.
31. Vitoria JC, Camarero·C, Sojo A. Enteropathy related to fish, rice and chicken. *Arch Dis Child* 1982;57:44–8.
32. Syme J. Investigation and treatment of multiple intestinal food allergy in childhood. In: Pepys J, Edwards AM, eds. *The Mast Cell: Its Role in Health and Disease.* Tunbridge Wells: Pitman Medical, 1979;438–42.
33. Katz AJ, Goldman H, Grand RJ. Gastric mucosal biopsy in eosinophilic (allergic) gastroenteritis. *Gastroenterology* 1977;73:705.
34. Rubin MI. Allergic intestinal bleeding in the newborn: a clinical syndrome. *Am J Med Sci* 1940;200:385–92.
35. Gryboski JD. Gastrointestinal milk allergy in infants. *Pediatrics* 1967;40:354–62.
36. Jenkins HR, Pincott JR, Soothill JF, Milla PJ. Cause of infantile colitis. *Arch Dis Child* 1984;59:326–9.
37. Chong SKF, Sanderson IR, Wright V, Walker-Smith JA. Food allergy in infantile colitis. *Arch Dis Child* 1984;59:690–1.
38. Walker-Smith JA. Prospective study of colitis in infancy in childhood. *J Pediatr Gastroenterol Nutr* 1986;5:352–8.
39. Gryboski J, Walker WA. *The Colon, Rectum and Anus in Gastrointestinal Problems in the Infant, 2nd edition.* Philadelphia: WB Saunders, 1953;524.
40. Wright R, Truelove SC. A controlled therapeutic trial of various diets in ulcerative colitis. *Br Med J* 1965;2:138–41.
41. Heatley RV. The gastrointestinal mast cell. *Scand J Gastroenterol* 1983;18:449–55.
42. Olives JP, LeTallec C, Bloom E, Agnese P, Familiades J, Ghisolfi J. Colitis and cow's milk protein sensitive enteropathy. *Pediatr Res* 1988 *(in press).*

Food Intolerance in Infancy: Allergology,
Immunology, and Gastroenterology, edited by
Robert N. Hamburger. Carnation Nutrition
Education Series, Vol. 1. The Carnation Co., Los
Angeles/Raven Press, Ltd., New York © 1989.

Cow Milk, Gastrointestinal Blood Loss, and Iron Nutritional Status of Infants

Ekhard E. Ziegler and Samuel J. Fomon

Department of Pediatrics, College of Medicine, University of Iowa, Iowa City, IA 52242

Gross melena or occult fecal blood loss is often present in patients with overt cow milk intolerance (1–5). However, a number of studies provide evidence that in infants and young children without signs of cow milk intolerance, the feeding of pasteurized cow milk is associated with development of iron deficiency. It has long been recognized that ingestion of large quantities of cow milk may result in extremely low intakes of other foods that contain more generous amounts of iron. In addition, there is considerable evidence that cow milk may induce gastrointestinal blood loss which may increase the requirement for absorbed iron, or even cause net loss of iron. A third possible contributor to development of iron deficiency in infants fed cow milk is that components of cow milk may inhibit iron absorption.

We shall review the literature on gastrointestinal blood loss and iron nutritional status of infants fed fresh cow milk in order to arrive at a recommendation concerning use of this food during infancy. As used here, cow milk refers to cow milk that has been pasteurized but not further heat-treated.

BLOOD LOSS BY ANEMIC INFANTS

That blood loss might be a contributing factor in iron deficiency anemia was recognized at least by the early 1960s (6,7). Wilson et al. (8–10), in a series of well-designed and executed studies, provided evidence that occult loss of blood is not uncommon in infants and small children with iron deficiency anemia, and demonstrated that the magnitude of the blood loss was sufficient to be of nutritional significance. In these studies, the investigators tagged the subjects' erythrocytes with ^{51}Cr and determined the extent of gastrointestinal blood loss from the radioactivity of the stools. Wilson et al. (10) presented clear evidence that in 17 of 34 anemic subjects, 6 to 25 months of age, blood loss occurred when cow milk was fed, and that blood loss was minimal when the infants were fed a soy flour-based formula or a milk-based formula. Mean gastrointestinal blood loss of the 17 subjects during intervals when they were fed fresh cow milk was 1.7 ml/day. When the subjects were fed infant formulas, mean blood loss was only 0.3 ml/day.

Assuming a mean hemoglobin concentration of 0.09 g/ml for these infants during the period of observation, blood loss of 1.7 ml would be equivalent to iron loss of 0.53 mg/day (1.7 ml/day $\times$ 0.09 hemoglobin/ml $\times$ 3.47 mg iron/g hemoglobin). The requirement for absorbed iron has been estimated to be 0.7 to 0.8 mg/day (11,12) (and our current estimate is even less). Therefore, a loss of 0.53 mg seems nutritionally highly significant.

Wilson et al. (10) systematically examined the effect of the quantity of cow milk ingested on the quantity of fecal blood loss in two children. In one child, daily intakes of 1,400, 1,500, 1,550, and 2,230 ml of milk were associated with losses of 4.0, 1.1, 4.7, and 9.3 ml of blood/day, respectively, whereas an intake of 300 ml of milk/day was accompanied by fecal loss of 1.2 ml of blood/day. In the other child, daily milk intakes of 930, 690, 990, and 497 ml were associated with fecal losses of 2.2, 0.2, 1.4, and 0.5 ml of blood/day. The data therefore suggest a dose-related response.

Elian et al. (13), using ^{51}Cr-labeled erythrocytes, demonstrated occult loss of blood by hospitalized infants, most of whom were anemic. Apparent blood loss averaged 0.59 ml/day by control infants and infants with acute infection not involving the gastrointestinal tract, and 1.85 ml/day by infants with acute gastroenteritis. The diets of these infants were not mentioned.

It is evident from the data reviewed so far that in anemic subjects gastrointestinal blood loss can be of sufficient magnitude to account for the development of the iron deficiency anemia. However, hypochromic anemia has been shown to be associated with decreased gastric acidity, impaired absorptive function, occult fecal blood loss, and histologic abnormalities of the gastrointestinal tract (14–16). Kimber and Weintraub (15) also demonstrated reduced intestinal absorption of iron by iron-deficient children. Treatment of the iron deficiency was in a number of cases associated with reversal of the functional and morphologic abnormalities of the gastrointestinal tract (14–16). Iron deficiency anemia per se has thus been alleged (14,17) to cause intestinal blood loss and to impair iron absorption in a self-perpetuating vicious circle. However, there is also considerable evidence that anemia or iron deficiency per se does not cause enteric bleeding (15,18). Therefore, observations in nonanemic infants are important for the understanding of the effect of cow milk on iron nutritional status.

BLOOD LOSS BY NONANEMIC INFANTS

The data of Wilson et al. (10) and the other reports we have mentioned thus far provide few clues about the relation of age to susceptibility to cow milk-provoked gastrointestinal blood loss. Neither do they provide information on gastrointestinal blood loss provoked by feeding cow milk to nonanemic infants. Initial information on the second of these points was provided by Woodruff et al. (18) as the result of a prospective study of normal infants. The infants were breast-fed or formula-fed to age 2 months and then fed whole cow milk (13 infants) or a noniron-fortified formula (25 infants). Presence of blood in the stools was detected by a guaiac test. The test was quite sensitive and a number of positive reactions were detected even in feces of fully breast-fed infants. Among formula-fed infants at 3, 6, 9, and 12 months of age, guaiac-positive stools were detected in 11 of 25, 13 of 25, 16 of 24, and 12 of 22 infants, respectively. Corresponding numbers for infants fed cow milk were 11 of 12, 9 of 13, 10 of 12, and 7 of 11. Thus, there was a greater percentage of guaiac-positive stools in infants fed whole cow milk than in infants fed formula, but it was not possible to judge the nutritional significance of the blood loss in either group. The study failed to provide evidence that younger infants are more susceptible than older infants to cow milk-provoked gastrointestinal blood loss.

A study somewhat similar to that of Woodruff et al. (18) was reported by Fomon et al. (19). Eighty-one normal infants were observed from 112 to 196 days of age in three feeding groups. One group was fed a low-iron milk-based formula, one group was fed homogenized whole cow milk heat-treated in the same manner as the infant formula, and one group was fed pasteurized, homogenized whole cow milk. All infants received a daily supplement providing 12 mg iron as ferrous sulfate. In most instances, a stool sample was collected each week and tested with the guaiac reaction. Figure 1 indicates the percent of subjects with guaiac-positive stools in each group at base line (112 days of age), from 119 to 140 days of age, from 147 to 168 days of age, and from 175 to 196 days of age. The number of infants with guaiac-positive stools and the total number of guaiac-positive stools during the first 28 days of the trial (i.e., from 119 to 140 days of age) were significantly ($p<0.01$ and <0.001, respectively) greater in the group fed whole cow milk than in the other groups. Differences in percent of subjects with guaiac-positive stools and in the total number of guaiac-positive stools in the three feeding groups were small and not statistically significant during the later periods. As is the case with the study reported by Woodruff et al. (18), the clinical significance of these observations is difficult to evaluate because guaiac tests do not yield quantitative data on blood loss.

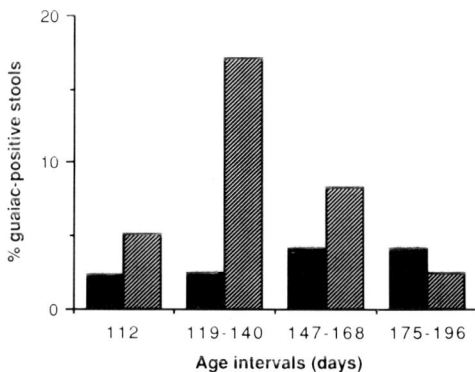

FIG. 1. Percent of stools with positive guaiac reaction of infants fed formula or heat-treated cow milk *(closed bars)* and of infants fed cow milk *(shaded bars)* after 112 days of age. (Data of Fomon et al., ref. 19.)

With the availability in recent years of more quantitative tests, it has become possible to determine the extent of blood loss. Thomas et al. (20) used an immunochemical method to detect fecal loss of hemoglobin in a study of 820 apparently healthy infants ranging from 2 weeks to 12 months of age: 354 breast-fed infants, 320 formula-fed infants (252 fed milk-based formulas and 68 fed isolated soy protein-based formulas), and 146 infants fed whole cow milk. The infants fed cow milk were more than 6 months of age. All infants were permitted to receive beikost. The fecal hemoglobin method was able to detect 1 mg of hemoglobin/g of wet feces. There was no difference in frequency of detectable fecal hemoglobin in the three groups: 7 of 338 stools of breast-fed infants, 6 of 314 stools of formula-fed infants, 4 of 140 stools of infants fed whole cow milk. In no instance was the concentration of hemoglobin >3 mg/g feces. Because the percentage of stools with more than 1 mg of hemoglobin/g of stool was low in each group, one can conclude that large losses of blood were uncommon. However, even a hemoglobin loss of <1 mg/g of stool may be nutritionally significant. If the wet weight of stool is 60 g/day, hemoglobin loss of 0.8 mg/g stool would represent an iron loss of 0.17 mg/day (0.8 mg hemoglobin/g stool × 60 g stool × 3.45 mg iron/g hemoglobin). With an estimated requirement for absorbed iron that is <0.7 mg/day, a loss of 0.17 mg of iron/day appears to be nutritionally significant.

In a study of normal infants fed either cow milk or a milk-based formula (Ziegler et al., *manuscript in preparation*), we have used a sensitive and specific method (21) for the quantitative determination of fecal loss of hemoglobin. With this method, it is possible to detect 0.01 mg hemoglobin/g wet feces. From 168 through 252 days of age, 26 infants were fed cow milk and 26 infants were fed a low-iron milk-based formula. Selected other foods low in iron content were permitted and we provided one jar per day of a specially prepared cereal-fruit combination providing 3.65 mg of iron in the form of ferrous sulfate. Before entering the trial, all infants had been fed a milk-based formula with 12 mg iron/liter for 28 days or more. Thirty-one infants had earlier been breast-fed, whereas 21 infants had never been breast-fed. Stool samples were collected before the start of the trial (i.e., at 140, 166, 167, and 168 days of age) and weekly during the trial for determination of hemoglobin concentration. In addition, stools were tested for occult blood with the guaiac reaction (Hemoccult, SmithKline Diagnostics, Inc., Sunnyvale, CA). Venous blood was obtained in most cases at 140 days of age and during the trial at 168, 196, 224, and 252 days of age for determination of hematocrit, hemoglobin concentration, erythrocyte protoporphyrin, serum iron, and ferritin.

Figure 2 indicates that the percent of guaiac-positive stools was significantly ($p<0.01$) greater in the group fed cow milk than in the group fed formula during the first 28 days of the trial (i.e., from 175 to 196 days of age). Differences in the percent guaiac-positive stools were smaller and not statistically significant during the two subsequent 28-day periods. Results of quantitative determinations of fecal hemoglobin are indicated in Fig. 3. It is evident that the group fed cow milk had much higher fecal hemoglobin losses than the group fed formula. The difference was statistically significant in each of the 28-day periods. Closer inspection of the data revealed that six infants fed cow milk showed no appreciable increase in fecal

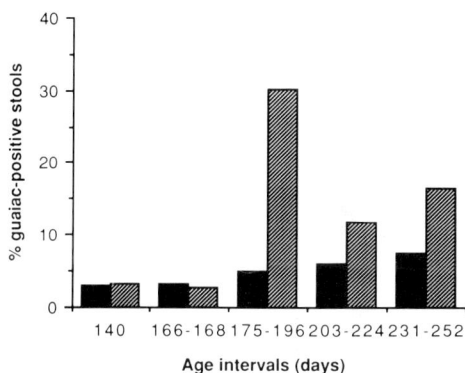

FIG. 2. Percent of stools with positive guaiac reaction of infants fed formula *(closed bars)* and of infants fed cow milk *(shaded bars)* after 168 days of age.

hemoglobin loss (nonresponders). Responses of the other 20 (responders) infants were highly variable, with the majority of infants showing increased hemoglobin loss even in the first stool sample obtained after starting on cow milk (i.e., at 175 days of age). In many infants fecal hemoglobin loss declined later, but a few infants had sustained high hemoglobin losses. In some infants, fecal hemoglobin loss did not increase until several weeks after initiation of cow milk feeding. Mean fecal hemoglobin of the 20 responders was 4,773 µg/g dry stool during the period 175 to 196 days of age.

Assuming a wet stool weight of 60 g/day with 20% dry solids, a fecal hemoglobin concentration of 4,773 µg/g dry stool represents an iron loss of 0.20 mg/day, a quantity we consider nutritionally significant.

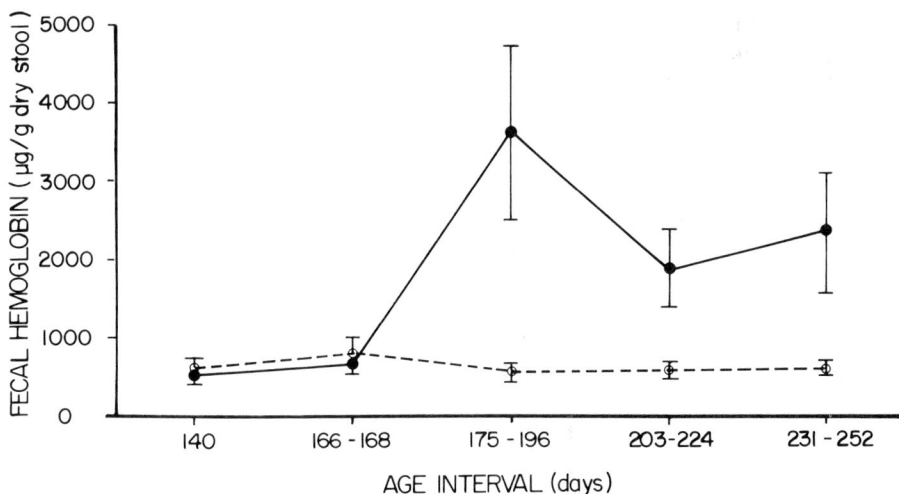

FIG. 3. Fecal hemoglobin concentration of infants fed formula *(open circles)* and of infants fed cow milk *(closed circles)* after 168 days of age. Bars indicate SE.

IRON NUTRITIONAL STATUS

When infants are fed cow milk, gastrointestinal blood loss is not necessarily the most important factor responsible for poor iron nutritional status. In the past, many pediatricians and hematologists believed that the major cause of development of poor iron nutritional status was the displacement by cow milk of other foods that were better sources of iron (17). The relative importance of this factor remains undetermined.

Less attention appears to have been paid to the possibility that components of cow milk may inhibit iron absorption and, in a way, contribute to the development of iron deficiency. Inhibition of iron absorption by dietary calcium and phosphorus has been demonstrated (22), and it seems possible that the relatively high intakes of calcium and phosphorus provided by cow milk might interfere with iron absorption.

Results of a study by Gross (23) are consistent with this possibility. In a study of the effect of feeding iron-fortified and noniron-fortified formulas on iron nutritional status, Gross (23) included 73 infants fed two milk-based formulas not fortified with iron. One formula provided 15 g protein, 650 mg calcium, and 500 mg phosphorus/liter. The other provided 24 g protein, 850 mg calcium, and 700 mg phosphorus/liter. The infants were enrolled at birth and followed until 18 months of age. Between 4 and 12 months of age, hemoglobin concentration, hematocrit, and serum iron concentration were generally less, and total iron-binding capacity was generally greater in the group fed the higher protein formula. Guaiac tests of the stools were consistently negative in both groups. Although it is possible that dietary intakes of iron were more satisfactory by infants fed the lower protein formula, there is no evidence that this was the case, and the possibility must be entertained that the formula with the higher protein and mineral concentrations somehow exerted an adverse effect on iron nutritional status.

The study by Gross (23) is of particular interest because it concerns comparison of two formulas that received the same heat treatment. The study by Fomon et al. (19) also included a comparison of infants fed formula and cow milk heat-treated in the same manner. Although no difference in iron nutritional status was detected between the various feeding groups (pasteurized cow milk, more extensively heat-treated cow milk, and formula), intakes of iron were generous and the period of observation was short.

Several other studies have compared iron nutritional status of infants receiving similar intakes of iron from diets that included either cow milk or a milk-based formula. Results of these studies do not permit evaluation of the relative importance of gastrointestinal blood loss and interference with iron absorption.

Smith and Hunter (24) studied 21 to 24 infants in each of three groups: one fed a commercially available iron-fortified milk-based formula (protein concentration 17 g/liter), one fed the same formula unfortified with iron, and one fed whole cow milk. The infants were observed from birth until 18 months of age. Comparison of results of feeding the noniron-fortified formula and whole cow milk is relevant to the present discussion. Iron intakes, as determined by 24-hr recall at intervals, were similar for the two groups. Anemia, defined as hemoglobin concentration <11 g/dl on two or more occasions at 6 months of age or older, occurred in 28% of infants fed the noniron-fortified formula and in 59% of infants fed whole cow milk. Between 6 and 18 months of age, percent saturation of transferrin of infants fed whole cow milk was less than that of infants fed the formula, but it is not stated whether the difference was statistically significant.

In addition to the investigation of gastrointestinal blood loss mentioned previously, Woodruff et al. (18) determined iron nutritional status of the infants enrolled in their study. Intakes of iron were similar by the infants fed the noniron-fortified formula and those fed cow milk. Blood samples were obtained at 3, 6, 9, and 12 months of age. In the group fed whole cow milk, hemoglobin concentration was significantly less at ages 9 and 12 months, and mean corpuscular volume and percent saturation of transferrin were significantly less at 6 and 9 months of age.

In our recent study (Ziegler et al., *manuscript in preparation*), indices of iron nutritional status did not differ between the group fed cow milk and the group fed formula. As indicated in Table 1, hematocrit and concentrations of hemoglobin, erythrocyte protoporphyrin, serum iron, and ferritin provided no evidence for deterioration of iron nutritional status among infants fed cow milk. There was also no difference in iron nutritional status between responders and nonresponders in the group fed cow milk. However, one infant with high fecal blood loss developed clear evidence of iron deficiency within 4 weeks after cow milk was introduced into the diet.

Three groups of preterm infants were studied by Halliday et al. (25). Mean birth weights of the groups ranged from 1,740 to 2,080 g. Whole cow milk was introduced into the diet at 40 weeks of age or less in Group 1 (14 infants), at 24 to 36 weeks of age in Group 2 (17 infants), and before 24 weeks in Group 3 (12 infants). At 54 weeks of age, iron intakes were estimated to be 2.15, 1.5, and 2.0 mg/kg per day, respectively. Mean hemoglobin concentration was 12.8 in Group 1, 11.8 in Group 2, and 11.7 in Group 3. The difference between Group 1 and Group 3 was statistically significant. Median transferrin saturations were not significantly different: 23, 20, and 14.5%, respectively. Median serum ferritin concentrations were 30.5, 21, and 11 ng/ml, the value for Group 3 being significantly different from that of Group 1.

In conclusion, the literature and our own studies provide convincing evidence that consumption of cow milk leads to increased gastrointestinal blood loss in the majority of normal, nonanemic infants. The data do not permit the conclusion that the response diminishes with increasing age during the 1st year of life, although the severity of the blood loss diminishes in most infants with the duration of feeding cow milk. A minority of infants experience quite a large blood loss, but the data are insufficient to estimate the prevalence of this phenomenon.

In our studies, few adverse effects on iron nutritional status have been evident, presumably because of the relatively short exposure to cow milk (i.e., 3 months). Studies with longer periods of cow milk feeding have generally demonstrated impaired iron nutritional status. Thus, there can be little question that the feeding of

TABLE 1. Indices of iron nutritional status

		Age (days)									
		140		168		196		224		252	
		Mean	SD	Mean	SD	Mean	SD	Mean	SD	Mean	SD
Hemoglobin (g/dl)	Cow milk	11.8	1.1	11.8	0.9	11.7	0.9	11.8	1.0	12.0	0.9
	Formula	11.9	1.0	12.1	1.1	11.8	1.0	11.9	1.0	12.1	0.6
Hematocrit (%)	Cow milk	35.2	2.6	35.4	2.9	35.9	2.2	36.1	2.5	36.4	2.7
	Formula	35.3	2.1	35.4	1.7	35.4	2.0	35.6	1.8	36.2	1.7
Serum iron (μg/dl)	Cow milk	46.1	17.8	55.8	21.4	47.9	16.7	41.1	14.5	49.5	25.1
	Formula	45.2	14.6	55.5	18.5	48.9	13.8	48.5	20.3	52.3	25.1
Ferritin (ng/ml)	Cow milk	64.9	51.0	36.4	34.8	33.7	32.1	20.9	11.9	25.1	13.6
	Formula	64.3	48.0	52.8	31.4	42.4	39.2	28.0	19.7	19.6	11.7
FEP[a] (μg/dl)	Cow milk	59.7	22.0	49.4	19.9	77.6	53.2	64.7	25.4	70.8	19.0
	Formula	89.2	31.4	63.2	20.5	67.4	15.0	58.9	15.4	60.2	17.0

[a]FEP, free erythrocyte protoporphyrin.

cow milk to infants and young children for a prolonged period is likely to lead to poor iron nutritional status and, in some infants, to frank iron deficiency. The relative importance of gastrointestinal blood loss, displacement by cow milk of more iron-rich foods, and inhibition of iron absorption remains to be determined. We conclude that cow milk is an unsuitable food during the 1st year of life.

ACKNOWLEDGMENTS

This work was partially supported by grant HD07578 of the United States Public Health Service, and by grants of Ross Laboratories of Columbus, Ohio; Mead Johnson Nutritional Division of Evansville, Indiana; and National Dairy Council of Rosemont, Illinois.

REFERENCES

1. Kravis LP, Donsky G, Lecks HI. Upper and lower gastrointestinal tract bleeding induced by whole cow's milk in an atopic infant. Experience and reason briefly recorded. *Pediatrics* 1967;40:661–5.
2. Gryboski JD. Gastrointestinal milk allergy in infants. *Pediatrics* 1967;40:354–62.
3. Kokkonen J, Similä S, Herva R. Impaired gastric function in children with cow's milk intolerance. *Eur J Pediatr* 1979;132:1–6.
4. Kokkonen J, Similä S. Cow's milk intolerance with melena. *Eur J Pediatr* 1980;35:189–94.
5. Coello-Ramirez P, Larrosa-Haro A. Gastrointestinal occult hemorrhage and gastroduodenitis in cow's milk protein intolerance. *J Pediatr Gastroenterol Nutr* 1984;3:215–8.
6. Rasch CA, Cotton EK, Harris JW, Griggs RC. Blood loss as a contributing factor in the etiology of iron-lack anemia of infancy. *Am J Dis Child* 1960;100:627 (Abstr).
7. Hoag MS, Wallerstein RO, Pollycove M. Occult blood loss in iron deficiency anemia of infancy. *Pediatrics* 1961;27:199–203.
8. Wilson JF, Heiner DC, Lahey ME. Studies on iron metabolism. Evidence of gastrointestinal dysfunction in infants with iron deficiency anemia: a preliminary report. *J Pediatr* 1962;60:787–800.
9. Wilson JF, Heiner DC, Lahey ME. Milk-induced gastrointestinal bleeding in infants with hypochromic microcytic anemia. *JAMA* 1964;189:122–6.
10. Wilson JF, Lahey ME, Heiner DC. Studies on iron metabolism. *J Pediatr* 1974;84:335–44.
11. Fomon SJ. *Infant Nutrition*. Philadelphia: WB Saunders Company, 1974.
12. Stekel A. Iron requirements in infancy and childhood. In: Stekel A, ed. *Iron Nutrition in Infancy and Childhood*. New York: Raven Press, 1984;1–10.
13. Elian E, Bar-Shani S, Liberman A, Matoth Y. Intestinal blood loss: A factor in calculations of body iron in late infancy. *J Pediatr* 1966;69:215–9.
14. Naiman JL, Oski FA, Diamond LK, Vawter GF, Shwachman H. The gastrointestinal effects of iron-deficiency anemia. *Pediatrics* 1964;33:83–99.
15. Kimber C, Weintraub LR. Malabsorption of iron secondary to iron deficiency. *N. Engl J Med* 1968;279:453–9.
16. Ghosh S, Daga S, Kasthuri D, Misra RC, Chuttani HK. Gastrointestinal function in iron deficiency states in children. *Am J Dis Child* 1972;123:14–7.
17. Diamond LK, Naiman JL. Letters to the editor. More on iron deficiency anemia. *J Pediatr* 1967;70:304–5.
18. Woodruff CW, Wright SW, Wright RP. The role of fresh cow's milk in iron deficiency. *Am J Dis Child* 1972;124:26–30.
19. Fomon SJ, Ziegler EE, Nelson SE, Edwards BB. Cow milk feeding in infancy: Gastrointestinal blood loss and iron nutritional status. *J Pediatr* 1981;98:540–5.
20. Thomas DW, McGilligan KM, Carlson M, Azen SP, Eisenberg LD, Lieberman HM, Rissman EM. Fecal α1-antitrypsin and hemoglobin excretion in healthy human milk-, formula-, or cow's milk-fed infants. *Pediatrics* 1986;78:305–12.

21. Schwartz S, Dahl J, Ellefson M, Ahlquist D. The "HemoQuant Test: A specific and quantitative determination of heme (hemoglobin) in feces and other materials. *Clin Chem* 1983;29:2061–7.
22. Monson ER, Cook JD. Food iron absorption in human subjects. The effects of calcium and phosphate salts on the absorption of nonheme iron. *Am J Clin Nutr* 1976;29:1142–8.
23. Gross MA. The relationship between milk protein and iron content on hematologic values in infancy. *J Pediatr* 1968;73:521–30.
24. Smith NJ, Hunter RE. Iron requirements during growth. In: Hallberg L, Harwerth H-G, Vannotti A, eds. *Iron Deficiency*. London, New York: Academic Press, 1970; 199–211.
25. Halliday HL, Lappin TRJ, McClure G. Cow's milk and anaemia in preterm infants. *Arch Dis Child* 1985;60:69–70.

*Food Intolerance in Infancy: Allergology,
Immunology, and Gastroenterology,* edited by
Robert N. Hamburger. Carnation Nutrition
Education Series, Vol. 1. The Carnation Co., Los
Angeles/Raven Press, Ltd., New York © 1989.

Skin Manifestations of Food Allergy

David J. Atherton

Pediatric Dermatology, The Hospital for Sick Children, London, United Kingdom

The skin appears to be a particularly frequent site for allergic reactions to foods. These reactions may follow ingestion, but in other cases, they may follow direct skin contact with the provocative food.

Like allergic diseases in other organs, allergic cutaneous reactions to foods are of two broad types: firstly, reactions of rapid onset after exposure and, secondly, reactions of slow onset. Rapid-onset reactions include contact urticaria and acute generalized urticaria. Slow-onset reactions include contact dermatitis and atopic eczema. However, it is frequent, perhaps even characteristic, for individual patients to be subject to combinations of these reactions, so that they tend not to be so well defined in clinical practice.

The skin is perhaps the most common organ to reveal symptomatic allergic reactions to foods. Some of these reactions follow oral ingestion of foods, but not uncommonly, foods may provoke reactions following direct skin contact. When these reactions are obviously provoked by food, the patient simply avoids the causative item and only rarely will seek medical advice. Therefore, this type of reaction, in which the causative link between food and an adverse cutaneous response is obvious to the patient, is probably more common than is generally recognized.

There are other cutaneous allergic reactions to foods in which the causative link is much less apparent, either to patient or to doctor. Thus, there may be disagreement as to the existence or relative importance of such a causative link, and, on occasions, this disagreement may be heated.

I find it helpful to divide food-allergic skin disease into two categories: (a) rapid-onset reactions, that is those in which the clinical reaction occurs very soon after appropriate exposure to the causative food, and in which the causative role of the food is usually obvious, and (b) slow-onset reactions, that is, those in which the clinical reaction develops more insidiously, and in which the causative role of food may be more or less concealed. In the first category, I shall consider contact urticaria, generalized acute urticaria, and protein contact dermatitis; in the second, contact dermatitis and atopic eczema.

RAPID-ONSET REACTIONS

Contact Urticaria

Allergic contact urticaria is arguably the purest of all type I hypersensitivity reactions. Direct skin contact with the relevant antigen provokes erythema and/or wealing within minutes, and may last for a period up to a few hours. Occasionally, contact urticaria may be accompanied by noncutaneous allergic reactions, such as bronchoconstriction and even by anaphylaxis (1). Contact urticaria may occur on previously normal skin, but it is probably more often elicited on damaged (e.g., eczematous) skin, and it may be a mechanism that is responsible for the chronicity of eczema in some individuals, such as caterers (2).

Food and food additives are among the most important causes of allergic contact urticaria, but other causes include insects and mites, animal saliva, dander and hair, cosmetics, plants, medicaments (particularly antibiotics), epoxy resin, and nickel (3).

Allergic contact urticaria may be particularly common in individuals with atopic eczema. When parents describe the appearance or worsening of skin lesions immediately after their eczematous child has eaten, they are usually describing contact urticaria to food antigens. A failure to be aware of allergic contact urticaria is probably the reason for medical skepticism of parental descriptions of skin reactions induced by foods in their eczematous children.

Nonallergic contact urticaria to food components is probably rather uncommon, but has been recorded with benzoic and sorbic acids, both of which are used as preservatives in foods, although such a reaction is probably more often seen following the application of topical medications containing them (4).

Generalized Acute Urticaria

Generalized urticaria (hives) is a pattern of skin reaction characterized by the development of itchy weals and/or lightly erythematous papules, that tend to become annular as they expand. Individual lesions are generally transient, lasting less than 24 hr, although crops of new lesions frequently occur side by side with resolving lesions. Angioedema is a term used to describe analogous lesions occurring deeper in the dermis and in subcutaneous tissue, taking the appearance of more diffuse cutaneous swelling, particularly in areas where the skin is looser, e.g., the periorbital area. Urticaria and angioedema may occur separately or together, and may occasionally be associated with systemic symptoms, either caused by visceral angioedema or to the distant effects of mediator release. They are also prominent and early manifestations of anaphylactic reactions.

Generalized urticaria is a very common problem, probably affecting 20% or more of the population at some time in their lives. It may occur as a single attack lasting up to a few days (acute urticaria), or it may take a more prolonged form, with lesions occurring for many weeks (chronic urticaria). Problems in distinguishing these two are: (a) the acute form is not infrequently recurrent, and (b) periods of remission may occur in the chronic form. In practice, the distinction between the two polar types is blurred, and it can be difficult to decide whether the patient has recurrent acute urticaria, or intermittent chronic urticaria. The point of attempting the distinction nevertheless is that the acute variety tends to have obvious allergic precipitating factors, whereas the chronic variety does not, suggesting that the two are pathogenetically distinct. This impression is strengthened by the association of the acute variety with atopic disease, in contrast to the absence of such an association in the chronic variety (5,6).

Although acute generalized urticaria is probably the most common of all types of urticaria, relatively few affected patients ever seek medical advice. This is likely to reflect the ease with which the patient can usually identify the provocative factor, whose avoidance relieves the problem. Classical type I hypersensitivity is the likely mechanism for the majority of such reactions, but other mechanisms can probably produce an almost indistinguishable clinical picture. For example, it is known that a variety of substances of relatively simple chemical structure can liberate histamine directly from mast cells (7), and it seems likely that many of the food additives that can provoke urticaria do so by nonimmunological means.

Foods and drugs are the agents that have been most frequently demonstrated as causes of acute generalized urticaria. Among the foods, those most commonly implicated include nuts, eggs, fish, shellfish, cow's milk, and tomatoes (8). More serious attacks associated with visceral angioedema and occasionally with anaphylaxis have been reported after the ingestion of nuts, fish, and shellfish, more rarely other foods including eggs and celery (5). Interestingly, anaphylactic reactions have also occurred with sunflower seeds (9) and chamomile tea (10), both of which are biologically related to ragweed. There is considerable suspicion that much food allergy reflects cross-reactivity between inhalant and food antigens. Perhaps the best established example is the cross-reactivity between birch pollen and apple (11,12).

Some urticarial reactions to foods reflect sensitization to traces of other antigens contained within the food: predominant among these is penicillin in milk (13).

Some foods appear likely to provoke acute urticarial reactions by direct histamine release rather than by specific immunological mechanisms. Lobsters, crayfish, mussels, egg white, and strawberries have been implicated in this type of reaction (14).

Food additives and preservatives have also attracted great interest as provocative factors in urticarial and other allergic reactions. Sulfites and metabisulfites used as antioxidants have been documented as causes of acute urticarial and anaphylactic reactions (15); these are probably able to do so by virtue of being antigenic. Additives such as azodyes and benzoate preservatives appear to be able to aggravate or provoke generalized urticaria (16), but the mechanism by which they do so is not likely to be an immunological one.

Protein Contact Dermatitis

Hand eczema occurs as an occupational hazard among caterers, many of whom describe the onset of pruritus soon after direct skin contact with particular foods.

Such individuals often fail to demonstrate classical 48-hr closed epicutaneous patch test reactions to the relevant foods, but they may instead demonstrate positive immediate-type reactions on intracutaneous or intradermal testing with the same foods (2,17), and some demonstrate contact urticarial reactions within minutes of the epicutaneous application of the same foods. These are usually patients with a personal history of atopic disorders (2). In some cases, epicutaneous application of the food to normal skin has caused no reaction, whereas an urticarial response has occurred if the food was applied to skin that was slightly eczematous (17,18). This difference presumably reflects greater antigen penetration through damaged epidermis.

A proportion of patients of this type have been shown to develop a vesicular reaction within approximately 20 min of the relevant food being applied directly to slightly eczematous skin (17). In such cases, biopsies taken at 30 min have shown the histological features compatible with an acute eczema (19). The pathogenetic significance of this reaction, which has been termed protein contact dermatitis, is unclear. However, overall, the implication of these findings is that immediate hypersensitivity reactions occurring at the site of food contact may lead to the maintenance of an eczematous reaction at the same site, but it must remain an unanswered question whether they could ever be responsible for its initial development. Perhaps the most plausible sequence of events is that these patients start off either with atopic eczema or with an irritant contact dermatitis, which is common in caterers (2), or with both. The damaged skin allows the penetration of food antigens to which the patient is already sensitized, or to which the patient thereby becomes sensitized, and an urticarial response is added to the eczema. Whether this can cause direct aggravation of the eczema is not established, but it will, at the very least, provoke unpleasant pruritus and increased excoriation. Studies with antigens applied directly to the skin of eczematous atopics certainly suggest that eczema itself can be provoked on currently unaffected skin in this way (20,21).

SLOW-ONSET REACTIONS

Contact Dermatitis

Classical delayed hypersensitivity contact dermatitis is a well-recognized occurrence in those who handle food professionally. One of the most common, and perhaps the best characterized example, is that of garlic contact dermatitis (2,17). The responsible allergen has been identified as diallyldisulfide (22), which, in common with most of allergens responsible for contact dermatitis, is a hapten. However, a very wide variety of other foods have been incriminated as causes of allergic contact dermatitis, and have been reported to have provoked positive 48-hr eczematous responses in classical epicutaneous closed patch tests (2,17,23). There are, however, considerable problems in the interpretation of such tests as raw foods are often able to provoke irritant reactions.

Atopic Eczema

Atopic eczema (atopic dermatitis) is principally a disorder of children and is now very common in developed countries, affecting as many as 15% of all children at some time in their lives. It is a rather persistent condition, with alternating periods of improvement and deterioration, but with an overall tendency to spontaneous resolution in the longer term. The etiology of the disease has not been established, but for many years, a more or less important role for foods has been suspected.

Children with atopic eczema have a high frequency of positive immediate skin-test reactions to foods (24), and high levels of circulating food-specific immunoglobulin E (IgE), as measured by the radioallergosorbent test (25). They commonly experience food-induced hypersensitivity reactions of rapid onset, both cutaneous (e.g., contact urticaria and acute generalized urticaria) and noncutaneous (e.g., vomiting). Double-blind, placebo-controlled food challenges have been used to demonstrate the frequency of these rapid-onset reactions to foods (26), their association with a concurrent rise in plasma histamine (27), and their close correlation with positive skin prick tests and circulating IgE antibody measurements (28).

When parents describe the appearance or worsening of skin lesions immediately after their eczematous child has eaten, they are usually describing contact urticaria to food antigens. A failure to be aware of contact urticaria is probably the main reason for medical skepticism of parental descriptions of skin reactions induced by foods in their eczematous children.

Children who experience contact urticaria, or other reactions of rapid onset induced by foods, should clearly avoid exposure to the causative items. However, the occurrence of such reactions does not establish a role for foods in the etiology of atopic eczema itself, although, as discussed previously in this article, it is possible that an eczematous reaction may follow contact urticaria locally. Thus, in some cases of atopic eczema, at least the eczema at sites exposed to contact with food may reflect such a sequence. However, this is extremely unlikely to explain the existence of eczema at sites not exposed to contact with foods, and it seems improbable that atopic eczema could be initiated in this way, not least because of the difficulty experienced by protein antigens in penetrating intact, noneczematous skin (18).

A number of authors have reported the successful dietary treatment of atopic eczema. The majority of these reports have described open studies of empirically selected elimination diets (reviewed in ref. 29). Unfortunately, the results obtained in such studies are likely to be highly subjective, and convincing demonstration of benefit from elimination diets requires placebo-controlled studies. Sadly, data are only available from two such studies.

The first study was that from our group (30). The trial diet comprised complete egg and milk avoidance, with the administration of soya formula as a milk substitute. The control diet comprised identical egg and milk avoidance, but each day the children were given a combination of dried egg and cow's milk in place of the soya formula. A double-blind, crossover design was used. Over half the children showed clear preference for genuine egg and milk exclusion. Of interest in our study was the finding that many children benefited from egg and milk avoidance in the absence of any previous parental suspicion that these foods could aggravate their children's eczema. Neither was there any association between response to diet and the presence or absence of positive immediate skin tests, or raised levels of IgE antibodies to egg or milk antigens (31).

The second controlled study (32) employed a similar experimental design, but included both adults and children. This showed a smaller overall response rate of 25%, although examination of the data shows that this reached 35% if only those under the age of 8 years were considered. This somewhat less striking response may reflect the increased exposure of babies to soya in recent years, which now makes it a less satisfactory milk substitute. However, a more important reason for the smaller proportion of responders in this study may relate to the fact that, today, few children attend a dermatology clinic whose parents have not already attempted unsupervised dietary therapy. Children responding to such manipulations are less likely to be referred, so that those now seen in the hospital setting will, to a degree, be selected for their unlikeliness to benefit from a simple elimination diet.

Others have addressed the possible provocative role of a wider variety of foods. For example, Hill and Lynch (33) used an elemental diet in an open, uncontrolled trial in 10 children with severe atopic eczema, and reported that 8 were substantially benefited, with the relapse on discontinuation of the diet. Hathaway and Warner (34) reported their experience in a group of 40 diet-responsive eczematous children. Those not helped by simple empirical diets have been given increasing restrictive diets until improvement occurred. Of the 40 children, 7 had responded to egg and milk exclusion alone, 30 responded to more restricted diets, and 3 improved only when placed on an elemental feed. An attempt was then made to identify the provocative foods, checked by double-blind challenges. In addition to milk and egg, frequently implicated foods included citrus fruits, colorings and preservatives, nuts, fish, wheat, tomatoes, lamb, chicken, and soya, demonstrating that unresponsiveness to a simple diet does not necessarily exclude a provocative role for foods in the individual case.

The evidence from the literature and our own experience suggest that a proportion of children with atopic eczema will show benefit from dietary elimination of selected foods. Several foods may need to be excluded, and currently available tests will not reliably identify these. The proportion of children likely to benefit is probably not less than 20% and not greater than 50%. Whether this response rate could be improved by the development of more accurate methods for the identification of provocative foods is an important but unanswered question. It is also unclear for how long the benefit of dietary modification is maintained. Our practice is to consider a trial of a simple, empirical exclusion diet in any children below the age of 8 years in which adequate topical treatment has provided insufficient benefit (35).

There is some evidence that the entry of intact food antigen after a meal is greater in those with atopic eczema than in normal individuals (36,37). This may reflect sensitization to food antigens, which has been shown to enhance their gastrointestinal absorption both in an antigen-specific (38) and in an antigen nonspecific way

(39,40). Furthermore, minor morphological abnormalities of the gastrointestinal tract have been demonstrated in some children with atopic eczema (41,42), which could be the effect of local hypersensitivity reactions. Indirect evidence for mucosal damage comes from the findings of increased gastrointestinal permeability to inert molecules such as lactulose, which are not normally absorbed in significant amounts from the gut lumen (43). There is some evidence that food antigens are handled differently in patients with atopic eczema once they have gained entry to the circulation. The formation of circulating IgA antibody-antigen complexes has been shown to occur in normal subjects after food administration (44,45); this is presumed to be a part of the normal mechanism for safe disposal of such antigens, and it takes place without the development of symptoms. However, under the same conditions, patients with atopic eczema characteristically also form complexes that contain IgG and IgM, and complexes that bind C1q (44). These complexes have been shown to contain food antigen (45). Prominent histological changes have been reported in the vessel walls of the superficial dermal venular plexus which include edema, endothelial cell hypertrophy, basement membrane thickening and reduplication, and pericyte hypertrophy (46). These changes reflect vessel damage compatible with the effects of antigen-antibody complex deposition. It is feasible that such deposition initiates a sequence of pathological events in the skin that result in the development of the typical lesions of atopic eczema (35). The precise cutaneous localization of such deposition might be determined by histamine release from cutaneous mast cells. This could occur as a sequel to antigen penetration from the skin surface. A very intriguing possibility is that scratching of the skin could itself induce mast cell degranulation, perhaps through the mediation of surface-bound IgE antibodies to tissue antigens that are released as a direct physical effect of excoriation. Some evidence for the existence of such antigens is provided by studies on dermographism (47).

On balance, the available evidence suggests that foods do play a role in the etiology of atopic eczema, but the relative importance of this role remains unclear. It may be that the role for foods is more connected with the initiation of the disease than with its long-term maintenance. Foods other than human milk provide the infant with its greatest antigenic challenge, and it may be no coincidence that approximately 75% of all those who will develop atopic eczema do so during the first 6 months of life. Some indirect support for this view is provided (a) by the finding that skin test reactivity to foods is particularly prominent in young children with atopic eczema, becoming less marked as the child grows (48), and (b) by the decreasing likelihood of a therapeutic response to simple exclusion diets as children grow older.

In conclusion, I have suggested that food allergic reactions in the skin can be broadly subdivided into those of rapid onset, in which symptoms occur within minutes of food exposure and are rather obviously linked etiologically to that exposure, and those of slow onset, where symptoms may not occur for hours, even days, after exposure, and where the causative link with the provocative food is more difficult, sometimes may be even impossible, to identify. Doctors see patients with both types of reaction. We see those with rapid-onset reactions when these are so severe that the patient is anxious that he may die, or when they occur in association with other compliants; they are, for example, common in children with atopic eczema. When rapid-onset reactions are mild and isolated, the patient does not bother to seek medical advice because it is so clear that appropriate treatment is avoidance. Paradoxically, the rarity with which these patients are seen by doctors has led to skepticism in the profession that such reactions occur very often, or at all.

A variety of pathological mechanisms may be involved in each type of reaction. Rapid-onset reactions probably all reflect mast cell degranulation, but there appear to be several routes, both immunological and nonimmunological, by which this common endpoint can be reached. The little known, but possibly clinically important, vesicular reaction known as protein contact dermatitis perhaps fits least happily into this category, and its pathogenesis may be completely different, perhaps involving antibody-dependent cellular cytotoxicity. Slow-onset reactions are perhaps even more likely than rapid-onset reactions to involve diverse pathogenetic mechanisms. Furthermore, not infrequently, there appear to be interactions between rapid- and slow-onset reactions, and the former may play a role in the sequence of pathogenetic events leading to the latter, as in the case of contact urticaria and atopic eczema.

REFERENCES

1. van Krogh G, Maibach HI. The contact urticaria syndrome: an update review. *J Am Acad Dermatol* 1981;5:328–42.
2. Cronin E. Dermatitis of the hands in caterers. *Contact Dermatitis* 1987;17:265–9.
3. Lahti A, von Krogh G, Maibach HI. Contact urticaria syndrome. In: Stone J, ed. *Dermatologic Immunology and Allergy.* St. Louis: CV Mosby, 1985;379–90.
4. Lahti M. Non-immunologic contact urticaria. *Acta Derm Venereol* [Suppl] *(Stockh)* 1980;60:91.
5. Golbert TM, Patterson R, Pruzansky JJ. Systemic allergic reactions to ingested antigens. *J Allergy* 1969;44:96–107.
6. Champion RH, Roberts SOB, Carpenter RG, Roger JH. Urticaria and angio-oedema: a review of 554 patients. *Br J Dermatol* 1969;81:588–97.
7. Paton WDM. Histamine release by compounds of simple chemical structure. *Pharmacol Rev* 1957;9:269–328.
8. Warin RP, Champion RH. Urticaria. In: *Modern Problems in Dermatology.* Philadelphia: WB Saunders, 1974, Vol. 1.
9. Noyes JH, Boyd GK, Settipane GA. Anaphylaxis to sunflower seed. *J Allergy Clin Immunol* 1979;63:242–4.
10. Benner MH, Lee HJ. Anaphylactic reaction to chamomile tea. *J Allergy Clin Immunol* 1973;52:307–8.
11. Hannuksela M, Lahti A. Immediate reactions to fruits and vegetables. *Contact Dermatitis* 1977;3:79–84.
12. Lahti A, Björkstén F, Hannuksela M. Allergy to birch pollen and apple, and cross-reactivity of the allergens studied with the RAST. *Allergy* 1980;35:297–300.
13. Ormerod AD, Reid TMS, Main RA. Penicillin in milk—its importance in urticaria. *Clin Allergy* 1987;17:229–34.
14. Paton WDM. Histamine liberation and lymphagogue action. *J Physiol (Lond)* 1954;123:58–9.
15. Prenner BM, Stevens JM. Anaphylaxis after ingestion of sodium bisulfite. *Ann Allergy* 1976;37:180–2.

16. Juhlin L. Recurrent urticaria: clinical investigation of 330 patients. *Br J Dermatol* 1981;104:369–81.
17. Hjorth N, Roed-Petersen J. Occupational protein contact dermatitis in food handlers. *Contact Dermatitis* 1976;2:28–42.
18. Maibach H. Immediate hypersensitivity in hand dermatitis. *Arch Dermatol* 1976;112:1289–91.
19. Krook G. Occupational dermatitis from *Lactuca sativa* (lettuce) and *Cichornium* (endive). *Contact Dermatitis* 1977;3:27–36.
20. Gondo A, Saeki N, Tokuda Y. Challenge reactions in atopic dermatitis after percutaneous entry of mite antigen. *Br J Dermatol* 1986;115:485–93.
21. Reitamo S, Visa K, Kahonen K, et al. Eczematous reactions in atopic patients caused by epicutaneous testing with inhalant allergens. *Br J Dermatol* 1986;114:303–9.
22. Papageorgiou C, Corbet J-P, Menezes-Brandao F, Pecegueiro M, Benezera C. Allergic contact dermatitis to garlic *(Allium sativum L.)*. *Arch Dermatol Res* 1983;275:229–34.
23. Veien NK, Hattel T, Justesen O, et al. Causes of eczema in the food industry. *Dermatosen* 1983;33:166–9.
24. Barnetson RStC. Hyperimmunoglobulinaemia E in atopic eczema (atopic dermatitis) is associated with "food allergy." *Acta Derm Venereol [Suppl] (Stockh)* 1980;92:94–6.
25. Turner MW, Brostoff J, Mowbray JF, Skelton A. The atopic syndrome: in vitro immunological characteristics of clinically defined subgroups of atopic subjects. *Clin Allergy* 1980;10:575–84.
26. Sampson HA. Role of immediate food hypersensitivity in the pathogenesis of atopic eczema. *J Allergy Clin Immunol* 1983;71:473–80.
27. Sampson HA, Jolie PL. Increased plasma histamine concentrations after food challenges in children with atopic eczema. *N Engl J Med* 1984;311:372–6.
28. Sampson HA, Albergo R. Comparison of results of skin tests, RAST, and double-blind, placebo-controlled food challenges in children with atopic dermatitis. *J Allergy Clin Immunol* 1984;74:26–33.
29. Pike M, Atherton DJ. Atopic eczema. In: Brostoff J, Challacombe SJ, eds. *Food Allergy and Intolerance*. London: Baillière Tindall, 1987;583–601.
30. Atherton DJ, Sewell M, Soothill JF, Wells RS, Chilvers CED. A double-blind controlled crossover trial of an antigen avoidance diet in atopic eczema. *Lancet* 1978;i:401–3.
31. Atherton DJ. Dietary antigen avoidance in the treatment of atopic eczema. *Acta Derm Venereol [Suppl] (Stockh)* 1980;92:99–102.
32. Neild VS, Marsden RA, Bailes JA, Bland JM. Egg and milk free exclusion diets in atopic eczema. *Br J Dermatol* 1986;114:117–23.
33. Hill DJ, Lynch BC. Elemental diet in the management of severe eczema in childhood. *Clin Allergy* 1982;12:313–5.
34. Hathaway MJ, Warner JO. Compliance in the dietary management of eczema. *Arch Dis Child* 1983;58:463–4.
35. Atherton DJ. Diet and atopic eczema. *Clin Allergy* 1988;18:215–28.
36. Dannaeus A, Inganas M, Johansson SGO, Foucard T. Intestinal uptake of ovalbumin in malabsorption and food allergy in relation to serum IgG antibody and orally administered sodium cromoglycate. *Clin Allergy* 1979;9:263–70.
37. Paganelli R, Levinsky RJ, Brostoff J, Wraith DG. Immune complexes containing food proteins in normal and atopic subjects after oral challenge, and the effect of sodium cromoglycate on antigen absorption. *Lancet* 1979;i:1270–2.
38. Byars NE, Ferraresi RW. Intestinal anaphylaxis in the rat as a model of food allergy. *Clin Exp Immunol* 1976;24:352–6.
39. Bloch KJ, Walker WA. Effect of locally induced intestinal anaphylaxis on the uptake of a bystander antigen. *J Allergy Clin Immunol* 1981;67:312–6.
40. Turner MW, Boulton P, Shields JG, et al. Intestinal hypersensitivity reactions in the rat. I. Uptake of intact protein, permeability to sugar and their correlation with mast cell degranulation. *Immunology* 1987;63:119–24.
41. McCalla R, Savilahti E, Perkkio M, et al. Morphology of the jejunum in children with eczema due to food allergy. *Allergy* 1980;35:563–71.
42. Kokkonen J, Simila S, Herva R. Gastrointestinal findings in atopic children. *Eur J Pediatr* 1980;134:249–54.
43. Pike M, Heddle RJ, Boulton P, Turner MW, Atherton DJ. Increased intestinal permeability in atopic eczema. *J Invest Dermatol* 1986;86:101–4.

44. Brostoff J, Carini C, Wraith DS, Paganelli R, Levinsky RJ. Immune complexes in atopy. In: Pepys J, Edwards AM, eds. *The Mast Cell—Its Role in Health and Disease*. London: Pitman, 1979;380–93.
45. Paganelli R, Levinsky RJ, Atherton DJ. Detection of specific antigen with circulating immune complexes. Validation of the assay and its application to food antigen-antibody complexes found in healthy and food allergic subjects. *Clin Exp Immunol* 1981;46:44–53.
46. Mihm MC, Soter NA, Dvorak HF, Austen KF. The structure of normal skin and the morphology of atopic eczema. *J Invest Dermatol* 1976;67:305–12.
47. Newcombe RW, Nelson H. Dermatographia mediated by immunoglobulin E. *Am J Med* 1973;54:174–80.
48. Van Asperen PP, Kemp AS, Mellis CM. Skin test reactivity and clinical allergen sensitivity in infancy. *J Allergy Clin Immunol* 1984;73:381–6.

Food Intolerance in Infancy: Allergology,
Immunology, and Gastroenterology, edited by
Robert N. Hamburger. Carnation Nutrition
Education Series, Vol. 1. The Carnation Co., Los
Angeles/Raven Press, Ltd., New York © 1989.

Interim Discussion for Section III

David J. Atherton, William Heird,
John A. Walker-Smith, and Ekhard E. Ziegler

Dr. Berman: Jim Berman from Illinois. I would like to ask Dr. Walker-Smith to comment on eosinophilic gastroenteropathy and its relationship to foods.

Dr. Walker-Smith: I think it's a very important differential diagnosis for gastrointestinal food allergy. Characteristically, in eosinophilic gastroenteritis there is not an adequate response to food elimination alone and steroids are required as well. Eosinophilic gastroenteritis is a major differential diagnosis of gastrointestinal allergy and it is quite a serious disorder. The histopathology may not be very different from the kind of eosinophilic infiltration in the colon that I demonstrated. However, the usual feature is that the eosinophilic infiltration is most marked, for example, in the upper gastrointestinal tract in the stomach and it actually gets less as you move down the gut.

Dr. Nandyal: Dr. Raja Nandyal, Racine, Wisconsin. I am a practicing neonatologist and have two questions for Dr. Walker-Smith. First, some growing premature infants who are on cow's milk formulas tend to develop a necrotizing enterocolitis-like syndrome without any radiological manifestations. They tend to have the symptoms even with repeated exposure to the same formula, and they improve with predigested casein formula. I wonder whether this is a case of cow's milk hypersensitivity in premature infants.

Dr. Walker-Smith: Yes, it may be on occasion, although not usually. We wrote a paper some years ago in *Acta Pediatrica Helvetica* (De Peyer and Walker-Smith, 1977;32:509) in which we did describe a similar case. I think there are some children allergic to cow's milk who may present like necrotizing enterocolitis (NEC). Although I would have reservations about the diagnosis of cow's milk allergy in a severe case of NEC with extensive air within the wall of the gut; however, I do think it is a possibility. This syndrome is much less common now since we use the modern, sophisticated adaptive milks. Such a syndrome was rather more common when I was a medical student in Australia and babies used to be fed with varying dilutions of ordinary cow's milk.

Dr. Nandyal: The second question is: One of your slides showed that acute gastroenteritis may induce a symptom complex similar to cow's milk allergy. Is it the same as the transient disaccharidase deficiency that we see in many children? If it is different, how do you differentiate it?

Dr. Walker-Smith: In patients who have cow's milk-sensitive enteropathy, there is depression of all disaccharidases, lactase in particular, and in some of these, depending upon the extent and severity of the lesion, there is lactose intolerance as well. There are two sorts of lactose intolerances in association with gastroenteritis; one, in fact, is due to rotavirus induced mucosal damage per se. This is brief and lactose intolerance disappears *pari passu* with healing of the mucosa. When there is delayed recovery with persistent lactose intolerance, this is a marker of persistent small intestinal mucosal damage. This could be persistent mucosal damage due, for example, to *Giardia lamblia* or enteropathogenic *E. coli,* but it could also be due to cow's milk allergy. The two (i.e., infection and allergy) may coexist, and we have shown some years ago by means of serial small intestinal biopsies. Lactose intolerance and cow's milk protein intolerance (i.e., cow's milk allergy) may coexist. I would feel that lactose intolerance occurring up to 2 weeks after acute diarrhea is related to the infection per se. When lactose intolerance is persistent for more than 2 weeks, then this is likely to be caused by cow's milk allergy. It's certainly a declining problem now.

Dr. Lifschitz: Carlos Lifschitz, Houston, Texas. This question is for Dr. Walker-Smith. In the bottle-fed infant who develops a noninfectious colitis, it is not difficult to recommend the use of a protein-hydrolyzed formula. However, that decision is not that easy when you are dealing with an exclusively breast-fed infant. I would like to know what is your approach to diagnosis and treatment of an infant who is exclusively breast-fed and develops a noninfectious colitis?

Dr. Walker-Smith: It depends on how severe the colitis is. Often it is relatively mild and the baby is basically well. Such children with cow's milk colitis are typically not nutritionally deficient like the enteropathic infants. They are well-nourished babies who have some blood in their stool and the mother is drinking a lot of cow's milk. In the first instance, we would put the mother on a strict cow's-milk-free, milk-elimination diet and see if the baby gets better. If that simple strategy doesn't work, we do a colonoscopy. It has been our experience that it's quite impossible clinically and also by using endoscopy to distinguish ulcerative colitis from cow's milk colitis until the histology of the colon is examined. When there is a dense infiltration of eosinophils, it is indicative of colitis caused by cow's milk. Usually the child will then recover with his mother on a cow's-milk-free diet. Quite often in Britain, mothers have been told to drink extra milk during lactation, and they are, in fact, taking more cow's milk than usual. I think that this has been an adverse factor. Nevertheless, now that we know this syndrome exists, we don't often do endoscopies. If cow's milk allergy is likely we just act clinically and eliminate cow's milk; we reserve endoscopy for those who do not respond.

Dr. McGeady: Steve McGeady, Philadelphia, Pennsylvania. A question for Dr. Walker-Smith. Two patients that we have seen in the last decade or so had what was diagnosed by us as enteropathy due to cow's milk sensitivity. Both of these children had rather significant gastroesophageal reflux and one of them even showed manifestations of the Sandifer syndrome. My question to you is how much of the protein and blood loss that we see in these children do you think is due to just nonspecific irritation of the gut as opposed to reflux esophagitis?

Dr. Walker-Smith: These cases are complicated. It has certainly been our experience, too, that vomiting is quite a major feature of children with cow's milk-sensitive enteropathy and that they may have associated gastroesophageal reflux. The ones in which we have seen gastrointestinal reflux seem to be undiagnosed cases, i.e., cases in which the symptoms have been persistent for some time. In fact, the main problem appears to have been the enteropathy and the resulting vomiting per se has been a factor in the development of gastroesophageal reflux. Nevertheless, I think they are associated features; there is no doubt that the esophagitis associated with blood loss is the cause for the blood loss in those circumstances. What I find so difficult to know in individual children is whether blood loss is actually coming from the colon or whether it is coming from the esophagus. When we have clear-cut evidence of gastroesophageal reflux as well as enteropathy, we treat the child with a protein hydrolysate to the enteropathy and with Metaclopromide and thickening of the feeds for the gastroesophageal reflux.

Dr. McGeady: Both of these cases occurred before that drug was clinically available in the United States, but I know that pylorospasm frequently is a feature of hypersensitivity and I have also had the same questions as to whether the reflux is not reflecting that.

Dr. Walker-Smith: Well, pylorospasm is also a feature of patients with a gastroesophageal reflux as well. So these cases are complicated.

Dr. Winter: Winter, Boston, Massachusetts. The 20-week human fetus has mostly CD-3 positive cells in lymphoid aggregates and very few cells in the epithelium. Could you comment on the response you found to pokeweed mitogen and if you believe that it is mediated by the small number of intraepithelial lymphocytes (IELs). Secondly, what is the role of gamma-delta thymus-derived cells (T cells) in the epithelium of patients with celiac disease or milk protein allergy?

Dr. Walker-Smith: We are not really suggesting that the IELs are themselves actually the major cause of pathology. The pathology is in the lamina propria itself. If you take the fetal organ culture and observe it over 3 days, the intraepithelial lymphocytes in fact disappear. They fall from about six down to zero. But in the activated T cell model where there is enteropathy, the lymphocytes actually slightly increase compared to control material and there is a rise in the CD-3 positive, CD-4, and CD-8 negative cells. This may represent an overflow from the lamina propria. We believe that the intraepithelial lymphocytes in this model have actually come from the lamina propria itself. It's technically difficult to quantify the cells within the lamina propria. We have analyzed those subjectively. We think that the major event is activation of T cells within the lamina propria. Now the gamma delta receptor T cells are a different population. They are increased in the epithelium of celiac disease and they are also increased in the lymphoma-associated enteropathy of celiac disease, but not in cow's milk sensitive enteropathy (Spencer et al. The development of gut associated lymphoid tissue in the terminal ileum of fetal human intestine. *Clin Exp Immunol* 1986;64:536). Thus, they all have the gamma delta receptor instead of the alpha beta. This is an intriguing observation but its significance is unknown.

Dr. Thomas: Dan Thomas, pediatric gastroenterologist from Los Angeles, California. I just want to make a point in regard to Dr. Ziegler's discussion of our work and point out that in the infants we studied, we also measured stool α_1 antitrypsin levels and found that these infants who were fed cow's milk did not have any abnormal excretion of stool α_1 antitrypsin. Also, I want to ask Dr. Ziegler, because perhaps I missed it, in the infants fed cow's milk, could you give me an idea of how much cow's milk or solid food they were consuming at the time of the study?

Dr. Ziegler: In response to your comment, of course I was aware that you measured α_1-antitrypsin. We measured the amount of cow's milk that these babies consumed and we also measured the amount of formula that the other group consumed and there were no appreciable differences between the two groups. So the sheer amount of milk or formula consumed could not be the explanation.

Dr. Thomas: The reason I asked is that the infants that we studied who were on cow's milk were taking less than 30 ounces a day of cow's milk, and there might be a discrepancy between our results and your results. We know, as we have heard in this discussion about cow's milk, and we've found in many infants who present to us with protein losing enteropathy or anemia, that they are usually taking excessive amounts of cow's milk in addition to perhaps starting at an earlier age. That might account for part of the discrepancy in our data.

Dr. Ziegler: That could well be the case. By the way, Wilson showed very nicely in two patients that the amount of blood lost in the stool was quantitatively related to the amount of cow's milk ingested. There was a very clear relationship. So that is a well-known phenomenon, but I don't think it explains the differences between your results and ours. I think it's the different assays we used for the fecal hemoglobin.

Dr. Thomas: May I ask what you consider a normal amount of blood lost in the stool for just the cross-sectional average for a population?

Dr. Ziegler: In our formula-fed group the average was around 500 micrograms per gram of dry stool, and the +2 sd was around 1,200. So that is 1.2 mg of hemoglobin per gram of dry stool, and I would consider that the upper limit of normal, and that is how we defined cow's milk responders versus nonresponders.

Dr. Thomas: The limit of sensitivity for a qualitative stool test is around 1 to 2 mg per gram of stool. So what you are saying is that the use of qualitative stool tests, even if they are accurate, is pretty much useless then?

Dr. Ziegler: Correct.

Dr. Thomas: So why use the qualitative tests at all?

Dr. Ziegler: Oh, you mean the guaiac test?

Dr. Thomas: The guaiac test or any test at all.

Dr. Ziegler: Well, I don't know in clinical practice how useful it is. What I showed is that among our infants, stools with very high hemoglobin concentrations were always guaiac positive, but there are always stools with low hemoglobin concentrations that for some reason test out positive in the guaiac test. In other words, you pick up all high hemoglobin stools, all of the bleeders, but you also pick up a number of nonbleeders with a guaiac test and these false positives really are the limitation of the guaiac test.

Dr. Devries: Jeffrey Devries from Detroit, Michigan. I have two questions, the first to Dr. Ziegler. In light of your finding of fecal blood loss associated with drinking cow's milk throughout infancy, would you recommend that cow's milk not be given at all during the entire first 12 months of life? Second, can a panel member describe the differences in allergenicity between cow's milk formula and cow's milk and what that difference can be attributed to? Is it primarily the heat-treating of cow's milk for use in the formula?

Dr. Ziegler: In answer to your first question, my personal opinion is that cow's milk is not a suitable food for infants below 1 year of age, and certainly not below 6 months. If the amount of cow's milk is limited, and I don't know exactly to where it should be limited, then maybe it's acceptable in the second 6 months of life, but it's very low on my list of acceptable foods. With regard to what might be the component of cow's milk that causes blood loss, Wilson did some very nice studies with bovine serum albumin which is present in cow's milk, and found that it was capable of inducing enteric blood loss, and it was inactivated by heat treatment. We also know that heat treatment of whole cow's milk takes away the capacity to induce blood loss. So, serum albumin is certainly a candidate, and whatever it is, it is heat-labile.

Dr. Walker-Smith: I would like to comment on the second question, too. Professor Coombs in Cambridge, England has used an anaphylactic shock model in guinea pigs to compare various milk formulas, ordinary untreated milk, evaporated milk, modern adapted feeding formula, the old feeding formula, casein hydrolysates, etc. Modern adapted feeding formulas are much less sensitizing, i.e., much less capable of inducing anaphylactic shock than the older feeding formula and certainly much less so than ordinary cow's milk. If you feed a guinea pig ordinary cow's milk and then put it in the trachea or give it intravenously, they invariably die. This happens less often with a modern adapted formula. Professor Coomb's view was that heat treatment was important in this phenomenon and also that perhaps the digestibility of the cow's milk was altered. Certainly it's been our clinical experience that the modern adapted formulas are much less sensitizing. This is why I emphasized in my talk that there is an unfortunate trend in East London for children to go back onto ordinary cow's milk when they are beyond 6 months for economic reasons. In fact, that is why in our deprived population we are still seeing cow's milk allergy. We are seeing children who have often had gastroenteritis in a deprived community who are being given cow's milk itself. If you live in an affluent community without gastroenteritis and are fed a modern adapted formula, I think the chance of developing cow's milk-sensitive enteropathy is much, much less.

Dr. Rhoads: Marc Rhoads, Chapel Hill, North Carolina. My question is directed to Dr. Walker-Smith. If approximately 3% of children that develop acute enteritis develop cow's milk protein intolerance, and given that the average child in the Third World develops about four episodes of enteritis per year, I guess one would have to assume that cow's milk protein intolerance would be a problem of major magnitude in the Third World, of much greater importance than it is as an entity in the developed world. If that is true, could we get your recommendations for how one might treat children with that condition in the Third World?

Dr. Walker-Smith: This I believe certainly to be the case. Dr. Peter Manuel, one of my clinical lecturers, went to Surabaja in Indonesia and we did a study, which we published, doing biopsies on children with chronic diarrhea on a milk-free diet and with milk challenge (Manuel P. Role of cow's milk protein intolerance in a developing community. In: Walker-Smith JW, McNeil AS, eds. *Diarrhea and Malnutrition in Childhood*. London: Butterworth, 1986). Certainly in urban bottle-fed babies in Surabaja, both from a private clinic and then a public hospital, it was very, very common. Now, you can't use modern sophisticated hydrolysates routinely in such communities, but what does work in the developing world is chicken-based formulas. You can make up a formula based on chicken as developed by Dorothy Francis at the Great Ormond Street Hospital in London. This is a relatively simple recipe which can be used among village people based on chicken where chicken is a staple food. Otherwise, of course, commercial formulas were far too expensive.

Dr. Rhoads: It's not a hydrolysate, so are the protein molecules in chicken meat less antigenic?

Dr. Walker-Smith: Yes, that's a curious thing. In fact, we found children who have failed on protein hydrolysates sometimes actually do quite well on chicken-feeding. I don't know quite why that is. Although egg allergy is quite common, chicken meat actually seems to be very low in the hierarchy of allergenicity. This is something I just don't understand, but it seems to work.

Dr. Siegel: Sheldon Siegel from Los Angeles, California. My question and comments are to Dr. Atherton. It's quite clear from Dr. Sampson's study and earlier studies that the elimination of foods that patients are sensitive to can benefit a child with atopic dermatitis. My experience has been, in the older child or adult who has atopic dermatitis, that the elimination of various foods from their diet has been rarely helpful in modifying their overall course. I would like your comment about that. In addition, you mentioned something about elimination of dyes, preservatives, and other substances from patients' diet as being helpful in the treatment of chronic urticaria. My associates have not found elimination of these substances very helpful in our management of patients. We recently reviewed 214 cases of urticaria and despite extensive investigative studies we were unable to detect the etiology in almost all of those cases that had chronic urticaria. I wondered if that has been your experience as well?

Dr. Atherton: In response to your first question about older children: it's certainly our impression now that dietary treatment really only works well in the very young. In fact, once the child is over about the age of 2, as I said, in cases where it would work most parents had already done it. But the number in whom it would work, I believe in any case, gets much smaller year by year. Certainly by the time you get older children and adults I think the chances of success with dietary treatment are probably very small. There may be a variety of reasons for that, and I'm sure one is that other allergens and other factors are playing an increasing role. Even within the area of foods, I'm sure that the number of allergen sources that is relevant in the older child is becoming so great that it's probably almost impossible really to identify them all. The only way we have of identifying them is by a trial and error system. As for additives, it's interesting that earlier on when we were playing around with the idea of doing double-blind food challenges in eczema, we found that the only thing we could produce, the only items in the diet which the parents could identify in this few-food diet protocol, where there did seem to be a reproducible provocation on a double-blind challenge, was actually with tartrazine and benzoic acid. In the last study that we did, which we are going to publish, it just so happened that those didn't really figure, but I'm quite sure they do play a role in some children and that is quite a reproducible thing. Certainly the intake now in our country, and I'm sure here as well, is very much less. I think it is very difficult to buy an orange drink in the United Kingdom that has artificial coloring in it.

Food Intolerance in Infancy: Allergology, Immunology, and Gastroenterology, edited by Robert N. Hamburger. Carnation Nutrition Education Series, Vol. 1. The Carnation Co., Los Angeles/Raven Press, Ltd., New York © 1989.

Sleep and Behavioral Changes in Milk-Intolerant Children: a Double-Blind Crossover Study

*A. Kahn, *M.J. Mozin, *E. Rebuffat, *M. Sottiaux, *G. Casimir, *J. Duchâteau, and **M.F. Muller

*Pediatric Sleep Unit, University Children's Hospital, Free University of Brussels; and **Clinique Universitaire Erasme, Brussels, Belgium

Approximately 10% of the children under 1 year of age present persistent settling and repeated awakening during the night. At 2 years of age, the rate of sleep disruption rises, and regular wakings occur in up to 20% of children (1,2), and it is reported for 10 to 15% of 3- and 4-year-old children (3,4). These sleep problems represent a challenge to both the parents and the pediatrician (5).

The sustained impossibility to initiate or to maintain sleep has been attributed to a variety of causes. Adverse environmental conditions, such as inadequate ambient noise or temperature (6,7), psychologic stress in the family (4), or inappropriate parental behavior (6,7), are among the most frequently reported causes for the development of abnormal sleep homeostasis in children.

In some children, constitutional sensitivity (7–9), the delayed effect of neonatal asphyxia (1,9), or the influence of breast-feeding (10) has also been suspected. Chronic physical discomfort caused by colic (7), recurrent episodes of upper airway obstruction, otitis (6), or gastroesophageal reflux should also be considered.

In 1985 we proposed that when no cause for persistent sleeplessness can be found in an infant, a tentative diagnosis of food intolerance should be made (11). All cow's milk is then excluded from the diet, even if no symptom of allergy is clinically present. We could show that the sleep characteristics of such infants cannot be differentiated from those of allergic infants (12), normalized within a few weeks after the withdrawal of all cow's milk from the diet, only to deteriorate again when the infants are orally challenged with cow's milk. As measured in the sleep laboratory, the number of arousals, the sleep latency and duration, and the percent of various sleep stages, are all closely related to the ingestion of cow's milk (13).

The preliminary report could suffer possible methodological shortcomings. One of these concerned the criteria used for the selection of the sleepless infants. By studying fairly young infants, we might have included subjects with symptoms of infantile colic. Another possible bias could be the open manipulation of the children's diet. These changes in regimen could have influenced the parents' attitudes, thereby inducing a placebo effect.

A new study was therefore undertaken, avoiding the possible shortcomings of the previous reports. Whereas our previous observation was limited to 8 infants, aged 14.8 weeks, we studied a new group of 17 sleepless children with a median age of 13.5 months. Their behavior difficulties were corrected by the exclusion of cow's milk from the diet. A double-blind, crossover milk challenge was then performed. The present study brings new evidence for the possible relationship between undiagnosed cow's milk intolerance and severe sleeplessness in children. It extends these observations to an older group of children, and better defines some of the possible limitations of our diagnostic and treatment procedures.

PATIENTS AND INVESTIGATIONS

From July 1986 to July 1988, 17 children (11.6%) with chronic sleeplessness, possibly related to intolerance to cow's milk, were studied in our University outpatient Sleep Clinic. They were selected from a total of 146 children under 5 years of age, referred by their physicians for continual waking and crying during sleep hours. They were studied according to a systematic protocol previously described (11). Interviews were conducted with the parents in the simultaneous presence of a pediatrician, psychologist, and a dietitian. Special attention was given to the description of sleep difficulties, allergy, and daily family life. The birth records and past history of the children were reviewed. A standard physical examination of the child was performed, and any sign of atopy was noted. A medical and psychologic protocol was followed to rule out the most frequent causes for chronic sleeplessness in children.

For 7 days the parents were asked to fill in a log describing the child's sleep and feeding schedule. It was discussed on a second visit. If any adverse environmental condition or inappropriate parental behavior seemed to contribute to the child's condition, it was discussed and appropriate counseling was given. If clinically indicated, further investigations were performed, such as ear, nose, and throat (ENT), blood, or urine studies; esophageal pH monitoring; or all-night polysomnographies. The sleep recordings were performed following usual procedures (11). Skin water evaporation rates were noninvasively monitored during quiet (nonrapid eye movement) sleep with the use of an evaporimeter. For ethical reasons, no control of the polysomnographies was made after the improvement of the children's sleep.

DETERMINATION OF MILK INTOLERANCE

For 17 children, no explanation for their sleep difficulties was found. To test the hypothesis that their continual awakening and crying could be related to cow's milk intolerance, all dairy products were excluded from their diet. The children were fed exclusively with a hydrolyzed whey protein mixture (NAN-HA, Nestlé) for 4 weeks. The dietitian explained to the parents the exclusion diet the child was assigned to, and gave the parents a list of items to be excluded from the diet, as well as a list of acceptable items. Procedures regarding compliance were discussed and general matters regarding food selection and recording were outlined. Follow-up interviews were done at 15-day intervals.

Prior to the initiation of the exclusion diet, assay kits for immunoglobulin E (IgE) paper radioimmunosorbent tests (PRIST, Phadebas), *in vitro* radioallergosorbent tests (RAST, Pharmacia Fine Chemicals), and antibodies against β-lactoglobulins were measured.

Placebo-Challenge Procedure

If the exclusion diet brought significant improvement of the children's sleep, a cow's milk challenge was then performed. The test was done double-blind. Two series of rice cream powder were given to the parents in coded boxes. One series contained rice cream (80%) and cow's milk powder (20%). The other contained rice cream powder only. The two cereals were indistinguishable by sight, smell, taste, or stain color. The placebo and challenge materials were developed and labeled by Nestlé (Belgium), and the codes were delivered to the dietitian under sealed envelopes. In no instance was it necessary to have access to the code assignment for medical or behavioral reasons. Parents were told that their child would try both rice powders, and that either might induce restlessness. They were told we were trying to confirm the need to pursue the exclusion diet. For 7 days 2 g of one of the powders was added to the children's last bottle of hydrolyzed milk mixture. Subjects were randomly assigned to one of the coded boxes of powder. To avoid any interaction between diet and diet order, a crossover design was established. Each child served as its own control. No parent or individual member of the study team knew whether a child was being challenged on a given day. The parents noted on the sleep logs the behavioral characteristics of their children, and any suspected dietary infractions. As soon as symptoms of intolerance (respiratory, cutaneous, or digestive symptoms) or insomnia appeared, feeding of the powder was interrupted. The next set of powder was started 7 days after the observed symptoms had disappeared, or after the completion of the first 7-day administration, if no symptom was noted. The code was broken when the administration of two series of powder was completed. Postexperimental interviews revealed that none of the parents correctly identified the placebo versus challenge materials during the investigation.

The diagnosis of milk intolerance was retained only if no symptom was seen during the feeding of the control powder, if the powder containing cow's milk was accompanied by signs of intolerance, and if all symptoms disappeared after the interruption of the challenge.

The same double-blind procedure was repeated at various intervals to determine whether the exclusion regimen was still mandatory. The tests were repeated at a median age of 18, 24, and 36 months, or at any other time when the parents questioned the need for maintaining the exclusion diet. If, in a previously intolerant child, the double-blind milk challenge did not induce adverse reactions, milk was admitted in the diet.

To appraise the children's progress, every family was interviewed during consultation or by telephone during the month of June 1988. The University Ethical Committee had given its approval for the study, and informed parental consent was obtained in each case. Statistical analysis was performed using the Chi-square and the Wilcoxon rank tests, with a level of significance of 0.05.

RESULTS

The main characteristics of the 17 infants whose sleeplessness was initially attributed to cow's milk intolerance are shown in Table 1. There were 11 boys and 6 girls, with a median age of 13.5 months (range 2.5 to 48 months). Two boys were twins. Eleven infants had been breast-fed for a median duration of 3 months. At the time of the study all infants were bottle-fed with a diet containing cow's milk.

A history of atopy was present in 10 families. In four, either a mother or father had suffered from hay fever or asthma. In six families, both the mother and father, or one of the parents and a sibling, had a history of nocturnal asthma or eczema.

Although no infant had been considered ill before entering the study, 7 had eczema on the face or trunk, 5 had at least three episodes of wheezing at night, and 10 had at least four episodes of rhinitis or otitis. Eight children had repeated diarrhea or vomiting. Plotting the weight by age of the infants on a local growth curve (Wach), it was found that the children had gained weight poorly. From birth, up to the start of the study, the children had fallen from percentile 75 for weight to percentile 25 (Wilcoxon rank test: $t = 158$; $p = 0.039$). On physical examination, 14 children looked pale and tired and 6 had serious rhinitis.

TABLE 1. *General characteristics of the 17 children initially suspected of cow's milk intolerance and sleeplessness*

Number of children	17	
Sex (M/F)	11/6	
Rank in the family	2	(1–3)
Gestational age (weeks)	40	(35–40)
No. of infants breast-fed	11/17	
Duration of breast-feeding (months)	3	(0.25–6)
Age (months) at:		
Beginning of insomnia	1.5	(0.25–18)
Diagnosis and challenge	13.5	(2.5–48)
Latest milk challenge test	15.0	(4–49)
Follow-up	21.0	(15–58)

The figures refer to absolute values, median values, and ranges.

Laboratory tests revealed abnormal IgE values in 1 out of 12 children tested (279 U/ml; normal value <100 U/ml), and a high level of antibodies against β-lactoglobulins in 9 out of 14 children (superior to 300 U). In 2 out of 10 children, the RASTs were positive to β-lactoglobulins and egg.

Severe sleep disruption had lasted since a median of 8 months (range 1.5–30 months).

Previous treatments included changes in family sleep habits in 15 infants, and the use of soya milk in 6 infants, sedative drugs in 4, and homeopathic or osteopathic treatments in 3. No marked improvement had been noted.

When they entered the study, five children were falling asleep within 15 min after being laid to bed, but 12 children took up to 1 hr to fall asleep (Table 2). During sleep all children were described as agitated, and eight were repeatedly found with drenching sweats. The bed covers were wet with sweat, and the pajamas of two children, aged 22 and 24 months, were frequently changed during the night because of the sweat. Loud snoring was reported for five children. A boy of 22 months had repeated body rocking during the night. The children's sleep was interrupted by a median of five complete arousals per night (range, 1 to 12 arousals). They usually awoke crying, and remained restless for a median duration of 30 min (range 20 to 180 min). During the night their median total sleep duration was 5.5 hr (range 2.5 to 8 hr), and they seldom slept during the day. Their total sleep time for 24 hr was 5.5 hr (range 3 to 8.5 hr). When awake, the children were described as fussy, demanding, and difficult to pacify.

TABLE 2. *Sleep characteristics of 17 children studied as reported by their parents' logs*

Characteristics	Before the diet	After 4 wk of diet	p
Data from parents' logs			
Time to fall asleep (min)	15.0 (15–60)	10.0 (10–15)	0.001
No. of complete arousals	5 (1–12)	0 (0–2)	0.001
Sleep duration (hr):			
Between 07.00–19.00	0 (0–3)	1.5 (0–2.5)	0.005
Between 19.01–06.59	5.5 (2.5–8)	11.0 (9–13)	0.001
Total sleep time (hr)	5.5 (3–8.5)	13.0 (10–14.5)	0.001
No. of children with night sweats	8	0	0.001
Data from sleep lab (n = 8)	Data from control children		
During the night (12 hr):			
No. of complete arousals	5 (1–12)	1 (0–2)	0.001
Sleep duration (hr)	5.5 (2.5–8)	9.1 (8.8–10.3)	0.001
Duration of arousals (min)	35.5 (10–60)	12.0 (0.5–32)	0.001
Transcutaneous water loss (g/m²·h)	32.0 (26–44)	14.0 (9–19)	0.001

The data collected from the logs are given before, and 4 weeks after, initiation of the diet. The observations from the sleep lab of 8 children are compared with those of 16 age- and sex-matched control children. The figures refer to absolute values, median, and ranges.

Because of frequent regurgitations or snoring, sleep was recorded in eight children. There were five boys and three girls, with a median age of 9 months (range 2.5 to 22 months). Despite frequent arousals and disrupted sleep patterns, no cardiorespiratory rhythm or esophageal acid reflux was found. Measurement of skin water evaporation showed high levels during nonrapid eye movement sleep. These sleep characteristics all closely matched the observations from the parents' logs, and were significantly different from those found in 16 age- and sex-matched control children.

Dietary compliance was excellent in all families, and no cow's milk was introduced during the 4-week test period. All children tolerated their artificial diet well. In 15 out of 17 children, the parents reported that their child's sleep schedule normalized after a median duration of 4 weeks (range 3 to 6 weeks). In one 12-month-old girl, sleep normalized within 4 days of the initiation of the diet. There was no apparent correlation between gender or age of the children and the rapidity of sleep normalization. During the night, the parents had no difficulty putting the children to sleep. The children slept 11 hr (range 9 to 13 hr), and awoke only occasionally. During sleep, they were reported to move less, and the drenching night sweats disappeared.

During the day, the babies' sleep lasted 1.5 hr (range 0 to 2.5 hr). During periods of wakefulness, the children were described as quieter and less demanding. The change in daytime behavior was seen after 2 weeks (range 1.5 to 4 weeks). The cutaneous symptoms had cleared up completely in four children and improved in three, and no infectious episode or digestive symptoms were reported. On physical examination, none looked pale or tired.

The sleep of one 12-month-old girl did not improve after 6 weeks of exclusion diet. Her sleep normalized only when the hydrolyzed hypoallergenic diet was interrupted. The child was fed a standard diet without cow's milk.

Cow's milk was reintroduced into the diet of all children 5 weeks after the initiation of the diet (range 4 to 6 weeks). The challenge was done double-blind, as already described. Postexperimental analysis of the test sequences revealed that the sequence placebo–challenge and challenge–placebo was equally represented. No difference was seen when the reactions were compared with the test order. No reaction was reported when the children received rice cream powder without cow's milk. Within 4 days of the introduction of cow's milk, 15 children demonstrated sleeplessness and agitated behavior. Their sleep was described as of poor quality similar to that seen before the exclusion diet. They slept a median of 5 hr (range 3 to 6 hr), and woke up five times per night (range 2 to 12 times). An 11-week-old boy and a 13-week-old girl had digestive symptoms, vomiting, or diarrhea. When the administration of milk was interrupted, the clinical condition and the behavior of these children normalized within 48 hr (range 24 to 120 hr).

The twin brothers showed a strikingly similar pattern of reaction. They were sleepless the same night of the challenge, and both slept normally again two nights after the termination of the test. The boy who rocked at sleep onset, and had showed a marked reduction of rocking duration and intensity 4 weeks after the initiation of the diet, resumed intense rocking and up to 10 arousals per night after the milk challenge.

Because of previous night crying, the parents of six children had picked up the habit of taking the child into their own bed. Now that their child's sleep was normalized, they were advised to have the child sleep in another room. Although this change in attitude did not bring any further improvement in sleep, it was considered advisable to prevent the possibility of new sleep complaints caused by inappropriate parental behavior.

In the girl whose sleep normalized after four nights of the exclusion diet, the milk challenge did not result in changes in behavior. During the exclusion diet, her total sleep time had increased from 6.5 to 11 hr, and the number of arousals had decreased from six to less than one per night. The parents had also been counseled not to allow the child to sleep in their bed. Because the child's sleep was not altered by the milk challenge, she was excluded from the milk-intolerant group and given a normal diet. Her previous sleep difficulties were retrospectively attributed to sleep mismanagement.

In seven children, only one milk challenge could be performed so far. In 10 children, the challenge was repeated at a later age. Nine children were tested twice, and one child three times. Challenges were done between 16 and 22 months in seven children, and between 25 and 57 months in three children. The type of reactions observed were comparable with that seen previously. In every child, the double-blind milk challenge was followed by a new deterioration of behavior, except in the 57-month-old girl. The child was being challenged because she began to refuse the hypoallergenic diet. As no obvious effect followed the new challenge, she was considered to have outgrown milk intolerance and was allowed a normal diet.

By June 1988, the follow-up period was 10 months (range 3 to 28 months). While still treated with the exclusion diet, 16 children were sleeping and growing normally. Their weight had increased from percentile 25 to pecentile 35 by age (range percentile 25 to 90). Weight percentile was not significantly different from that noted at birth (Wilcoxon rank test: $t = 124.5$; $p = 0.07$). No cutaneous, respiratory, or digestive symptoms of atopy were reported. In seven children, accidental introduction of cow's milk into the diet in the form of cheese, biscuits, or ice cream was immediately followed by nighttime restlessness and repeated arousals that subsided within one to five nights. A significant increase in the intensity and duration of bedrocking was noted for the 50-month-old boy following accidental cow's milk ingestion.

During follow-up visits, the children and parents were systematically interviewed for possible physical discomfort that would favor arousals and agitation. We could not find any evidence for abdominal, head- or earaches, or for skin itching.

The girl who had been excluded, because of her lack of response to the milk challenge and who had been placed on a normal diet, had an eventless growth at the age of 17 months.

DISCUSSION

The children investigated in our University Clinic were referred by pediatricians and family practitioners for continuous waking and crying at sleep time. They had failed to respond to various forms of treatments such as changes in sleep habits or the use of sedative or homeopathic drugs. Despite this preliminary selection, sleep could be normalized through appropriate counseling in 58% of the children. Appropriate management of the children's sleep habits has rightly been advocated as the most efficient form of treatment for continuous restlessness during sleep hours (6,7).

For 20.5% of the children, a physical problem could be considered as the origin of sleep disturbance. Undiagnosed middle ear otitis, inguinal hernia, or esophageal reflux was found in children whose sleep normalized after treatment of the condition.

Undiagnosed cow's milk intolerance represented the problem of 11.6% of the children referred. The prevalence of allergy-related sleeplessness in the general population cannot be evaluated from our data. The prevalence of milk allergy is reported to be as high as 3% (14). Some pediatricians and practitioners have long been known to eliminate cow's milk from the diet of a cranky baby, particularly when there is a family history of atopy or other clinical manifestations of allergy. Only a community survey could establish the prevalence of the association between sleep quality and food intolerance.

The state of milk intolerance was not confirmed through skin tests, RAST, or antibodies against cow's milk. The laboratory studies were done only to illustrate a possible state of immunologic reaction in some of the children. The tests are reported not to be clinically indicative of food intolerance (15).

Additional counseling was given to several parents concerning possible mismanagement of their children's sleep schedules and habits. We cannot exclude that such changes in behavior contributed in resolving some of the sleep problems (4,6,7). Likewise, the exclusion of milk from the diet, or the daily filling-in of the sleep diary, could have induced a placebo effect in some parents. Their anxiety could have been diminished by the expectation of the elimination diet's positive effect, or by the ritual completion of the sleep log (7). This possible bias cannot be completely rejected by arguing that previous treatments with soya milk, sedative, or homeopathic drugs had failed to normalize the children's sleep.

Double-blind crossover placebo versus offending food challenges were the best available methods to exclude such methodological bias.

The challenges gave evidence for cow's milk intolerance in all children, except in a 12-month-old girl. We excluded the child from the milk-intolerant group of patients, and tentatively attributed her improvement in sleep behavior to better parental management of sleep. The results of the double-blind challenges were eventually supported by the effects of the accidental reintroduction of small quantities of cow's milk into the diet. In seven children, restless nights and agitation were reported following the ingestion of cheese, biscuits, or ice cream. In children old enough to reach for food, the compliance to the exclusion diet can become a problem, as the offending foods are often those patients like most.

The diagnosis of cow's milk intolerance was maintained for the 12-month-old girl who did not improve after 6 weeks of exclusion diet, whose sleep normalized when the hydrolyzed hypoallergenic diet was interrupted, only to deteriorate again during challenge. The observation only presents further evidence about the difficulty of selecting an adequate milk substitute in a young child. Soya can be well tolerated, but did not favor any improvement in the behavior of six infants.

The age at which cow's milk avoidance can be interrupted remains to be determined. The clinical manifestations of cow's milk intolerance usually improve after the 3rd year of age (14). In the present group, double-blind milk challenges still induced insomnia at 2.5 and 3 years of age, and only at 57 months could one girl be safely allowed a normal diet, after an eventless milk challenge. Further follow-up of the children will help to determine the age at which milk-induced insomnia disappears.

We cannot explain why cow's milk intolerance induces insomnia in some children. The disturbance in sleep homeostasis cannot be ascribed to an immediate, reaginic type of allergic reaction. Metabolic, pharmacological, or immunological mechanisms could all contribute to the development of restlessness. Blood IgE levels were in the normal range for 11 out of 12 children tested.

It could be argued that our observations only describe common colic, with resulting abdominal discomfort and paroxysmal crying. Infantile colic is found in up to 20% of infants (7), mainly under 4 months of age, and rarely persists beyond this age. Colic has been attributed to a variety of factors, including hypersensitivity to cow's milk (3), although a scientific demonstration of causality is still lacking (3,7). Only occasionally does a change in diet prevent further attacks of colic. The children described in this report could hardly be considered as colicky babies. Their median age when referred for consultation was 13.5 months (range 2.5 to 48 months), and cow's milk-induced insomnia was still present in 16 children at the age of 21 months. This age range does not fit with the classical definition of colic, nor did the close relationship seen between the changes in behavior and the modifications of the diet. Skin itching, abdominal ache, gastroesophageal reflux, and respiratory distress were all excluded as potential causes for insomnia, either by medical history, questioning of the older children, or through laboratory investigations.

The association between insomnia and food intolerance could be genetically mediated, as illustrated by the history of atopy in 10 out of 17 families, or by the similar evolution seen in the twin brothers. The manifestations of agitated behavior, and of drenching night sweats in eight children that normalized with milk exclusion, could argue in favor of an autonomic nervous system involvement. Its contribution in the clinical manifestation of food intolerance has already been evoked (16). It is impossible, though, to evaluate its role in inducing arousals.

In conclusion, this report adds further evidence for the possible relationship between chronic sleeplessness and the presence of an undiagnosed intolerance for cow's milk in children. At this point of the study, whereas our data indicate the major importance of a biological factor in the polysymptomatic syndrome of the children investigated, we cannot rule out the presence of an interactive psychological component.

Because most insomniac infants respond successfully to changes in sleep routine, and to behavioral approaches, only the most persistent and severe cases should be considered potential candidates for the diagnosis of milk intolerance. When no other form of treatment is found for a chronically sleepless child, food intolerance should be suspected. An exclusion diet, managed under competent medical supervision, could within a few weeks bring the family the relief long awaited. Whenever possible, a double-blind, controlled provocation test with the offending food should be done to confirm the diagnosis of food intolerance.

ACKNOWLEDGMENTS

We thank Professor H.L. Vis for constant encouragement. This work was supported by the Fondation Nationale de la Recherche Scientifique (Grant 3.4543.83).

REFERENCES

1. Bernal JF. Night waking in infants during the first 14 months. *Dev Med Child Neurol* 1973;15:760–9.
2. Blurton-Jones N, Ferreira RMC, Farquar-Brown M, et al.The association between perinatal factors and later night waking. *Dev Med Child Neurol* 1978;20:427–34.
3. Jenkins S, Owen C, Bax M, Hart H. Continuities of common behavior problems in preschool children. *J Child Psychol Psychiatry* 1984;25:75–89.
4. Richman N. A community survey of characteristics of one to two-year-olds with sleep disruptions. *J Am Acad Child Psychiatry* 1981;20:281–91.
5. Bax MCO. Sleep disturbance in the young child. *Br Med J* 1980;5:1177–9.
6. Ferber R, ed. *Solve Your Child's Sleep Problems*. New York: Simon and Schuster, 1985.
7. Weissblut M, ed. *Healthy Sleep Habits, Happy Child*. New York: Fawcett Columbine Book. Ballantine Books, 1987.
8. Carey WB. Night waking and temperament in infancy. *J Pediatr* 1974;84:756–8.
9. Moore T, Ucko LE. Night waking in early infancy: Part I. *Arch Dis Child* 1957;32:333–42.
10. Elias MF, Nicolson NA, Bora C, et al. Sleep/wake patterns of breast-fed infants in the first two years of life. *Pediatrics* 1986;77:322–9.
11. Kahn A, Mozin MJ, Casimir G, Montauk L, Blum D. Insomnia and cow's milk allergy in infants. *Pediatrics* 1985;76:880–4.
12. Kahn A, Rebuffat E. Blum D, Casimir G, Duchâteau J, Mozin MJ, Jost R. Difficulty in initiating and maintaining sleep associated with cow's milk allergy in infants. *Sleep* 1987;10:116–21.
13. Kahn A, François G, Sottiaux M, Rebuffat E, Nduwimana M, Mozin MJ, Levitt J. Sleep characteristics in milk-intolerant infants. *Sleep* 1988;11:291–7.
14. Bahna SL, ed. *Allergies to Milk*. New York: Grune and Stratton, 1980.
15. Frick OL. What tests should a clinician ask for? In: Brostoff J, Challacombe SJ, eds. *Food Allergy and Intolerance*. London: Baillière Tindall, 1987;907–16.
16. Moneret-Vautrin DA. Food intolerance masquerading as food allergy: false food allergy. In: Brostoff J, Challacomber SJ, eds. *Food Allergy and Intolerance*. London: Baillière Tindall, 1987;836–49.

Food Intolerance in Infancy: Allergology, Immunology, and Gastroenterology, edited by Robert N. Hamburger. Carnation Nutrition Education Series, Vol. 1. The Carnation Co., Los Angeles/Raven Press, Ltd., New York © 1989.

Cow's Milk Proteins as a Cause of Infantile Colic

*Iréne Jakobsson, **Tor Lindberg, and *Lasse Lothe

*Departments of *Pediatrics, University of Lund, Malmö General Hospital, S-214 01 Malmö, Sweden; and **University of Umeå, Umeå, Sweden S-90185*

Infantile colic is a common and troublesome disorder for the infant and its parents. In spite of this, the nature of the disorder is still open for discussion (1).

Infantile colic is defined (2–7) as intermittent, unexplained excessive crying many times a day for at least 4 days a week and continuing for 1 week or more. Each episode lasts from 30 min to 2 hr and the infant cries for a total of approximately 3 hr or longer per day. The crying occurs at approximately the same time each day for the same infant. Although crying is generally regarded the major symptom in infantile colic, one or more of the following symptoms are often present: gas formation, hiccuping, vomiting, diaper rash, and disturbed sleep.

It is important to distinguish colic from normal or physiological crying. There are different opinions about normal crying time in infants of this age group. From various studies it seems to be around 1 hr/day (8–11). The overall frequency of infantile colic in the city of Malmö, Sweden, is around 20%.

Most probably there are several causes of this disease. In recent years psychosocial factors and/or a failure in the parent-infant interaction have been suggested as dominant primary causes (5–7,10).

Since 1978 we have published results of several studies indicating that cow's milk can elicit symptoms of infantile colic in certain infants, whether they are formula-fed or breast-fed.

INFANTILE COLIC IN FORMULA-FED INFANTS

Infantile colic is well known as a symptom in infants with cow's milk protein intolerance (12,13). In 1982 (3) our first study was published, indicating that cow's milk formula could be a cause of infantile colic.

Recently the results of another study (14) have been accepted for publication.

Twenty-seven term-born, Swedish infants aged 2 to 12 weeks (mean age 6.4 weeks), fed a cow's milk-adapted formula, were admitted during a period of 6 months, because of infantile colic according to definition. Clinical examination showed a group of well-nourished infants without diarrhea and with no signs of infection.

All 27 infants were put on a cow's milk-digested diet with a formula based on hydrolyzed casein (Nutramigen®). The symptoms of infantile colic vanished completely or diminished noticeably in 24 of the 27 infants, mostly within 2 days (Fig. 1). Twelve infants did not cry at all on Nutramigen. The other 12 infants who still cried had markedly decreased their crying time. The time of crying (Table 1) per day decreased significantly from the mean value of 5.6 hr on cow's milk-based formula to 0.7 hr on cow's milk-digested formula.

All 24 infants entered a double-blind crossover trial. Capsules were used containing either 135 mg bovine whey protein powder or 135 mg of human albumin powder as placebo substance. Challenge was done on the 6th and on the 10th day after introduction of cow's milk-free formula. One capsule was added to the bottle with formula five times a day. The amount of whey protein in five capsules corresponded to the amount in approximately 70 ml of whole cow's milk.

Eighteen of the 24 infants reacted with colic when challenged with capsules containing whey protein. Two infants reacted on placebo capsules and four showed no reaction on either capsule. The crying time was significantly longer after whey protein capsules than after placebo capsules.

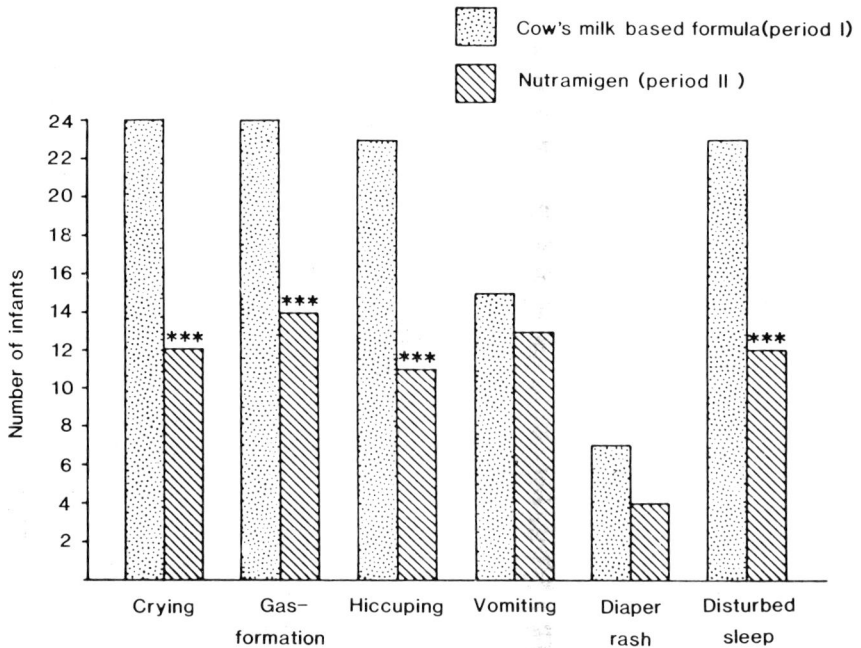

FIG. 1. Symptoms in colicky infants (N = 24) on cow's milk-based formula and on cow's milk-digested formula (Nutramigen®).

TABLE 1. *Crying in 24 infants with infantile colic on cow's milk-based formula (Period I), on cow's milk-free formula (day 3–5) (Period II), and when double-blind challenged with bovine whey protein (Period III)*

N = 24	Period I[a]	Period II[a]	Period III[a]	
			Whey protein	Placebo
Mean value ± SD (hr/day)	5.6 ± 2.0	0.7 ± 0.9	3.2 ± 2.4	1.0 ± 1.6
Paired *t* test (two-tailed)		$p < 0.001$	$p < 0.01$	$p < 0.01$
Mann-Whitney U-test		$p < 0.001$	$p < 0.001$	$p < 0.001$

INFANTILE COLIC IN BREAST-FED INFANTS

It has been recognized for approximately 50 years that substances can pass from mother to infant via the breast milk and cause adverse reactions in the infant (15–17). We know that infantile colic is as common in breast-fed as it is in formula-fed infants. The hypothesis that cow's milk proteins given to the mother could reach the infant via the breast milk, thus causing colicky symptoms of colic, was tested in 18 mothers with 19 totally breast-fed colicky infants (18). Cow's milk was totally eliminated from the mothers' diets. The colic disappeared within 1 to 2 days in 13 of the infants of this preliminary study. Figure 2 illustrates the symptoms in one infant in relation to the diet of mother and infant.

The patient is a girl with a family history of allergy. She was fed only human milk since birth. Colic started at age 3 to 4 weeks. When cow's milk was eliminated from the mother's diet, the colic promptly disappeared. Several challenges (a glass of milk to the mother) resulted in symptoms of colic within ½ hr after a breast-feed. At 3½ months, while still on breast milk, she did not react when challenged, and

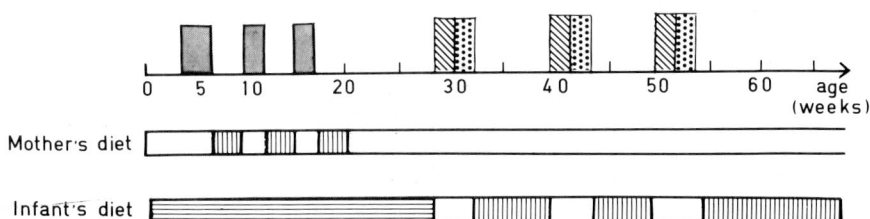

Fig. 2. Symptoms in relation to diet in a breast-fed colicky infant. ⊟ human milk, ☐ cow's milk, ▥ free of cow's milk, ■ colic, ⦂⦂ skin rash, ▨ diarrhea.

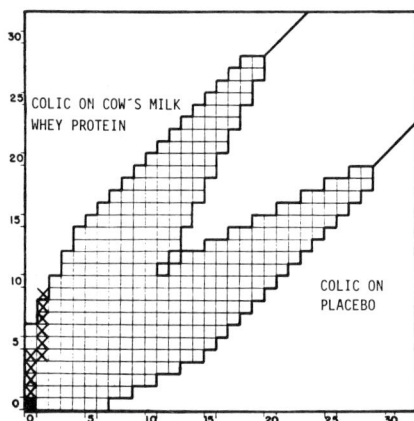

FIG. 3. Double-blind crossover trial of effect of cow's milk whey proteins, given to 10 mothers, on appearance of colic in their breast-fed infants.

the mother was able to take cow's milk again. When she was weaned at 6 to 7 months, she had diarrhea and skin rashes when given cow's milk and soy-based formula. The symptoms disappeared when she was given a formula containing hydrolyzed casein. Challenges on four occasions produced skin and gastrointestinal reactions each time. At age 10 months she also became intolerant to wheat. A small intestinal biopsy showed a slight mucosal damage.

In 1983, we reported (4) our extended experience on infantile colic in breast-fed infants and included a double-blind crossover challenge with bovine whey protein capsules. We observed 66 mothers with 66 breast-fed infants. The elimination of cow's milk from the mothers' diet resulted in disappearance of the colic in 35/66 infants (53%). After reintroduction of cow's milk into the mothers' diet, the symptoms reappeared within 8 hr in 23/35 infants (35%). The mothers of the remaining 12 infants could return to a normal cow's milk-containing diet without their infants showing any symptoms.

The group of 23 infants with relapse of colic after the mothers' intake of cow's milk constituted the group further studied. Challenge was done with capsules containing 200 mg bovine whey protein or potato starch as placebo. The capsules were taken by the mothers, three capsules four times a day according to a certain scheme.

Challenge was done in 10 mothers and infants. Results were analyzed with sequential analysis (Fig. 3). Nine infants reacted with colic after their mothers had ingested the capsules containing cow's milk whey protein. One infant had colic on the placebo capsules.

The conclusion drawn from the sequential analysis is the existence of evidence of a connection between bovine whey proteins and infantile colic.

BOVINE β-LACTOGLOBULIN IN THE HUMAN MILK

Since the beginning of this century up to 1985, several clinical investigations have shown a distinct correlation between mothers' intake of cow's milk and allergic symptoms in their breast-fed infants (4,15–18), but without any direct analysis on content of bovine milk proteins in the human milk.

Using animal models, a transmission of dietary protein has been shown to occur across the placenta to the fetus, and via milk to the suckling animal (19,20).

We have developed a radioimmunological method to analyze content of bovine β-lactoglobulin in human milk (21).

Out of the various bovine milk proteins, β-lactoglobulin was analyzed because several authors have shown that it is this protein that most often provokes symptoms in cow's milk-allergic infants (22,23).

Human milk samples were obtained from three mothers whose infants had infantile colic, which disappeared after the mothers changed to a diet free from cow's milk. Milk samples were collected with the mothers on a normal diet and on a diet free from cow's milk (Fig. 4). When placed on a cow's milk-free diet, two of the mothers had no measurable amounts of β-lactoglobulin in the milk whereas the third mother had 6 μg/liter. All three infants became free from colic within 5 days after change of diet.

To find out when β-lactoglobulin appears in the breast milk after intake of cow's milk, we studied one mother on a cow's milk-free diet (Fig. 5). At time 0 hr she drank 250 ml of cow's milk. Breast milk samples were then collected at every breast

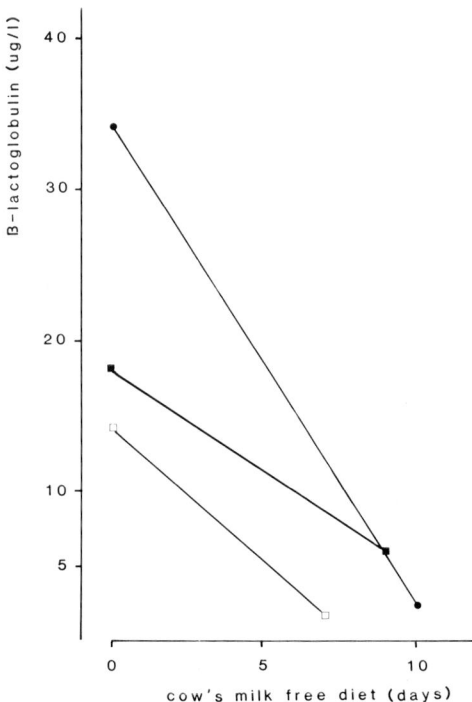

FIG. 4. Influence of a cow's milk-free diet on the content of β-lactoglobulin in the human milk from three mothers with colicky infants.

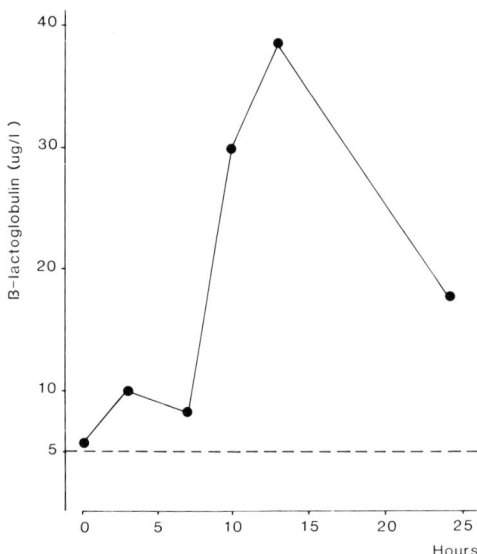

FIG. 5. Content of β-lactoglobulin in the breast milk of one mother after drinking 250 ml cow's milk at time 0 hr.

meal the next 24 hr when she continued on a cow's milk-free diet. As seen in Fig. 5, β-lactoglobulin had a peak concentration 8 to 12 hr after the cow's milk intake.

We have also done a longitudinal study (24) with determinations of bovine β-lactoglobulin content in human milk samples collected during the whole lactation period in mothers with allergic and nonallergic history. We have tried to correlate the amount of β-lactoglobulin in the human milk with cow's milk intake in the mothers and with presence of symptoms in the infants. Bovine β-lactoglobulin was detected in 93 out of 232 milk samples (40%) collected by 25 mothers. Six mothers (32 samples) had no detectable β-lactoglobulin in their breast milk on any occasion. Two mothers had measurable β-lactoglobulin in all their milk samples ($N = 27$). The content of β-lactoglobulin varied greatly between samples from one mother to another and also between samples from the same mother.

There was no correlation between daily cow's milk intake and concentration of β-lactoglobulin in the breast milk samples.

Seven mothers had more than 50 μg β-lactoglobulin/liter in at least one sample. Six of these seven mothers complained that their infants had diarrhea, vomiting, colic, or exanthema. Of the 18 mothers with β-lactoglobulin below μg/liter, the same symptoms occurred in five infants. This difference is significant.

It has been reported that intestinal permeability to macromolecules is increased in allergic patients (25). Therefore it seems plausible to assume that mothers with the highest amounts of β-lactoglobulin in their milk would have an allergic disease or a family history of allergic diseases. However, we did not find such a correlation in our study. However, the mother with high concentration of β-lactoglobulin in all her milk samples had a pronounced family history of allergy.

Other investigators have also shown content of food antigens in the human milk.

Stuart et al. (26) measured content of β-lactoglobulin with an enzyme-linked immunosorbent assay (ELISA) technique and found that 18% (compared to our results = 40%) of mothers had detectable β-lactoglobulin in their milks. Cant et al. (27) have studied cow's milk and egg proteins in the human milk in relation to eczema in the infants. They found concentrations of ovalbumin in the milk of the same magnitude in both mothers with and without infants with eczema.

One side of the problem of food antigens in the human milk is the risk of sensitization and development of food allergy already when the infant is fed only breast milk. Maybe this is a minor part of the problem, maybe development of intolerance is an exception rather than a rule. The content of food antigens in the human milk might be of importance for development of a proper immunologic response to common food antigens in the very young infant, i.e., a development of tolerance.

In mice (28) it has been shown that intraperitoneal injection of human gamma globulins to lactating mice did result in systemic tolerance in the nursing offspring, specific to these proteins. It has also been shown that the specific protein content in the diet of the pregnant and lactating animal (29,30) is of importance for the immunologic response of the offspring, i.e., the offspring becomes immunologically tolerant to proteins included in their mothers' diet.

INFANTILE COLIC AND MOTILIN

Intestinal hyperperistalsis has often been stated to play an important role in the pathogenesis of infantile colic. In recent years it has been stated that several of the gut hormones are involved in the regulation of gut motility (31). We were therefore interested in investigating some of these hormones in the serum of colicky infants (32). Motilin, vasoactive intestinal peptide, and gastrin were analyzed preprandially in infants with colic, in infants with other gastrointestinal disease, and in healthy infants. Interesting results were found concerning motilin (Fig. 6). The serum motilin

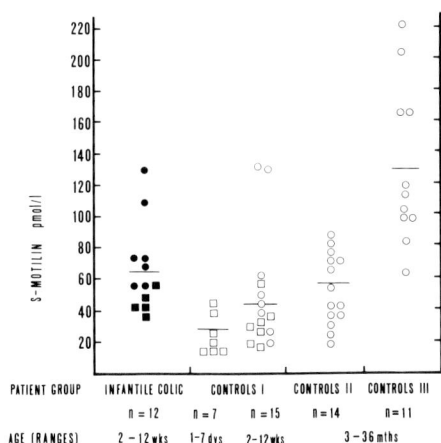

FIG. 6. Serum concentration of motilin (picomoles/liter) in infantile colic (closed symbols) and control groups (open symbols). Breast-fed infants (squares), formula-fed infants (circles).

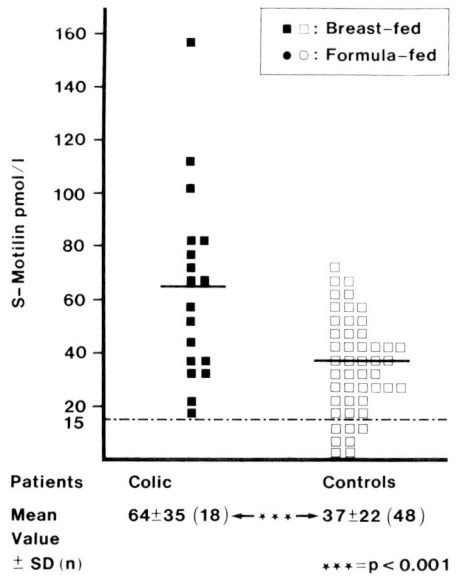

FIG. 7. Serum concentration of motilin (picomoles/liter) in term neonates who developed colic *(closed squares)* and in term neonate controls *(open squares)*.

levels were higher in infants with infantile colic compared with age-matched controls (Controls I were infants at the maternity ward or infants coming for control to the out-patient clinic. Controls II were infants admitted because of nongastrointestinal disorders. Controls III were infants admitted because of vomiting, prolonged diarrhea, or failure to gain weight).

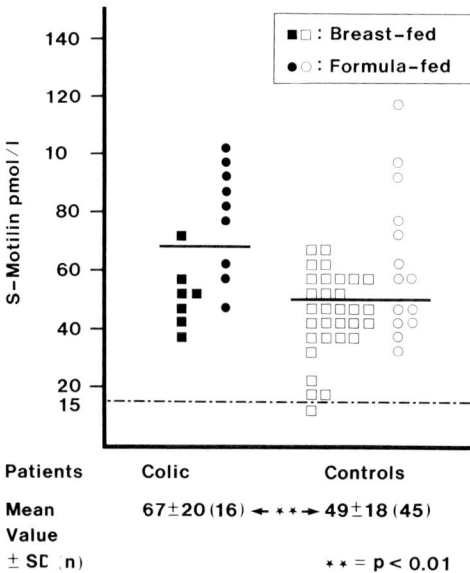

FIG. 8. Serum concentration of motilin (picomoles/liter) in 12-week-old colicky infants *(closed symbols)* and in age-matched healthy controls *(open symbols)*.

It could be speculated upon whether the increased motilin levels are a primary or a secondary phenomenon in infantile colic. An increased motilin level observed in other gastrointestinal disorders supports the latter hypothesis.

For further clarification, a prospective study was recently performed (Lothe et al., *manuscript in preparation*). Serum motilin has been analyzed in cord blood and in infants less than 24 hr of age (before being fed for the first time), at 6 weeks, and at 12 weeks of age. The study group consisted of 78 term infants. Nineteen developed infantile colic. Serum motilin level was increased in both cord blood and in serum from newborns (Fig. 7) in those infants who later developed infantile colic. The same difference was also seen at 6 and 12 weeks of age (Fig. 8).

This study could also conclude that formula-fed infants (with or without colic) had higher basal serum motilin levels than breast-fed infants. This difference between formula-fed and breast-fed infants has been reported earlier by Lucas et al. (33).

The increased level of serum motilin in infants with colic might be a primary phenomenon of importance in the development of infantile colic.

MACROMOLECULAR ABSORPTION IN INFANTS WITH INFANTILE COLIC

Several methods have been used to study gut permeability in man. Heterologous food proteins such as bovine serum albumin, ovalbumin, and cow's milk proteins have been used as markers (34,35). When serum concentrations of heterologous proteins are measured, local intestinal and systemic immune responses must be considered. The molecules used in most permeability studies are not proteins but, for example, lactulose or polyethylene glycols with relatively low molecular weights (25,36,37). The transfer of these substances through the gut membranes does not reflect the situation for transfer of food proteins (38).

We have developed a new method for measuring macromolecular absorption by using a human protein as a marker (39).

We have chosen human α-lactalbumin (mol wt 14,000), the dominant whey protein of human milk. This protein is not present in blood except in pregnant and lactating women and in infants after a human milk feeding.

Human α-lactalbumin has been purified from human milk. The purified protein has been used to develop a radioimmunological method for measuring content of human α-lactalbumin in serum.

Serum samples are analyzed for content of human α-lactalbumin 30 and 60 min after intake of a certain amount of human milk. Results are expressed as micrograms α-lactalbumin per liter serum per liter human milk given per kilograms body weight.

Serum α-lactalbumin has been analyzed in 40 breast-fed infants with infantile colic (Lothe et al., *manuscript in preparation*). Breast-fed colicky infants had increased absorption of human α-lactalbumin compared with breast-fed control infants of corresponding ages (Fig. 9).

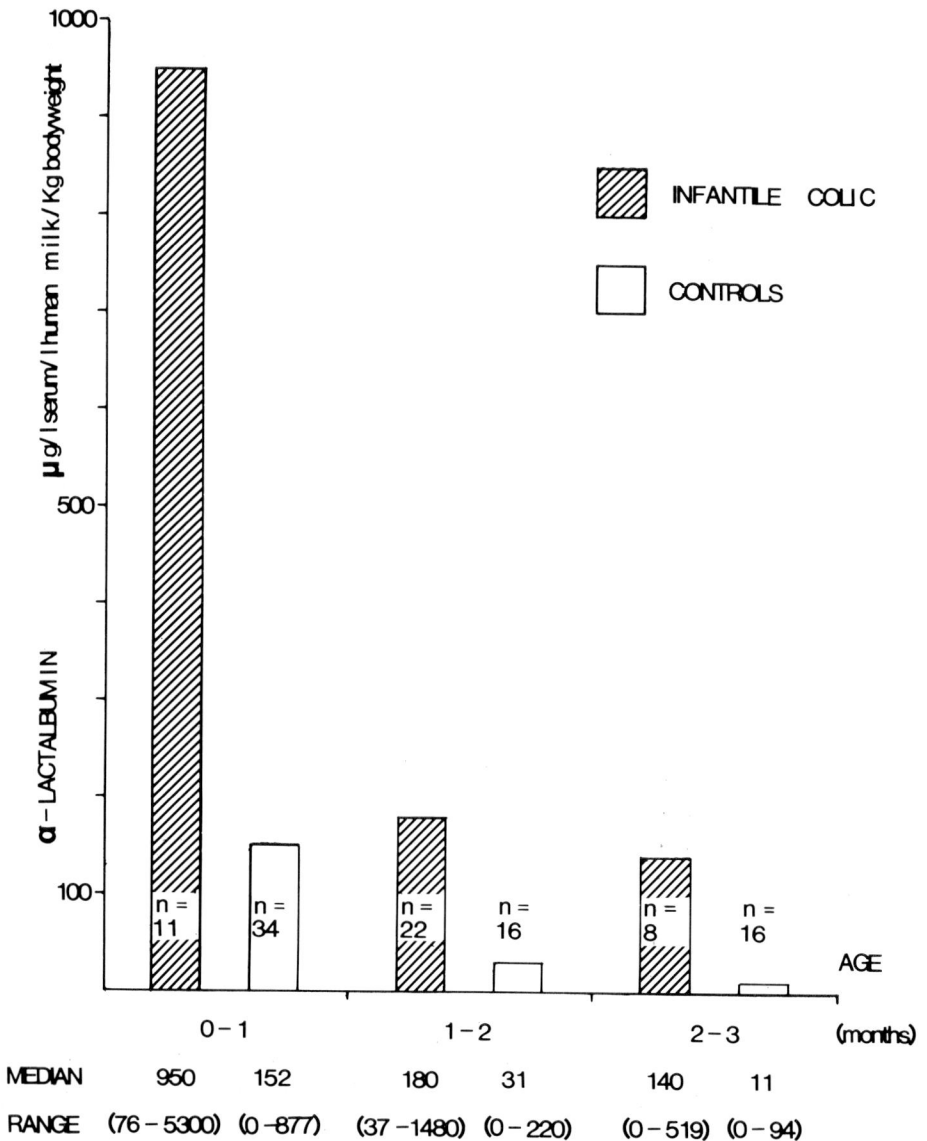

FIG. 9. Content of human α-lactalbumin in serum (micrograms α-lactalbumin/liter serum/liter human milk/kilograms body weight) in 40 breast-fed infants with infantile colic compared with aged-matched healthy controls.

Serum analyses were also done in 24 formula-fed infants with infantile colic. Colicky formula-fed infants had increased absorption of human α-lactalbumin compared to control infants (Fig. 10).

In conclusion, the analyses showed that infants with infantile colic have increased absorption of the macromolecule human α-lactalbumin. The increase was most pro-

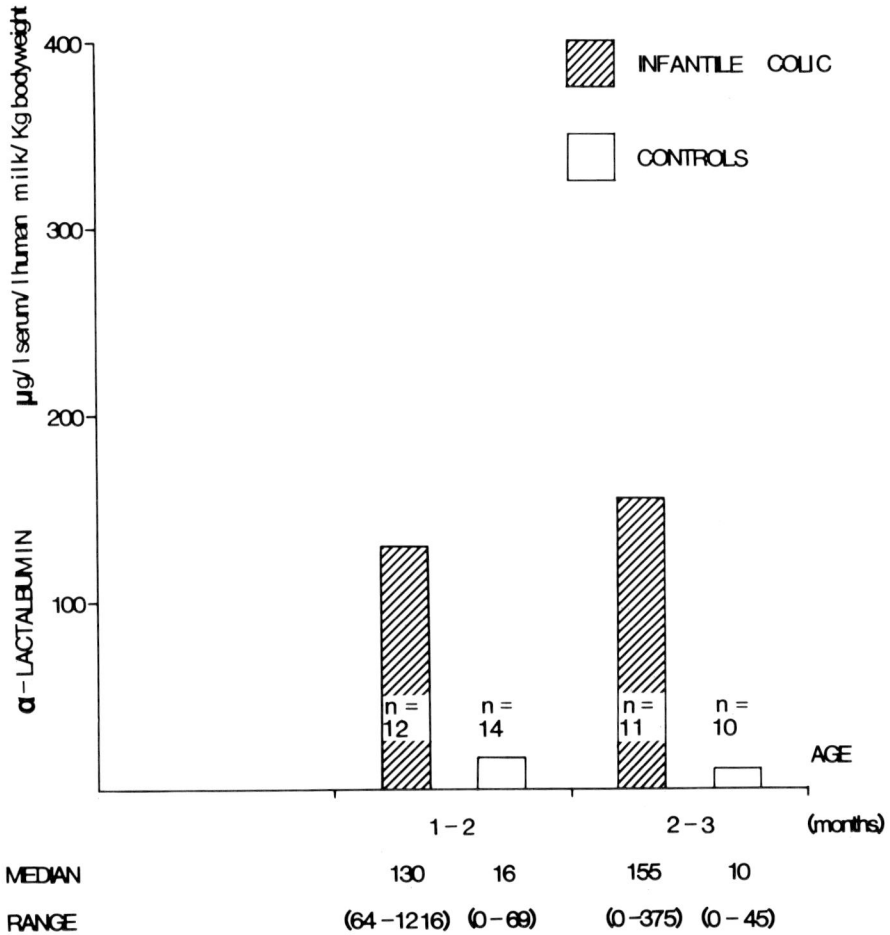

FIG. 10. Content of human α-lactalbumin in serum (micrograms α-lactalbumin/liter serum/liter human milk/kilograms body weight) in 24 formula-fed infants with infantile colic compared with age-matched healthy controls.

nounced in breast-fed infants. These findings might suggest that the gut mucosa is in some way affected in infants with infantile colic.

REFERENCES

1. Illingworth RS. Infantile colic revisited. *Arch Dis Child* 1985;60:981–5.
2. Wessel MA, Cobb JC, Jackson JB, et al. Paroxysmal fussing in infancy, sometimes called "colic." *Pediatrics* 1954;14:421–34.
3. Lothe L, Lindberg T, Jakobsson I. Cow's milk formula as a cause of infantile colic: A double-blind study. *Pediatrics* 1982;70:7–10.
4. Jakobsson I, Lindberg T. Cow's milk proteins cause infantile colic in breast-fed infants: a double-blind cross-over study. *Pediatrics* 1983;71:268–71.

5. Carey WM. "Colic"—primary excessive crying as an infant-environment interaction. *Pediatr Clin North Am* 1984;31:993–1005.
6. Schmitt BD. Colic: excessive crying in newborns. *Clin Perinatol* 1985;12:441–51.
7. Taubman B. Parental counselling compared with elimination of cow's milk or soy milk protein for the treatment of infant colic syndrome: A randomized trial. *Pediatrics* 1988;81:756–61.
8. Aldrich CA, Sung C, Knop C. The crying of newly born babies. I. *J Pediatr* 1945;26:313–26.
9. Brazelton TB. Crying in infancy. *Pediatrics* 1962;29:579–88.
10. Taubman B. Clinical trial of the treatment of colic by modification of parent-infant interaction. *Pediatrics* 1984;74:998–1003.
11. Hunziker UA, Barr RG. Increased carrying reduces infant crying: A randomized controlled trial. *Pediatrics* 1986;77:641–8.
12. Gerrard JW, MacKenzie JWA, Golnboff N, et al. Cow's milk allergy: Prevalence and manifestations in an unselected series of newborns. *Acta Paediatr Scand [Suppl]* 1973;234.
13. Jakobsson I, Lindberg T. A prospective study of cow's milk protein intolerance in Swedish infants. *Acta Paediatr Scand* 1979;68:853–9.
14. Lothe L, Lindberg T. Cow's milk whey protein elicits symptoms of infantile colic in colicky formula-fed infants. A double-blind cross-over study. *Pediatrics* 1989;83:262–6.
15. Talbot FB. Eczema in childhood. *Med Clin North Am* 1918;1:985–6.
16. Shannon WR. Demonstration of food proteins in human breast milk by anaphylactic experiments on guinea pigs. *Am J Dis Child* 1921;22:223–31.
17. Gerrard JW. Allergy in breast-fed babies to ingredients in breast milk. *Ann Allergy* 1979;42:69–72.
18. Jakobsson I, Lindberg T. Cow's milk as a cause of infantile colic in breast-fed infants. *Lancet* 1978;2:437–9.
19. Hemmings C, Hemmings WA. The transmission of dietary IgG to the milk and sucklings in rats. *IRCS (Int Res Commun Syst) Med Sci Libr Compend* 1977;5:247–8.
20. Dahl GMK, Telemo E, Weström BR, Jakobsson I, Lindberg T, Karlsson BW. The passage of orally fed proteins from mother to foetus in the rat. *Comp Biochem Physiol* 1984;77A:199–201.
21. Jakobsson I, Lindberg T, Benediktsson B, Hansson BG. Dietary bovine β-lactoglobulin is transferred to human milk. *Acta Paediatr Scand* 1985;74:342–5.
22. Bleumink E, Young E. Identification of the atopic allergen in cow's milk. *Int Arch Allergy* 1968;34:521–43.
23. Freier S, Kletter B, Gery I, Lebenthal E, Geifman M. Intolerance to milk protein. *J Pediatr* 1969;75:623–31.
24. Axelsson I, Jakobsson I, Lindberg T, Benediktsson B. Bovine β-lactoglobulin in the human milk. A longitudinal study during the whole lactation period. *Acta Paediatr Sand* 1986;75:702–7.
25. Jackson PG, Lessof MH, Baker RWR, Serrett J, McDonald DM. Intestinal permeability in patients with eczema and food allergy. *Lancet* 1981;1:1285–6.
26. Stuart CA, Twiselton R, Nicholas MK, Hide DW. Passage of cow's milk protein in breast milk. *Clin Allergy* 1984;14:533–5.
27. Cant A, Marsden RA, Kilshaw PJ. Egg and cow's milk hypersensitivity in exclusively breast-fed infants with eczema and detection of egg protein in breast milk. *Br Med J* 1985;291:932–5.
28. Halsey JF, Benjamin DC. Induction of immunologic tolerance in nursing neonates by absorption of tolerogen from colostrum. *J Immunol* 1976;116:1204–7.
29. Parhirana C, Goulding NJ, Gibney MJ, Jennifer M, Gallagher PJ, Taylor TG. Immune tolerance produced by pre- and post-natal exposure to dietary antigens. *Int Arch Allergy Appl Immunol* 1981;66:114–8.
30. Telemo E, Jakobsson I, Weström BR, Folkesson H. Maternal dietary antigens and the immune response in the offspring of the guinea pig. *Immunology* 1987;62:35–8.
31. Creuzfeldt W, ed. Gastrointestinal hormones. In: *Clinics in Gastroenterology*. London, Philadelphia, Toronto: WB Saunders, 1980;9:3.
32. Lothe L, Ivarsson SA, Lindberg T. Motilin, vasoactive intestinal peptide and gastrin in infantile colic. *Acta Paediatr Scand* 1987;76:316–320.
33. Lucas A, Adrian TE, Sarson DL, et al. Breast vs. bottle: endocrine responses are different with formula feeding. *Lancet* 1980;1:1267–9.
34. Dannaeus A, Inganäs I, Johansson SGO, Foucard T. Intestinal uptake of ovalbumin in malabsorption and food allergy in relation to serum IgG antibody and orally administered sodium cromoglycate. *Clin Allergy* 1979;9:263–70.
35. Roberton DM, Paganelli R, Dinwiddie R, Levinsky RJ. Milk antigen absorption in the preterm and term neonate. *Arch Dis Child* 1982;57:369–72.

36. Beach R, Menzies JS, Clayden GS, Scopes JW. Gastrointestinal permeability changes in the pre-term neonate. *Arch Dis Child* 1982;57:141–5.
37. Fälth-Magnusson KE, Kjellman N-IM, Sundqvist T. Intestinal permeability in healthy and allergic children before and after sodium-cromoglycate treatment assessed with different-sized polyethylene glycols (PEG 400 and PEG 1000). *Clin Allergy* 1984;14:277–86.
38. Weström B, Svendsen J, Tagesson C. Intestinal permeability to polyethylene glycol 600 in relation to macromolecular "closure" in the neonatal pig. *Gut* 1984;25:520–5.
39. Jakobsson I, Lindberg T, Lothe L, Axelsson I, Benediktsson B. Human α-lactalbumin as a marker of macromolecular absorption. *Gut* 1986;27:1029–34.

Food Intolerance in Infancy: Allergology, Immunology, and Gastroenterology, edited by Robert N. Hamburger. Carnation Nutrition Education Series, Vol. 1. The Carnation Co., Los Angeles/Raven Press, Ltd., New York © 1989.

General Discussion for Section III

David J. Atherton, William Heird, Iréne Jakobsson, André Kahn, Russell J. Merritt, John A. Walker-Smith, and Ekhard E. Ziegler

Dr. Goldstein: Paul Goldstein, Chicago, Illinois. I have several questions for Dr. Kahn. With regard to the response time of the infants with insomnia, your present protocol calls for about a 4-week trial of milk elimination before giving up on a response, but the response time in the handout on the 17 infants investigated states a range of 4 to 6 weeks with an average response time of about 5 weeks. Secondly, in the placebo segment challenge of your investigation, you used a 7-day span in providing the milk and then a placebo and then the milk to determine the response, which I understand was the response being fairly unequivocal in those patients in that particular time span. Was there a washout period that you're hypothesizing in the patient seen *de novo* that wasn't necessary for the patients that were somehow purged of the milk protein in their system, and that is why they responded in that short time unequivocally as opposed to the 4 to 6 week range initially in your work? And, finally, poorly sleeping, cow's milk protein-sensitive infants, presumably colicky infants, respond very rapidly, 1 to 2 days after elimination of that particular protein. Would you speculate on what may be happening pathophysiologically that might account for the 4- to 6-week response time in your work?

Dr. Kahn: I will try to answer all of your questions. First, indeed by looking backwards to the time needed for children who improved, to really improve, a 4-week period was the time needed. Some children improved much earlier, and much earlier means after 2 weeks, and we never saw a child who improved in less than that period of time. Turning to the physiopathologic part of your question, I have no explanation. Of course, it is very tentative to think that something is happening that needs to be eliminated. That time needed for natural elimination, would it be related to some type of antibodies and would 4 weeks be suitable for such a delay? I only can speculate. I have no data. As for the washout period, when you opened the double-blind placebo procedure, either the patient had no medication and no possible antigenic substances or the patient had it. If he didn't have it, we did not think it was necessary to have a washout period after the 7th day of administration. I turn to another of your questions. Seven days seems to be sufficient. I only can argue on a pragmatic basis because of observation. We have no theoretical documentation for seven days. On the other hand, if a child was being given by chance the allergenic cow's milk, then in that case we waited until the child was completely cleared of any manifestation once the challenge was interrupted, and then started on the other challenge without milk. In that case, yes, we had a washout period based on the clinical aspects of the child.

Dr. Goldstein: Dr. Atherton, in your work did you eliminate dairy products altogether, including yogurt, or just milk itself?

Dr. Atherton: Yes, all sources of milk protein completely; it is a complete dairy product elimination.

Dr. Zucker: Preston Zucker from New Jersey. Dr. Kahn, it has been my clinical impression that there is no difference in the sleep disturbance incidence between breast-fed and formula-fed babies. Could you comment on that question, and have you done similar studies with breast-fed mothers who restricted their milk intake?

Dr. Kahn: Let me start from the daily discussion we had with parents. Indeed, parents with breast-fed infants complain of more frequent arousals than parents with non-breast-fed infants, and that is the usual observation and I think it is a classical observation as well. Now, concerning real sleep disturbances, those infants who really cry out 4 or 5 hr per night and sleep less than 5 hr a night, in those cases we had no difference in breast-fed and non-breast-fed infants. We did indeed have some breast-fed infants who improved their behavior once the mother was put on an elimination diet. That was also reported for babies with colic.

Dr. Zucker: For Dr. Jakobsson, one of the old pseudoacademic names for colic was periodic irritability, the most common period being the late afternoon or early evening. Can you somehow correlate that with your findings?

Dr. Jakobsson: Could you restate the question, please?

Dr. Zucker: Yes. The most common period for irritability reported in colic is in the late afternoon and early evening. How can you explain that observation if at least a portion of colic is dietary and the diet remains the same during the entire day?

Dr. Jakobsson: I actually can only speculate. I have no real explanation, but we know that several substances in the body circulate in ups and downs, like waves, for instance, and maybe this is literally true for gut hormones. So I think it's possible to explain why colic could occur during some hours of the day and not during others.

Dr. Sturner: Sturner from Durham, North Carolina. Dr. Kahn, have you tried the hydrolyzed formula on normal babies or babies who are colicky without allergies? What is the effect on sleep in normal babies?

Dr. Kahn: I don't remember having tried it, I haven't tried it on babies without any symptoms apart from that child I reported to you where I was wrong when diagnosing the possible relationship between sleeplessness and milk tolerance. That in fact was just a behavior problem, a management problem. In that case that was one of the normal children with the hypoallergenic diet. In a previous study, we did measure prealbumin because we were very concerned about the growth curves of those children. The growth curves were perfect.

Dr. Sturner: What I was wondering about is whether the effect is due to elimination of some protein or possibly to something such as a neuropeptide in the hydrolyzed formula that could have a beneficial effect?

Dr. Kahn: It's a very good question and I can't answer it. The only argument would be on the chronology of the presentation of the symptoms, and once milk is reintroduced in the diet it's extremely fast. The response is extremely fast. So my presumption would be that something in the milk induces a series of reactions that may be related to something else in the central nervous system, whether it be a histamine liberation or whatever, I do not know. This is the way I view the phenomenon.

Dr. Sturner: Dr. Jakobsson, you noted that 24 out of 27 of the babies responded to the formula change to the hydrolyzed formula. I may have missed the response rate to the rechallenge. How many babies then were rechallenged and were positive of that group?

Dr. Jakobsson: If I remember correctly, I think 18 responded to the double-blind challenge, to the subsequent challenge with the whey proteins.

Dr. Sturner: You started out by saying that colic is multifactorial. Are there some predictive characteristics of babies that will tell you, apart from rechallenge, that they will be responders? And I'm wondering if you have a referral clinic that has more gastrointestinal (GI) flavor or something of that sort?

Dr. Jakobsson: A small group of these infants are atopic. They continue with atopic symptoms further on, like eczema. But most of the infants of this group are quite healthy afterwards.

Dr. Puglise: Puglise from Northern Virginia. Dr. Jakobsson, do you have any data about women who drank scalded or boiled fresh milk and its effect on the pickup or secretion of the α-lactalbumin?

Dr. Jakobsson: Actually I have not tested having the mothers drink boiled milk. It was possible for some mothers to take small amounts of foods containing cow's milk, but most of the mothers couldn't take anything at all containing cow's milk. So I think boiled milk would be a possibility for only a few of them.

Dr. Merritt: I am Dr. Russell J. Merritt, Associate Professor of Pediatrics at U.S.C., Childrens Hospital of Los Angeles and I would like to insert a comment on *The Importance of Subject Selection in Studies of Colic.* The etiology of infantile colic has been and remains a controversial question. There seems to be a developmental component to the colic syndrome since it resolves over time and it, and the developmental pattern of normal infant crying behavior, overlap. Some studies have concluded that the problem of colic and excessive crying is a behavioral disorder, while other studies suggest an allergic component.

Analysis of the differences in sample selection between some of these studies provides insight into the mechanism by which apparently disparate conclusions have been reached. Investigators interested in colic have studied crying behavior in samples of normal newborns in samples of infants with the colic syndrome. It is instructive to divide the studies of crying and symptomatic colic as to whether infants with possibly atopic symptoms are (a) specifically excluded, (b) included along with nonatopic infants, or (c) selectively included. When normal newborns are prospectively studied or potentially atopic infants are excluded from the study, behavioral interventions for colic appear effective. However, when potentially atopic infants are included along with other colicky infants, feeding interventions appear to be helpful, at least for some patients. When atopic infants are selectively included, feeding interventions appear to be even more effective. As these feeding interventions involve a change in milk or formula antigens, they suggest an allergic, or at least food-related, component to infantile colic.

This analysis of selection criteria suggests that patient or subject entry criteria may largely determine the conclusions that will be drawn. Infants without an allergic diathesis are likely to respond to behavioral interventions. On the other hand, colicky infants with atopic features respond to a change in their formula or in their mother's diet in breast-fed infants. Infants who develop the colic syndrome are probably from at least two populations. In feeding studies, as well as in clinical practice, we need to clearly define the crying or colicky group under evaluation and attempt to identify those infants with and without markers for allergic diathesis or acquired hypersensitivity.

Dr. Schmitz: I am Dr. Schmitz from Paris. I would like to ask a general question to the panel. We heard yesterday that the cow's milk protein intolerance was mainly due or related to the immaturity both of the gut and of the immunological system. This means that we expect cow's milk protein intolerance or other food intolerance to happen very early in the life of the baby. This morning we heard different reports on that. First, Dr. Walker-Smith said that in his experience cow's milk protein intolerance or food allergy begins later than it used to, between 6 months and 18 months of age, which is very late in the life of a baby. Then we heard Dr. Kahn say that his babies were around 1 year old, and at the end we heard Dr. Jakobsson say that her colicky children were less than 3 months old. So my question is are all these children affected by the same disease?

Dr. Hamburger: I would like to respond. There is a somewhat humorous clumping of observations in that question, but it actually reflects much of the confusion with which I am confronted by both parents and by pediatricians. My response, first of all, should have been "yes" when asked a question like that because, in fact, there was nothing incompatible with any of those statements. They all fit exactly the data that most pediatricians are familiar with. Infantile colic is a disease or syndrome which starts in the first few weeks of life and lasts for 3 or 3½ months; many of those babies are milk-intolerant and some of those are milk protein atopic. Dr. Walker-Smith stated very clearly that he sees them later because they are breast-fed or on modern heat-treated formulas. If they were on old-style milk or milk formulas they would start their symptoms just like the colics do. Other forms of milk intolerance such as colitis (not colic), or Heiner's syndrome are rarely seen before several months of age, yet Dr. Kahn's babies continued their symptoms well into the first year and later. I just wanted to say that those statements were all correct, and that you are obviously a very good listener, but none of them were incompatible with each other.

Dr. Jakobsson: I also would like to say I don't think we have talked against one another this morning. I think you can be intolerant to foods at any age, actually. As I told you, I have been very interested in studying permeability, gut permeability at different ages, and that is very important for the development of food allergy. If you recall my data on macromolecular absorption in breast-fed infants, and if we do a comparative analysis on preterm infants, we find that they have about 30 times higher absorption as the term infants. Then what will influence if the child will become tolerant or intolerant? That depends on a lot of factors, not only on gut absorption but, for instance, on heredity, atopic heredity, and many other things.

Dr. Steele: Marilyn Steele, Oklahoma City. I have a question directed to both Dr. Jakobsson and Dr. Walker-Smith. In this country we have three cow's milk formulas available. Two are whey-predominant and one is a casein-predominant formula. In your opinion, does that affect the outcome in terms of food allergy? In other words, is one more allergenic than the other?

Dr. Jakobsson: I think it could be important. A few years ago we did some studies on digestibility of different cow's milk proteins, and we found maybe a surprise for both ourselves and others that it is much easier to hydrolyze the casein fraction of the proteins than the whey proteins.

Dr. Walker-Smith: In the kind of patients that I see, I don't think it makes a difference. The thing that makes a difference in our experience is having a modern adaptive formula. It was when the older formulas and ordinary cow's milk were used that there was a higher incidence of problem. In responding to Professor Jacques Schmitz' comments, I think the specific milk formula is of some importance, but there is an intriguing unanswered question in all of this. We have heard about all of these different syndromes that I had mentioned in my talk, but why is it there is organ specificity. What is it that induces a particular syndrome? There is a broad spectrum of clinical features. I find it difficult to understand why a child has a small intestinal enteropathy at one particular stage of his or her life, and then, at another point in life another organ is affected. It's very, very complicated.

Dr. Nandyal: I am Raja Nandyal from Racine, Wisconsin. In premature infants, who are essentially growing premature infants, we rarely see colic. Sometimes our babies stay for 3 or 4 months and as far as I know, the incidence of colic in those babies even when they are fed with formulas made from cow's milk is very minimal. I was wondering, is there any study showing the difference in incidence of colic between babies who stay in the hospital for 3 to 4 months versus babies who are brought up at home?

Dr. Jakobsson: Actually, I don't think we see any difference between premature infants and full-term infants concerning colic, but I haven't done a study and I don't know if anyone else has. I can say one thing because there was one study reported not long ago to see if the incidence of cow's milk allergy was higher in premature infants, and they couldn't prove that.

Dr. Machtinger: Machtinger, San Francisco. My question is primarily for Dr. Kahn. Doctors Deamer and Crook and other researchers and clinicians have reported over a period of time a syndrome termed tension fatigue syndrome, which is often related to food allergy. I wonder if you would comment on the similarity or dissimilarity between that clinical syndrome and the patients whom you are describing?

Dr. Kahn: Indeed, that syndrome was described as early as 1916 if I am not wrong. What we see in our children, and I have no experience with patients above

5 years of age up to now, what we see in our children is a daytime fatigue which is manifested by agitation, by crying, and by difficulty in concentration, and that does not always appear evident until the child is taken off milk. At that time, what usually occurs is after a couple of weeks, after 2 weeks the parents enter your consultation ward smiling where they were crying before. They are smiling and they say, oh, doctor, that's wonderful, my child is not the same child any more. So you feel very proud and you say, well, he is sleeping well? And they say, oh, no, not at all, that hasn't changed, but the daytime behavior changed a lot, tremendously. Then if you are not wrong, after 2 more weeks the child starts to sleep; say in 2 or 3 more weeks, the child starts to sleep. What I mean is that the tension fatigue syndrome defined during the daytime seems to be also evident in our young patients and their behavior is perhaps not only related to what happens during the nighttime. It might be a direct effect during the daytime as well. We don't know whether there is headache and we don't know whether there is any sense of depression, or whatever it is. We don't have any available analysis, but what occurs seems to be evident in the daytime behavior. So I would agree with that definition. The point is that it is difficult to prove it, and therefore the procedure of exclusion and challenge seems to be necessary.

Dr. Fleisher: I'm David Fleisher from Los Angeles, California. The term, colic, implies pain emanating from a hollow viscus, like the colon. I am someone who has grave doubts that what we are calling infantile colic is 3-months colic or paroxysmal nocturnal fussiness, or whatever pseudoacademic term you want to apply to it, has very little to do with abdominal pain. Regardless of the pathogenesis of this crying, does anybody on the panel know of any data to suggest that this crying is due to somatic pain in the abdominal area versus somatic pain in the elbow versus inner tension having nothing to do with somatic pain?

Dr. Jakobsson: I think this is a very good question or comment because there is a discussion going on as to where the pain actually comes from. Maybe it actually comes from the head. The studies which I reported to you tell us that there is something going on in the gut, but if that is where the pain comes from or if it comes from somewhere else, I can't tell and I think no one else today knows. We know that the intestinal hormones are in the intestine, but they are also in the brain.

Dr. Kahn: I would like to comment on that question. It is not exactly related to your question, but I would like to comment nevertheless. I have been surprised by the sweating activity of the babies who are sleepless and agitated. Of course, if they cry and if they move a lot, they may sweat, but the increased sweating activity was possible, or evaporational activity at least was possible, to measure during nonagitation periods in non-rapid eye movement (non-REM) sleep. Whereas when they were in deep sleep we could not measure higher sweating activity in those infants. Does that implicate the autonomic nervous system and does the autonomic nervous system have anything to do with colic and with sleeplessness? I don't know.

Question: Is there a temperamental style that goes together with an autonomic style?

Dr. Kahn: I cannot answer. It's just a matter of observation.

Dr. Hamburger: I would like to make a comment about pediatricians and hollow viscus pain. We, like veterinarians, tend to "read" our babies, and interpret their behavior. When I see a baby passing flatus with a bloated stomach or a bloated belly and writhing, I read in pain; I interpret that as gas cramps. I think some of our colicky babies do indeed look as though they are having real hollow viscus cramps.

Dr. Fleshood: Lee Fleshood from Nashville, Tennessee. In the general population among term infants, what would be the prevalence or percentage of infants that would not do well on any one of the standard formulas, if you had a choice between milk and soy base formulas? What percentage of children at birth, if they were term infants, and then how would that change at 4 to 6 months?

Dr. Walker-Smith: Well, there are no data to answer that question. I would think a relatively small percentage of babies. In fortified formulas we are seeing highly selected children. These are children who are referred to us with problems from general practitioners to our tertiary referral centers. So we are actually seeing relatively small numbers in a westernized society. To answer your question I believe it would be in a very small percentage.

Dr. Fleshood: What would be the maximum percentage?

Dr. Walker-Smith: Again, it would be a pure guess. It might be 1%. If you add in other events, for example, if you are in a community where there is a lot of gastroenteritis, you would then see a higher incidence. However, if you continue on the modern adapted formula, I think the chances of becoming sensitized to cow's milk are still fairly low, but I wouldn't like to hazard a guess of how low. The percentage would be larger if you were in a community where there was much infection.

Dr. Fleshood: Is it safe to say that it would be less than 5%?

Dr. Walker-Smith: Yes, I should think so.

Dr. Kahn: Just a comment. Maybe some of the later speakers this afternoon will try to answer that question, but without hard data right now I would certainly not go above 1 or 2%. I understand Dr. Parkinson in London is going to run a field study to know what percentage of children with insomnia, chronic insomnia, have insomnia related to the problems we are dealing with right now. We are presently doing the same type of corroborative study in Belgium. But we have no data yet, but I expect it to be very low, a very small figure.

Dr. Erdman: Steve Erdman, Loma Linda, California. Many of the infants, particularly those older than 4 months of age that are referred to us for presumed milk and/or soy protein intolerance, have been exposed to a variety of other antigenic materials, particularly in the form of infant foods. The raging question our parents ask after you've had an acceptable response to a hypoallergenic formula is when can I feed the baby solids. This presents two issues, and I would like to ask the panel as a whole: when do you feed your babies that you have had an acceptable clinical response in, and what do you feed them?

Dr. Walker-Smith: Well, in the very special circumstance with the kind of babies that I see on various food elimination diets, we would introduce solids which were free of the particular antigen at the appropriate time. In England we recommend that solids come into the diet from the age of 6 months. If you are asking the question of how long should they remain on the elimination diet in general, we in fact challenge babies after 3 to 6 months on the elimination diet. This is usually between the age of 1 year and 18 months going up to 2 years.

Dr. Erdman: Any feel for what you would introduce first, as far as cereals, vegetables, or fruit?

Dr. Walker-Smith: Rice and potato are the ones which we particularly favor using at first.

Dr. Deckelbaum: Richard Deckelbaum, New York. In considering food intolerance and colic, one of the problems that colicky babies might have would be associated nausea. Since we don't know what colic is due to, why not put nausea in as well as a cause of colic? Gas retention certainly is associated with nausea and adults can describe that and document it. When changing formulas we are also changing lipid sources and fat sources in the different formulas. Has anyone looked at the effect of changing lipids in food intolerances and particularly or independently, has anyone looked at the relationship of gastric emptying time to food intolerance?

Dr. Jakobsson: I don't know of any study like that actually, but you don't change the fat content if you continue on breast milk, but of course you could do it if you change one formula to another. Of course, vomiting is quite a common symptom of food intolerance as well.

Dr. Walker-Smith: Certainly gastric stasis is seen with children where vomiting is a major feature, and this certainly is a major clinical manifestation of some of the children that we see with cow's milk intestinal enteropathy.

Dr. Fish: I am Lloyd Fish from Minneapolis, Minnesota. I would like to address my question to Dr. Walker-Smith. It is in regard to the cow's milk-sensitive enteropathy that you spoke about so elegantly earlier. Is the cow's milk an effective mitogen either on the biopsy specimen or on the lymphocytes from those individuals?

Dr. Walker-Smith: Well, it's speculation. The speculation that I have made is based on the work of Dr. Tom MacDonald (MacDonald TT, et al. JEEM 1988;167:1361–9) is that cow's milk antigens pass across the epithelium and they then in some way activate sensitized thymus-derived cells (T cells). Thus, the pathology is related to activation of T cells in the mucosa. The actual precise mechanism required to produce an enteropathy isn't clear. One guesses that some kind of lymphokines are then produced from the lymphocytes.

Dr. Fish: One would suspect that if your rodent model was analogous to what is going on in humans, you might be able to show that in tissue culture from the biopsy specimen.

Dr. Walker-Smith: Oh, right. I see what you mean, using it directly in the *in vitro* system. Yes, we are planning to actually do that. Clearly we need to add a number of dietary food antigens/antibody complexes into the fetal organ culture system. One of the striking things about the fetal organ culture system is that the epithelium is absolutely normal when you look at it under the electron microscope. This is clearly different from celiac disease where the epithelium is very abnormal. So activation of the T cells per se is causing lamina propria events, but it is not actually damaging the enterocyte. As a generalization in cow's milk-sensitive enteropathy, the epithelium is much less damaged than in celiac disease. So the model in some ways fits much more with the situation found in cow's milk-sensitive enteropathy, where the epithelium is much less damaged than in celiac disease. I don't believe that activation of the T cells per se can be the only thing. It would be too simplistic, and nature and biology are so much more complicated. There must be other factors that are going on as well. We've been talking about these 3 allergic mechanisms of injury classified by Gell and Coombs as types 1, 3, and 4. It may be that there is an element of all 3 of these mechanisms involved in the pathogenesis of the enteropathy. For example, that immune complex deposition is a factor which is having a pathological role as well. I think the *in vivo* situation is extremely complicated. John Soothill, London, England, talked about the adjuvant role of bacterial infection either by toxins produced by bacteria or various bacterial products. These may have a role, too.

Dr. Seker: Dr. Seker from Illinois. My question is addressed to Dr. Kahn. I was interested in his studies of sleep disturbance as associated with milk intolerance. I want to know if you have extended your studies to see if milk intolerance is related to learning disability and hyperactivity in the older kids.

Dr. Heird: Is the question, is milk intolerance related to learning disabilities?

Dr. Seker: I wanted to know if you have any experience to see if milk intolerance is related to symptoms in older kids. I know there is a lot of controversy about diet and hyperactivity and all those things.

Dr. Kahn: Well, I honestly cannot answer your question. We have pieces of evidence concerning school performances in children with insomnia and chronic insomnia at a later age, but we are not dealing any more with the same type of pathology. The environmental conditions are so much different and the study designs are so far away from what has been done in what I have reported to you that I would hate to join the conclusions of the two studies. So to be honest, I cannot answer your question now.

Dr. Robberecht: Robberecht from Belgium. I have a question for Dr. Walker-Smith. There is growing evidence as you showed for the frequent occurrence of colitis in cow's milk protein allergy. In at least one center I know, they turn it the other way around and use it as the method for diagnosing cow's milk protein intolerance. In fact, they perform proctoscopy in every child suspected of having a cow's milk protein allergy and look whether they find something or not. Could you comment on that?

Dr. Walker-Smith: Jean Pierre Olives has done endoscopies in children with cow's milk-sensitive enteropathy. In fact, in that study the majority of children with cow's milk-sensitive enteropathy had histological changes in the colon. I'm struck as a clinician by the two distinct patterns in general presentation of cow's milk allergy. First, children with cow's milk-sensitive enteropathy are usually babies presenting with failure to thrive and malnutrition, i.e., clearly having a small bowel problem. Second, children with cow's milk colitis very often are well-nourished children whose only abnormality is that they pass bloody stools. The two disorders have quite different clinical pictures. Pathologically there may be some overlap as there are histological changes in the colon in some of the children with the cow's milk-sensitive enteropathy as referred to above. Recently we had an international celiac symposium in London at St. Bartholomew's Hospital and data were presented that biopsy of the rectum of patients with celiac disease quite often showed a proctitis. So in practice I think you have to biopsy the organ that seems to be affected clinically. In clinical practice as a gastroenterologist, we are not just thinking of cow's milk-sensitive enteropathy in a bottle-fed infant with chronic diarrhea and malnutrition, but we are thinking of giardiasis, postenteritis enteropathy, sucrase and maltase deficiency, and autoimmune enteropathy, hypogammaglobulinemia, and even AIDS. There are indeed a whole series of other investigations that might be relevant as well as a small bowel biopsy. So I think you have to be guided in your diagnostic approach by the organ which you think in fact is involved.

Dr. Cohen: Stan Cohen from Atlanta, Georgia. This is directed to Doctors Kahn and Jakobsson. We have been talking here predominantly about intact proteins and their effect. Yet we have accumulated data some time ago about the use of carbohydrates, their altering colic-type symptoms and direct effect on gastric motility. My first question is whether other components besides the proteins have been looked at in affecting both vasoactive intestinal peptide (VIP) and motilin. Then, secondly, I want to ask whether Dr. Kahn has looked at taurine or tryptophan regarding symptoms such as sleep?

Dr. Jakobsson: The only answer I can give you is that we actually did double-blind studies using proteins, but we have not studied changes in other types like carbohydrates and fats.

Dr. Kahn: As for my part, we try to supplement some of those children, I must confess it's a limited number of cases, but we tried to supplement them with tryptophan. The idea behind tryptophan is to induce sleep through the metabolism of *serotonin*. We saw no difference when we tried to do that on a control/placebo basis. Tryptophan versus placebo made no difference in those children.

Dr. Walker-Smith: Could I ask Dr. Atherton to comment on the role of disodium chromoglycate in the treatment of the children he described?

Dr. Atherton: We did a study, a double-blind controlled trial of oral disodium chromoglycate in a completely unselected group of children with atopic dermatitis. They weren't selected for the presence of suspected food allergy or anything like that. In fact, there was absolutely no difference at all; it was clearly not therapeutically beneficial in unselected children. I must confess that at that time we rather lost interest. If we had had a group of children where there was well-documented aggravation of atopic dermatitis by foods, and those children are very few and far between; if you have such a group, then they would justify some kind of study, but I always felt that the correct treatment for food provocation of atopic dermatitis was food elimination and not some attempt to mask it with medication. But as some of you well know, there have been studies, and particularly one from Rome, which did suggest that children with atopic dermatitis could relax their dietary measures. With children who benefited from diet if they then had disodium chromoglycate they could on occasion relax their diet. But I must confess that I wasn't by myself terribly convinced by that because, as I said, those sort of children are very few—the sort of children who have very regular exacerbation of atopic dermatitis by food are relatively few and far between.

Dr. Heird: How high was the dose of cromalyn that you used? Luisa Businco, in the study that you're talking about from Rome, used enormous doses to get that effect, that blocking effect.

Dr. Atherton: As a matter of fact, I can't actually remember the dose we used. I think it was about 200 mg 4 times a day. So they were high, but slightly higher than standard doses.

Dr. Sandberg: My name is Sandberg from Miami, Florida. I have a question for Dr. Kahn about the formula which you were using, a formula that was a whey protein-based formula; is that correct?

Dr. Kahn: Yes.

Dr. Sandberg: I was just wondering whether there might be some relationship with endorphin-like molecules. As I remember correctly, the exorphin-type molecules from milk were casein-related, β-caso-morphin. Do you have any thoughts about that?

Dr. Kahn: We have been thinking about the effect of milk administration. Would that be enhanced by the industry manipulation of milk? I cannot answer. That's something that should be looked into. I have only an indirect argument, and my indirect argument is that the only thing enhancing sleep effect might not be only the aspect that we have been studying. I'm referring to the speed with which those infants deteriorate again when they are challenged. But that does not put aside your question, which also should be looked into.

Dr. Heird: Dr. Atherton would like to make one more comment before we take the next question.

Dr. Atherton: With reference to the earlier question about disodium chromoglycate, we have done some studies on topical disodium chromoglycate, and the interesting thing is that it doesn't actually block cutaneous mast cells at all. Thus, you can inject disodium chromoglycate into the skin and do a prick test and then you inject disodium chromoglycate into the skin and it doesn't inhibit the skin test reaction. So the question is, if it works obviously, what is the mechanism? It would have to be some other effect on the gastrointestinal tract.

Dr. Kerzner: Dr. Walker-Smith, I am concerned that there are going to be many mothers who are going to be deprived of cow's milk and other sources of protein to treat poorly defined entities such as breast milk colitis, sleep disorders, and colic. I wonder if we can select the relevant infants a little more carefully. In the area of cow's milk colitis, you mentioned that eosinophils in the colonic mucosa are an index. I would think isn't it eosinophils penetrating the basement membrane into the crypt; the mere presence of eosinophils in the lamina propria is too nonspecific.

Dr. Walker-Smith: Well, I'm not so sure about that actually. Some of these cases of cow's milk colitis in infancy that have responded to milk elimination do have only a generalized increase of eosinophils within the lamina propria. However,

I do share your general concerns. I hope people are not going to go away thinking that cow's milk colitis is a terribly common disorder which in fact requires endoscopy and mucosal biopsies in every case. This is in contrast to suspected cow's milk-sensitive enteropathy where, in my view, because they are severely ill such children with chronic diarrhea and failure to thrive do require a small bowel biopsy in every case to make a diagnosis. The child with suspected milk colitis, in the first instance, if it's mild, warrants a therapeutic trial of a milk-free diet, in our practice, and at most just a simple proctoscopy. It is only when there is a failure to thrive or the child is more seriously ill with very severe bloody diarrhea that ones goes ahead to perform a colonoscopy to include chronic inflammatory bowel disease. It's difficult to generalize about these matters. I think when you see individual patients, you use your clinical judgment. But I don't want to exaggerate the need for endoscopy. Nevertheless, total colonoscopy is what we recommend in any child in whom we suspect chronic inflammatory bowel disease or enterocolitis as a diagnosis.

Dr. Kahn: I think that I must answer your comment, and I think it's a very important comment. What I tried to do this morning is to limit the field of application. This is what I have been telling you at the beginning as well as at the end of the presentation, and I am again going to repeat that aspect. I have been repeating that this is only a limited number of children I was dealing with, less than 10% or 11% of all of my own clinical referrals, and certainly more than 55% of the cases can be easily treated with a change in feed, but you are right to stress that point again.

Dr. De Vlieger: Hugo De Vlieger from Belgium. I have a question to Professor Walker-Smith. Enteritis may induce or precipitate cow's milk intolerance. I would like to have your comment on that statement in view of your experience in intestinal biopsies.

Dr. Walker-Smith: Well, we certainly see children who have had gastroenteritis, rotavirus gastroenteritis, or entrapathogenic *Escherichia coli* enteritis who then fail to recover and continue to have diarrhea. We then find an abnormal small intestinal mucosal biopsy. The minimum time is 3 weeks after the acute gastroenteritis before we biopsy these children. Those who have an abnormal mucosa and then respond to a milk elimination diet we would diagnose as cow's milk-sensitive enteropathy. In the past, we proved in some of these children that this was so by means of serial biopsies related to elimination and challenge. Whether gastroenteritis actually unmasks preexisting cow's milk sensitization or whether in fact such sensitization is the cause by damaging the mucosa and permitting an increased amount of antigen to enter the mucosa is not certain. Increased antigen in the mucosa per se is not enough to cause cow's milk sensitization because it has been shown some years ago by Gruskay and Cook that most children during acute gastroenteritis have excess antigen entry. There is a group of these children who are selected out, and I don't understand why exactly that is. I wonder if it is related to the antigenicity of the proteins, as I have said earlier, but I'm also wondering whether there is some particular vulnerability of the small intestine in these children. It may be related to the immaturity of the T cell system, the T4:T8 ratio, i.e., the helper/suppressor ratio. Whether there is some disequilibrium or some immaturity of the T cell system, I don't know.

Question: Is there any difference in milk-associated symptoms in children whose mothers have high concentrations of milk during pregnancy versus those with low concentrations of milk during pregnancy?

Dr. Jakobsson: I think Dr. Kjellman should answer that question because he did a study where they varied the diet during pregnancy and found no differences. Actually, we are just now doing a study where I come from, Malmö, Sweden, and maybe in 1 or 2 years I can give you the results. We have just started. We are studying the families during pregnancy, but we are doing nothing to foods in the diet of the mother. But when the children are born, we are varying their intake during the first 3 days of life. One group is given breast milk, one group is given a common adapted cow's milk formula, and a third group a hypoallergenic formula, and then all children are breast-fed again. Those children we will follow up concerning the absorption of macromolecules in the gut and the immunological development.

Dr. Hamburger: We asked the same question that you did but looked at it in a different way. We measured the amount of immunoglobulin G (IgG), maternal IgG anti-cow's milk, which is a crude measure of the amount of cow's milk mother is drinking during pregnancy. We looked at it in the cord, which is mother's IgG, and looked for a correlation between the amount of the IgG and the amount of response in terms of IgE sensitization. That is, whether they were tolerized or sensitized, and we saw no correlation. That was only in 60 babies of several hundred in our prophylaxis study. So we could have missed it, but at least with a quick look, we didn't see tolerization in human infants. That type of study done in animals (rodents) does clearly show tolerization.

Food Intolerance in Infancy: Allergology, Immunology, and Gastroenterology, edited by Robert N. Hamburger. Carnation Nutrition Education Series, Vol. 1. The Carnation Co., Los Angeles/Raven Press, Ltd., New York © 1989.

Introduction to Section IV

Samuel J. Fomon

Department of Pediatrics, Division of Pediatric Nutrition, College of Medicine, The University of Iowa, Iowa City, IA 52242

I should like to present my estimate of the frequency of adverse reactions to milk-based or isolated soy protein-based formulas in young infants. Our experience presents a sharp contrast to that of the pediatric allergists. Their patients are highly selected for adverse reactions or family history of adverse reactions, whereas, in the case of our normal infants, there may be some self-selection in the opposite direction, with the possibility that families with strong history of atopy may rather infrequently volunteer to enroll their infants in our formula studies. We enroll apparently healthy infants by the 9th day of life and follow them closely until 112 or 196 days of age, depending on the nature of the studies and the parents' willingness for the infant to continue in a study beyond 112 days of age. We know in each instance the stated reason for discontinuing participation in the study. Some of the reasons are unrelated to feeding (e.g., moving away from the city). Some parents suspect that objectionable infant behaviors such as fussiness or spitting up are caused by an experimental milk-based formula, and report that the problem is solved by feeding a commercially available milk-based formula. If we exclude all dropouts for whom there is little likelihood that the cause of withdrawing from the study was formula-related, we are left with 2 or 3% of the total number enrolled who might have experienced adverse reactions to the formula. If these infants had been subjected to double-blind placebo-controlled testing, it would be remarkable to be able to confirm diet-related adverse reactions in one-third of the infants. Thus, my guess is that of the infants enrolled in our studies, less than 1% demonstrate adverse reactions to milk-based or isolated soy protein-based formulas during the early months of life.

REFERENCE

Ziegler EE and Fomon SJ, *this volume*.

Food Intolerance in Infancy: Allergology, Immunology, and Gastroenterology, edited by Robert N. Hamburger. Carnation Nutrition Education Series, Vol. 1. The Carnation Co., Los Angeles/Raven Press, Ltd., New York © 1989.

The Melbourne Milk Allergy Study, 1976 to 1988

David J. Hill and C.S. Hosking

Allergy-Clinical Immunology Unit, Royal Children's Hospital, Melbourne 3052, Australia

The multiplicity of poorly defined illnesses and the variability of pathological lesions caused by milk ingestion in children have led to difficulties in the diagnosis of cow's milk allergy (CMA). Several well-defined syndromes (1–6) have been associated with CMA (Table 1) but it is our experience these affect <5% of all children with this disorder. Difficulties in the recognition of CMA probably stem as much from a healthy cynicism regarding various aspects of allergic diseases as from a failure to appreciate the nonanaphylactic or delayed-onset manifestations of this disorder.

In this review, the effects of a controlled milk challenge in young children suspected of suffering from CMA are described to emphasize the diversity of this disorder. In addition, the relationship between these diverse clinical forms of CMA and various markers of different immune hypersensitivity mechanisms is explored and the natural history of the disorder examined. This report is based on studies at our center over a 12-year period.

We have defined CMA as an adverse reaction to cow's milk protein; other causes of milk intolerance (e.g., lactase deficiency as a cause of gastrointestinal disturbance, and milk aspiration as a cause of bronchitis) have been excluded. In this paper the terms CMA, cow's milk protein intolerance (CMPI), and cow's milk enteropathy (CME) have been used interchangeably. Specific immunological sensi-

TABLE 1. *Syndromes associated with cow's milk allergy*

Milk-induced pulmonary disease (1)	(Heiner & Sears, 1962)
Allergic gastroenteropathy (2)	(Waldemann et al., 1967)
Iron losing enteropathy (3)	(Wilson et al., 1964)
Neonatal thrombocytopenia—TAR (4)[a]	(Whitfield & Barr, 1976)
Neonatal thrombocytopenia (5)	(Jones, 1977)
Milk-induced colitis in infancy (6)	(Gryboski et al., 1966)

[a]TAR, thrombocytopenia-absent radius (syndrome).

tivity, not exclusively immunoglobulin E (IgE) associated, to one or more milk antigens is assumed to be the basis of the adverse clinical response to cow's milk described.

CLINICAL MANIFESTATION OF COW'S MILK ALLERGY

The 100 patients with CMA who made up the initial cohort were challenged with cow's milk in a specialized hospital unit for the first 2 days (7). If this volume of milk was tolerated, the challenge was continued at home but patients were reviewed subsequently at the time of any suspected adverse reaction, as well as 1 week and 1 month after commencement of milk ingestion. On Day 1: 10, 20, 30, and 60 ml of cow's milk were ingested at 30-min intervals. On Day 2: 120 ml was given as a sin-

TABLE 2. *Clinical features of 100 infants with proven cow's milk allergy*

Clinical feature[a]	Incidence
Gastrointestinal	
Vomiting	41
Diarrhea	48
Colic	14
Colitis[b]	4
Functional intestinal obstruction[b]	3
Generalized anaphylaxis[b]	
Stridor, collapse	2
Dermatological features	
Urticaria (general)	10
Angioedema	13
Circumoral lesions	26
Morbilliform eruptions	6
Eczema	13
Perianal eruptions	1
Respiratory	
Stridor (recurrent)	4
Rhinitis	21
Cough, wheeze	29
Tachypnoea	1
Nervous system	
Irritability[b]	40
Syncope—collapse alone[b]	12
Convulsion[b]	2
Other manifestations	
Anemia[b]	2
Osteoporosis[b]	1
Severe failure to thrive[c]	22
Gross gastroesophageal reflux (radiological)[b]	6

[a]All symptoms elicited by challenge unless otherwise indicated.
[b]Features attributed to milk ingestion prior to formal challenge.
[c]Weight < 3rd percentile.

gle morning dose. On Day 3: 240 ml as a single morning dose, and from Day 4: a normal intake (>300 ml per day) was ingested.

Every effort was made to follow this schedule but in some cases of suspected profound hypersensitivity, or where parents were reluctant to increase milk intake rapidly, a slower incremental dose was used. The precise volume of milk ingested, and the time of onset of specific reactions from the time the challenge commenced, was documented. There were 64 boys and 36 girls (median age 16.2 months); 5 children were older than 3 years at the time of diagnosis in the first study.

In Table 2, the symptoms elicited by milk challenge as well as some clinical features of these patients are recorded. Most skin lesions developed rapidly within an hour of commencing milk. However, some patients developed eczema rapidly, whereas others took hours or days to develop these lesions (Fig. 1). Relatively small volumes of milk precipitated vomiting symptoms in some children, but larger vol-

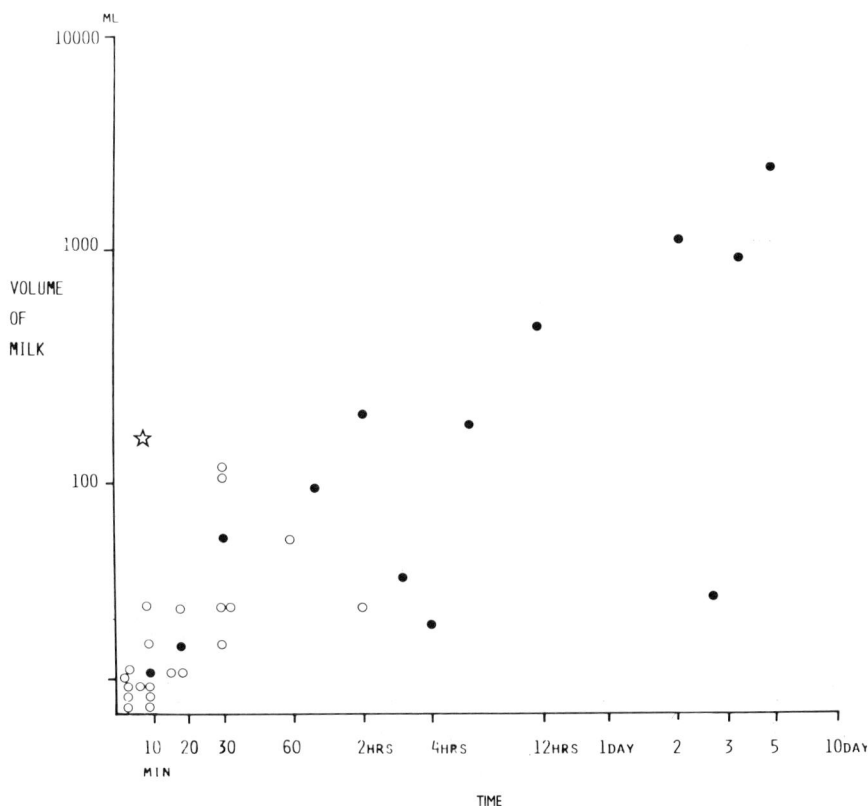

FIG. 1. Development of cutaneous lesions after cow's milk challenge. The vertical axis shows the volume of milk given up to the time of development of symptoms, and the horizontal axis shows the time after beginning formal milk challenge for the first signs of shock *(star)*, urticaria *(open circle)*, or eczema *(closed circle)*.

umes of milk were ingested before diarrhea developed (Fig. 2). Nearly a third of the patients developed respiratory symptoms on challenge. Small volumes of milk precipitated acute stridor or wheeze, in association with skin eruptions in some patients, whereas others ingested larger volumes of milk before coughing and bronchitic symptoms developed (Fig. 3). More than half the patients with respiratory symptoms had cutaneous manifestations of CMA and a third demonstrated some gastrointestinal disturbance, usually diarrhea. Respiratory manifestations of CMA remain one of the more controversial aspects of this disorder; of the patients in this study, 5% displayed respiratory symptoms alone as the sole manifestation of CMA. None demonstrated rhinitis as the only adverse clinical response to milk ingestion.

The results of these initial studies highlighted: (a) the different rates of evolution of various manifestations of CMA as elicited by the challenge protocol followed, and (b) the multisystem effect of CMA in most patients. These findings emphasized

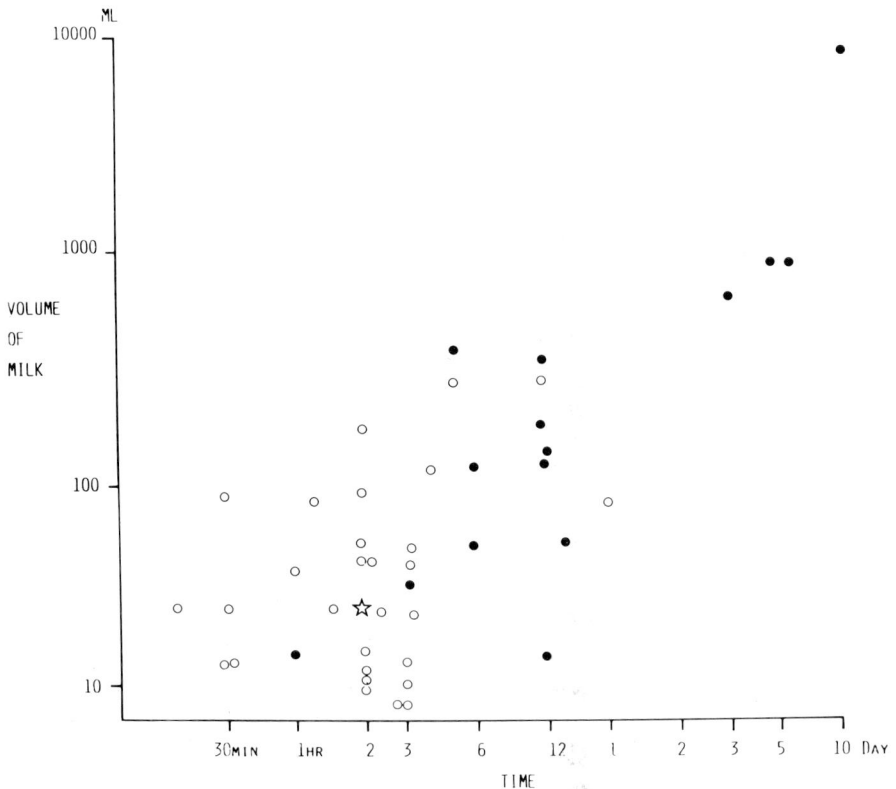

FIG. 2. Development of gastrointestinal symptoms in individual patients after cow's milk challenge. The vertical axis shows the volume of milk given up to the time of development of symptoms and the horizontal axis shows the time after beginning formal milk challenge for first signs of either vomiting *(open circle)*, shock *(star)*, or diarrhea *(closed circle)* to develop.

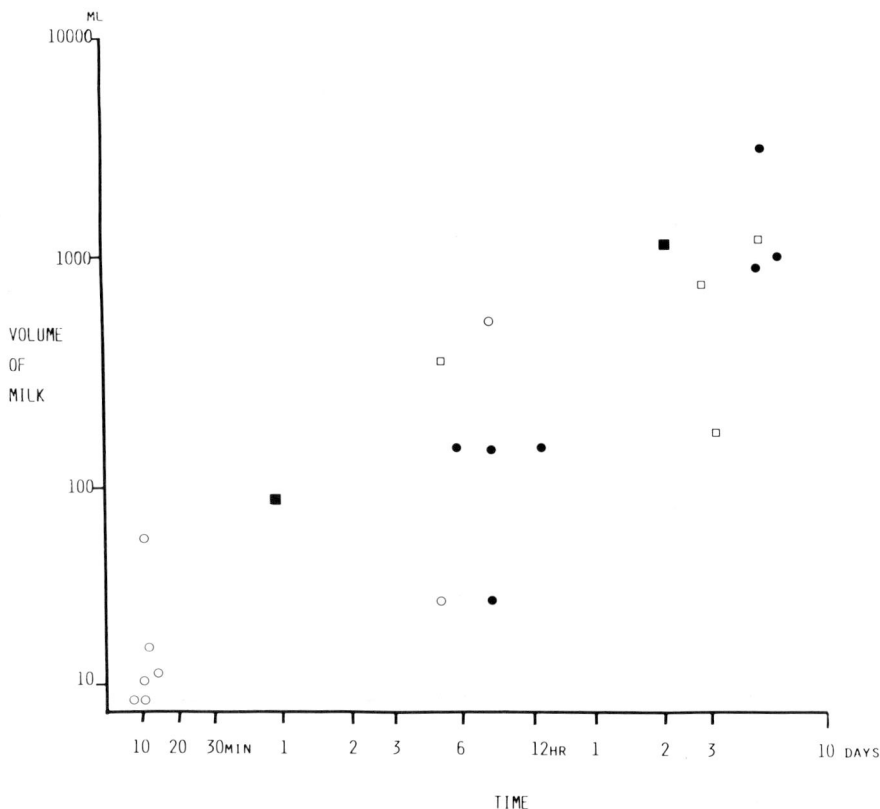

FIG. 3. The development of respiratory tract symptoms after cow's milk challenge in individual patients. The vertical axis shows the volume of milk given up to the time of development of first symptoms and the horizontal axis indicates the time of the development of rhinitis *(closed box)*, lower respiratory tract symptoms only *(open box)*, lower respiratory and cutaneous symptoms *(open circle)*, or gastrointestinal manifestation *(closed circle)* of CMA.

the difficulty in trying to identify groups of patients with patterns of disease which could be recognized clinically.

RECOGNITION OF CLINICAL PROFILES IN COW'S MILK ALLERGY

In an attempt to group patients with common features, 30 items of historial data and information relating to milk challenge on the initial cohort of 100 patients were entered into a computer data base (8). The historical details included acute or chronic skin, gastrointestinal, respiratory, and behavior disorders that may or may not have been related to milk ingestion. Data regarding the effect of milk challenge included the volume of milk ingested as well as the nature and the time of onset of symptoms provoked by this challenge.

A K-means algorithm was used to identify groups of patients with common features. In the initial analysis, symptoms at presentation and those elicited by milk challenge were the variables used. This analysis revealed that patients appeared to cluster naturally into three groups: one with skin eruptions, another with gastrointestinal disturbance, and a third with gastrointestinal, respiratory, and skin symptoms. In Tables 3 and 4 the frequency of presenting symptoms as well as the symptoms induced by milk challenge for each of these three groups is shown. In a subsequent analysis it was found that the time of onset of symptoms in the three groups was different; the first group of patients responded within 45 min of commencing milk challenge, the second between 45 min and 20 hr, and the third more than 20 hr.

In summary, these investigations identified three groups of patients with the following characteristics:

Group 1 developed rapid onset of symptoms within minutes of ingestion of small volumes of milk. Urticaria, angioedema, and eczema were frequently seen, but gastrointestinal and respiratory symptoms, as features of mild systemic anaphylaxis, were also documented. The patients in this group demonstrated positive skin prick test (SPT) to a milk allergen extract.

Group 2 patients developed symptoms confined to the gastrointestinal tract. Vom-

TABLE 3. *Presentation features in cow's milk allergy*

	Group 1	Group 2	Group 3	p Value
Patients	27	53	20	
Age—median (months)	10[a]	10[b]	17[ab]	a = 0.015 b = 0.002
Urticaria—acute	20[ab]	11[ac]	0[bc]	a = < 0.001 b = < 0.001 c = < 0.001
Eczema—chronic	5	6[a]	9[a]	a = 0.003
Vomiting—episodic	10[a]	27[b]	2[ab]	a = 0.036 b = 0.006
—persistent	1	10	3	
Diarrhea—episodic	2[a]	21[ab]	3[b]	a = 0.002 b = 0.04
—persistent	9	17	9	
Wheeze—episodic	7[a]	2[a]	2	a = 0.006
Wheeze/bronchitis— persistent	6[a]	7[b]	11[ab]	a = 0.02 b = < 0.001
Weight < 3rd percentile	4[a]	10	8[a]	a = 0.05
Height < 3rd percentile	1	4	1	

Frequency of symptoms at presentation in Groups 1, 2, and 3. Level of difference indicated if $p < 0.05$ by Chi-squared analysis and Fischer's exact test. There was no significant difference in frequency with which persistent vomiting, persistent diarrhea, or height < 3rd percentile occurred at presentation between the groups (Data not shown.). Differences in age at presentation analyzed by Mann-Whitney U-test and two-tailed test.

[a, b, c] Indicate level of statistical difference between groups 1, 2, and 3 for each parameter.

TABLE 4. *Effect of milk challenge in cow's milk allergy*

	Group 1	Group 2	Group 3	p Value
Patients	27	53	20	
Angioedema (urticaria)	21[ab]	6[a]	2[b]	a = < 0.001 b = < 0.001
Eczema	3	2[a]	7[a]	a = 0.001
Morbilli	1	4	0	
Vomiting	9[ab]	32[ac]	0[bc]	a = 0.02 b = 0.003 c = < 0.001
Diarrhea	4[ab]	32[a]	12[b]	a = < 0.001 b = 0.001
Colic (irritable)	10	24	10	
Cough (wheeze)	8[a]	2[ab]	10[b]	a = 0.002 b = < 0.001
Stridor	2	0	0	
Rhinitis	2	4	6	

Frequency of symptoms induced by formal milk challenge in Group 1, 2, and 3. Level of difference indicated if $p < 0.05$ by Chi-squared analysis and Fischer's exact test. There was no significant difference in frequency of morbilliform eruptions, colic, stridor, or rhinitis between each of the groups (Data not shown.).
[a, b, c] Indicate level of statistical difference between groups 1, 2, and 3 for each parameter.

iting and/or diarrhea developed several hours after ingestion of modest volumes of cow's milk. Most of these patients were skin test negative to a cow's milk extract. These patients have been described as suffering from CME or CMPI.

Group 3 patients developed gastroenteritic symptoms with or without respiratory and/or eczematous reactions more than 20 hr after commencing milk ingestion. These patients were ingesting large volumes of milk at the time symptoms developed. Positive SPT to milk was confined to those with eczema.

Thus, the patients in Group 1 had relatively uniform atopic features, whereas those in Group 2 demonstrated gastrointestinal symptoms. These findings contrasted with the heterogeneous symptoms of the Group 3 patients in whom multisystem disease was common. In addition the patients in Group 1 and Group 2 were of similar age (10 months) whereas the Group 3 patients were significantly older (median age 17 months) at the time CMA was diagnosed.

IMMUNOLOGICAL FEATURES ASSOCIATED WITH COW'S MILK ALLERGY

Serum Immunoglobulin Levels

Studies of serum immunoglobulin levels in the initial cohort of CMA patients documented a high incidence of relative immunodeficiency (8). A third of all the infants had a serum IgA level below the 5th percentile, but IgG and IgM percentile values were also low compared to a normal population. IgA deficiency was not confined to the atopic Group 1 patients but also occurred in the Group 2 nonatopic patients with milk enteropathy. The patients in Group 1 had elevated total IgE levels as well as a high incidence of positive SPT to milk (Table 5).

TABLE 5. *Immunoglobulins in cow's milk allergy*

	Group 1	Group 2	Group 3	p Value
IgG percentile	23	32	33	—
IgA percentile	16	13[a]	40[a]	a = 0.034
IgM percentile	29[a]	33[b]	65[ab]	a = 0.019 b = 0.019
IgE, IU/ml	77[a]	12[ab]	48[b]	a = 0.012 b = 0.012

Median IgG, IgA, IgM percentiles and IgE (international units per milliliter) levels for Groups 1, 2, and 3. Differences between each group are indicated only where $p \leq 0.05$ using Mann-Whitney U-test and Fischer's two-tailed test for significance.

The role of IgA deficiency in relation to mucosal handling of dietary antigens has received considerable attention in the past but these findings identified a relative immunodeficiency of the serum IgG, IgA, and IgM classes in patients allergic to cow's milk. Thus, any defect in handling of dietary antigens in CMA need not be confined to the mucosal level but may also occur at the systemic level through IgG-, IgA-, and IgM-dependent mechanisms.

Anti-Cow's Milk IgE Antibodies

Serum was available from some of the patients from the three groups with CMA to study the detailed humoral immune response to cow's milk at the time of initial diagnosis (9). These studies confirmed an association between elevated IgE milk antibodies and the Group 1 patients with rapid onset of clinical reactions to milk ingestion. In Fig. 4, the anti-cow's milk IgE antibody levels in the three patient groups as

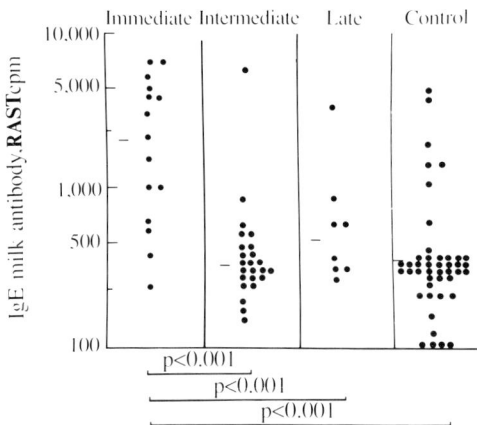

FIG. 4. Immunoglobulin E (IgE) milk antibody levels in the three patient groups at diagnosis and in a group of age-matched controls. Significant differences between the groups are indicated.

well as an age-matched control population are indicated. The IgE milk antibody levels were clearly elevated in the immediate-reacting patients. These levels were significantly higher than in the controls. The IgE antibody level in both the intermediate-reacting Group 2, and late-reacting Group 3 patients was not significantly different from those in the age-matched control population. The association of elevated IgE milk antibodies in the rapidly reacting Group 1 patients points to the involvement of an immediate Type 1 hypersensitivity reaction in this disorder.

Anti-Cow's Milk IgG, IgA, and IgM Antibodies

In these patients the levels of anti-cow's milk IgA and IgM antibodies were similar in all patient groups to that of an age-matched control population (9). However, the IgG isotype response to whole cow's milk was significantly lower in the CMA patients compared to an age-matched control group (Fig. 5). The possibility that increased levels of IgG antibodies in soluble IgG-containing immune complexes, which would not be detected by enzyme-linked immunosorbent assay (ELISA), cannot be excluded but we believe it more likely that this finding reflects prolonged milk avoidance. Our patients were on a milk-free diet for at least 4 weeks prior to testing. Recently Burgin-Woolf et al. (10) have demonstrated a decline in milk antibody titers after milk exclusion in CMA patients.

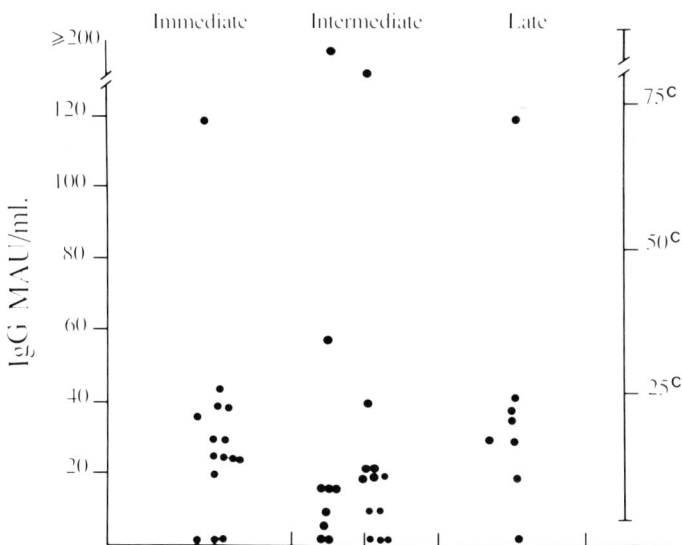

FIG. 5. Immunoglobulin G (IgG) milk antibody levels at the time of diagnosis in the three patient groups. Percentile values from a control group of similar age are shown.

Delayed-Type Hypersensitivity in Cow's Milk Allergy

The role of delayed-type hypersensitivity (DTH) in food allergy is controversial because of the difficulty in accurately documenting nonimmediate reactions to food, and the difficulty of performing reliable assays of DTH. In a separate study of 51 children with CMA, 32 patients developed immediate rapid-onset reactions (median age 26 months), 9 children (median age 18 months) were found to be milk tolerant, and 10 were late reactors of whom 9 developed adverse responses several days after commencing milk ingestion (11).

In this study the effect of milk ingestion was assessed clinically and from information recorded on diary score cards which patients completed in the week prior to commencing milk ingestion and continued in the following week while undergoing the milk challenge procedure. Parents recorded the volume of milk formula given, the number of bowel actions and vomit episodes each day, the presence of colic/irritable behavior, wheezing/cough, rhinitis, skin rashes, and episodes of waking each night. Symptom frequency during the period on cow's milk was compared with the similar period without cow's milk in the prechallenge week. The classification of patients into late reactors or milk tolerant was based on a standard clinical history and the diary score cards.

The clinical scores before and after milk challenge were compared between the late-reacting milk-allergic and nonallergic groups. No significant difference was demonstrated in the change in incidence of skin rash, vomiting, wakeful nights, and cough before and after the milk challenge between these two groups. However, differences were observed with irritability ($p = 0.01$), the number of bowel actions ($p = 0.02$), rhinitis ($p = 0.01$), and the sum of differences ($p = 0.001$) between the groups, indicating a worsening of symptoms during milk ingestion for the CMA late reactors. In Table 6 the clinical and immunological features of these late-reacting CMA patients are recorded.

When leukocyte inhibition factor (LIF) production to α-lactalbumin, α-casein, and β-lactoglobulin was compared between the milk-tolerant and late-reacting CMA patients, it was noted that the patients with late-onset CMA demonstrated greater production of LIF to each of the milk proteins studied. However, there was no difference in the level of LIF production to these proteins for the milk-tolerant patients and patients with immediate-type hypersensitivity to milk ingestion (Fig. 6).

Based on these findings, one hypersensitivity immune mechanism alone cannot explain the whole spectrum of CMA. It would appear an array of antibody and cell-mediated immune responses operate in this disorder. In the immediate Type 1 hypersensitivity reactions, IgE-sensitized mast cells probably interact with milk proteins causing release of mediators eliciting urticaria, angioedema, eczema, and anaphylaxis within minutes of exposure to small volumes of milk. It is possible to speculate that in the Group 2 CMA patients with milk enteropathy, asymptomatic gut and mucosal IgE hypersensitivity might lead to enhanced absorption of milk antigen, increased production, and local deposition of immune complexes and

TABLE 6. *Clinical and immunological features in late-reacting cow's milk allergy patients*

Patient number	Age, months	Milk ingested	Irritable days[a]	Number of bowel actions[b]	Rhinitis days[a]	α-Casein[c]	β-Lactoglobulin[c]	α-Lactalbumin[c]
10	13	2,300 ml in 5 days	3	5	4	84.2	95.0	104.4
11	9	1,200 ml in 7 days	6	3	0	77.8	64.3	53.5
12	68	3,100 ml in 6 days	6	0	6	57.8	62.8	71.3
13	66	1,100 ml in 5 days	0	7	0	71.5	66.3	64.6
14	57	4,000 ml in 7 days	6	2	3	92.9	65.0	68.0
15	36	550 ml in 7 days (intermittent)	2	6	4	108.7	107.3	94.4
16	92	2,000 ml in 6/7	4	5	3	—	86.8	74.6
17	17	1,200 ml in 5 days	0	5	5	98.5	90.8	83.7
18	100	90 ml in 3 hr	1	1	0	86.8	64.4	59.5
19	8	500 ml in 5 days	1	— 2	3	82.8	77.5	75.8

[a][Days of symptoms postchallenge] — [Days of symptoms prechallenge]
[b][Number of bowel actions postchallenge] — [Number of bowel actions prechallenge]
[c]Leukocyte inhibition factor score (percent of control migration) to individual milk proteins.

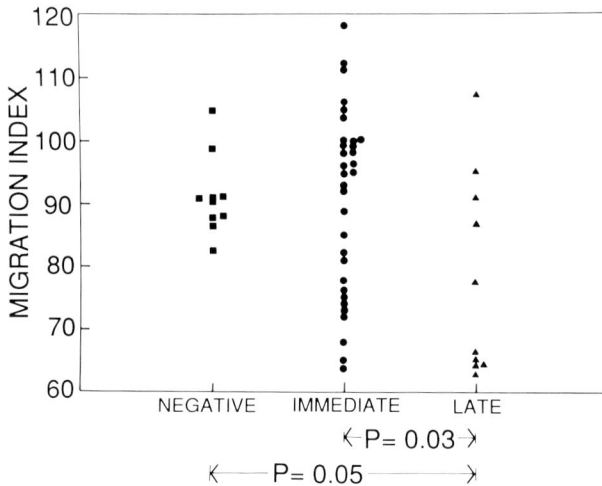

FIG. 6. Results of testing leukocyte inhibition factor (LIF) production to β-lactoglobulin in patients clinically tolerant to cow's milk (negative patients) and those with immediate or late-reacting cow's milk allergy.

complement, with the subsequent recruitment of lymphoid cells, leading to cell-mediated damage in target tissues. It has been suggested that high levels of IgG milk antibodies are responsible for some symptoms in CMA caused by the production of immune complexes, but we have been unable to confirm these findings. However, we cannot exclude the possibility of soluble IgG complex formation as these are not specifically detected by our assay. In some patients with late-onset CMA, we envisage that sensitized lymphocytes exposed to milk antigen *in vivo* generate a range of lymphokines leading to the clinical manifestations of this form of CMA. This is supported by the demonstration of milk antigen in the systemic circulation following ingestion of cow's milk (12), and our demonstration of circulating milk antigen-sensitized lymphocytes (11).

FACTORS ASSOCIATED WITH THE DEVELOPMENT OF DIFFERENT SYNDROMES OF COW'S MILK ALLERGY

The Effect of Antigen Load on Development of Milk Antibodies in Infants with Cow's Milk Allergy

We investigated the possibility that the different immune responses in children with distinct clinical features of CMA might be related to their degree of exposure to milk protein (13). The feeding history of 24 children with challenge-proven CMA was examined in relation to their humoral immune response to whole cow's milk.

Two groups of patients were identified: Group A consisted of 10 patients in whom the first known cow's milk exposure, of <60 ml, developed rapid onset of vomiting, diarrhea with or without acute angioedema, and/or urticaria. Group B consisted of 13 children who had received substantial volumes of cow's milk >60 ml on at least two occasions or had received frequent small feeds of cow's milk at intervals over months.

Both groups of infants were of comparable age and had been breast-fed for similar lengths of time and were comparable with an age-matched control population being investigated for nonallergic conditions.

The results showed that children with CMA who had minimal exposure to whole cow's milk had lower levels of IgG, IgA, and IgM antibody isotype to cow's milk compared to those patients who had been fed substantial volumes of milk prior to diagnosis. In addition, the patients with minimal exposure to cow's milk showed markedly increased total IgE levels and milk-specific IgE antibodies to cow's milk compared to those fed larger volumes. These results are shown in Fig. 7.

These findings challenge the assumption that the first significant immune contact with dietary antigen is at weaning. Possibly sensitization occurs either antenatally via bovine antigen-containing soluble immune complexes crossing the placenta, or postnatally during supplementary feeds in the neonatal nursery, or via cow's milk excreted in breast milk during the postnatal period. The findings support the concept that low-dose antigen exposure favors development of IgE hypersensitivity to cow's

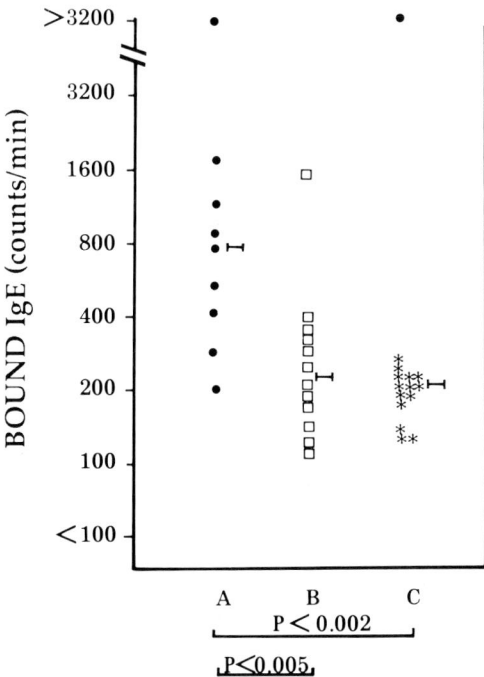

FIG. 7. Milk-specific immunoglobulin E (IgE) antibodies in the two patient groups and controls measured by radioallergosorbent test. Low cow's milk exposure *(closed circle)*; high cow's milk exposure *(open box)*; control *(asterisk)*.

milk, whereas high-dose antigen exposure suppresses this immune response. Jarrett (14) described similar findings in rodents.

A Possible Role for Rotavirus in the Development of Cow's Milk Enteropathy in Infants

Frick (15) produced evidence that viral infection induced dysregulation of thymus-derived cell (T-cell) function leading to increased IgE synthesis. This led us to hypothesize that early infection with rotavirus could lead to the development of IgE hypersensitivity to a bystander antigen, namely, cow's milk.

To test this hypothesis, we compared the incidence of rotavirus sero-conversion in the Group 1 (IgE-sensitized) with the Group 2 (gut-reacting) patients (16).

The results showed a higher incidence of antibodies to rotavirus in the nonatopic patients with milk enteropathy than those in Group 1 with atopic features ($p < 0.05$) (Fig. 8). Although the atopic patients had significantly higher levels of total and

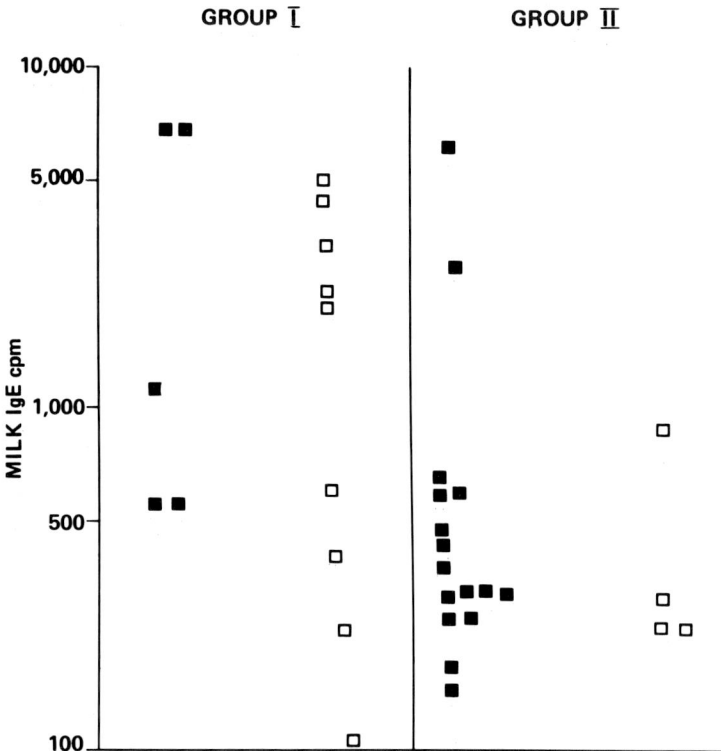

FIG. 8. Levels of immunoglobulin E (IgE) antibodies to cow's milk in Group I and Group II patients according to rotavirus IgG antibody status. Rotavirus + *(closed box);* rotavirus − *(open box).*

milk-specific IgE antibodies to cow's milk than those of the second group, both patient groups had lower levels of total serum IgG, IgA, and IgM than an age-matched control population.

It is possible that rotavirus infection during a period of immune vulnerability leads to an alteration in gut permeability thus enhancing absorption of milk antigen inducing a disturbance in normal immunological priming to milk antigen, and ultimately leading to milk enteropathy. However, this will require prospective studies of the outcome of rotavirus infection. Such a study would have to take account of the role of genetic factors and the age of first exposure to milk antigen.

TESTS FOR THE DIAGNOSIS OF MILK ALLERGY

Skin Tests

In a recently completed investigation of 135 consecutive milk challenges in children with a good clinical history of CMA (median age 24 months), only half the patients were challenge positive (17). The SPT was performed with a commercially available cow's milk extract and the size of the skin weal elicited by the extract was compared with that produced by 1% histamine acid phosphate and a control solution. The results were graded according to the histamine reference standard. The skin reactions were scored so that patients whose weal diameter was twice that of histamine or more were graded at 4 or >4, respectively. Radioallergosorbent test (RAST) analysis was conducted and scored from 0 to 4 according to the manufacturer's directions.

All the patients whose skin reactivity to cow's milk was equal to or greater than twice the histamine standard reacted to the milk challenge. In a statistical evaluation of the diagnostic value of skin test and RAST, it was shown that in patients with a history suggestive of CMA and an SPT >4 to the milk extract being used, the probability that patients had CMA was 1 (i.e., all children with these findings will react positively to milk challenge). Although all the patients with the RAST score of 4 had CMA, this represented <10% of all our milk-allergic children, suggesting that it is not as useful as skin testing in this age group.

Based on the results of our previous investigations, approximately 25% of all children with CMA have an immediate-type hypersensitivity reaction which may be identified with the use of a simple SPT used in this investigation. In most children with this pattern of CMA, the diagnosis will be clear from the clinical history but there are two clinical situations in which the SPT may be of assistance. Firstly, in the occasional infants who present with anaphylactic or severe hypersensitivity reactions with the cause of the allergen unknown, a strongly positive SPT to milk may identify that cause. Secondly, in infants with a history of anaphylactic reaction to cow's milk where there is a reluctance to rechallenge for several years, SPT may be used to follow the natural history of the disease. Based on the results of this study, it would seem unwise to milk challenge a child who has a previous history of anaphylaxis if the SPT remains >4.

The findings of this study are only valid for the population of patients investigated and the agents used. However, these findings highlight the potential diagnostic value of SPTs.

In Vitro Measurements of the Immune Response to Cow's Milk

Based on the investigations described previously, an association was established between the patients who developed rapid-onset reactions of urticaria and eczema after milk ingestion and elevated IgE milk-specific antibodies (8). However, in subsequent investigations it was found that although RAST assays did discriminate allergic from nonallergic children, the test was not superior to SPTs using a commerically available whole cow's milk allergen extract (17). Furthermore, the levels of IgG, IgA, and IgM antibody responses to whole cow's milk did not distinguish milk allergic from nonallergic patients across the broad spectrum of the clinical disorder. Indeed, our studies showed that the IgG isotype response to whole cow's milk was significantly lower in patients with CMA than age-matched controls, a phenomenon we attributed to milk exclusion (9).

One parameter of DTH, the level of LIF produced in response to individual milk proteins, was higher in patients with slowly evolving reactions to cow's milk ingestion when compared to control and immediate-reacting patients (11). However, considerable overlap in the results was noted between the three patient groups for the protein α-casein, β-lactoglobulin, and α-lactalbumin (Fig. 6). Thus the assays' poor sensitivity and specificity make it unlikely that further exploration of this method will lead to the development of a diagnostic test of value in the identification of non-immediate-reacting CMA patients.

Evaluation of Gastrointestinal Function in Cow's Milk Allergy

Two separate studies from this laboratory have examined gastrointestinal function in children with CMA. In the first (18), sequential biopsies immediately prior to and within 24 hr of the onset of symptoms of milk challenge were undertaken. In Table 7 the results of these studies are shown. The structural changes were graded according to whether they showed normal appearance, mild, moderate, or severe changes as described by Townley et al. (19). From Table 7, three children showed significant changes on biopsy after a positive response to milk challenge. However, more than half of those who showed an adverse clinical response to milk ingestion did not show any significant lesion on the postchallenge biopsy specimen. In subsequent studies we have identified a number of children with chronic diarrhea and essentially normal duodenal histopathology who respond to milk avoidance.

In a separate study from this laboratory Ford et al. (20) identified 36 children who had gastrointestinal symptoms attributed to CMA. They were investigated before and after milk challenge by one or more of four tests of gastrointestinal function. The following conclusions were reached.

TABLE 7. *Effect of milk ingestion on duodenal histopathology in cow's milk allergy*

Clinical group	Patient	Challenge symptom[a]	Histological abnormality[b]		Lactase ($N > 1.1$ U/g wet wt)	
			Before	After	Before	After
1	A	U,AE	Mild	Mild	2.4	2.6
1	B	AE	N	Mild	3.7	5.8
1	C	U,AE,V,D	N	N	1.9	2.9
1	D	Rash, D	Mild	Mild	1.5	2.0
1	E	V	N	N	3.2	2.4
2	F	D	Mild	Moderate	3.3	1.3
2	G	V,D	N	N	2.1	1.1
2	H	V,D	N	Severe	2.1	0.3
2	I	V,D	N	Moderate	3.6	1.6
3	J	D	N	N	4.3	4.7
3	K	V,D	N	N	4.5	5.0
3	L	D	N	N	3.2	4.5
3	M	Wh,C,D	M	M	1.0	0.5

[a]Challenge symptoms: U, urticaria; AE, angioedema; V, vomiting; D, diarrhea; Wh, wheezing.
[b]Histological abnormality: Mild, moderate, or severe according to Townley et al. (19).

Confirming the earlier study, most of the children who showed CMA clinically had normal duodenal biopsies following a positive challenge although a few showed minor changes. The incidence of these changes was not significantly different from those patients who were milk-tolerant. There was no significant difference in the incidence of changes in duodenal biopsy, lactase, sucrase, or maltase levels in the patients who were milk-tolerant compared to those with CMA. Furthermore, the 1-hr blood xylose test was not useful in identifying patients with CMA. Although a few children with CMA developed a positive breath hydrogen test with lactose challenge following milk ingestion, some patients with milk tolerance also showed this abnormality. Based on these studies, which were conducted exclusively on children with major gastrointestinal responses to milk ingestion, we concluded it was unlikely that measurements of lactose breath hydrogen and 1-hr blood xylose tests would be useful in the identification of patients with CMA. One possible reason for these conclusions is that these tests only show abnormalities when there is extensive bowel damage. However, duodenal biopsies still have an important role in excluding other causes of gastrointestinal symptoms in children with milk-induced gastrointestinal disease.

ASSOCIATED FOOD ALLERGIES

The incidence of intolerance to various foods as reported by parents of children with CMA is shown in Table 8. Many patients elected to withhold these substances

TABLE 8. *Associated food intolerance in 100 children with cow's milk allergy*

Egg	40/77	Chicken	7/75
Orange	27/56	Lamb	2/45
Soy	32/75	Beef	9/79
Chocolate	14/22	Fish	6/69
Wheat	12/88	Tomato	5/31
Casein hydrolysate	11/54		
Peanut	13/26		

during the period of follow-up study because they were concerned that hypersensitivity reactions might occur. This was particularly so for oranges, chocolate, peanut, fish, and tomato. Although some of these patients had positive skin tests and elevated IgE antibodies to these substances as measured by RAST, the possibility that many of these responses may have been caused by nonimmune mechanisms cannot be excluded. In particular, the high incidence of diarrhea induced by fruit which is probably caused by some forms of sugar intolerance warrants consideration. This possibility is strengthened by our studies which identified a high incidence of abnormally elevated sucrase/isomaltase ratios in duodenal biopsies of some children with CMA suggesting they may be sucrose-intolerant. Some formulas contain sucrose raising the possibility that adverse gastrointestinal reactions to them may be caused by the biochemical abnormality.

It is worth noting the relatively high incidence of hypersensitivity reactions to cow's milk substitute formulas in our highly selected population. Many infants appear to tolerate both soy and casein hydrolysate preparations initially but hypersensitivity reactions developed usually within a few weeks. A few patients appear to tolerate these special formulas for months, and in one case years, before clinical features consistent with acute hypersensitivity responses developed. The true incidence of hypersensitivity reactions to these commonly used cow's milk substitutes cannot be judged from this study because of patient selection.

Our preliminary observations suggest that the three broad patterns of adverse clinical response to milk ingestion in CMA is also seen in children with hypersensitivity reactions to egg, soy, wheat, and casein hydrolysate preparations.

Some children with the slow-onset type non-IgE-associated hypersensitivity reactions to cow's milk demonstrated an IgE-associated immediate-type hypersensitivity reaction to egg. The frequency with which such disparate clinical and immunological responses to these different food antigens occur is unclear, but these observations suggest the possibility of separate immune responses to different proteins in individual patients. Thus, the assumption that a child who shows an immediate-type IgE hypersensitivity to one food allergen will respond with a similar clinical and immune response to an unrelated food allergen is incorrect. The precise frequency with which these disparate clinical and immune responses to different food antigens occur is unclear.

CLINICAL OUTCOME OF COW'S MILK ALLERGY

A follow-up study of 94 of the first 100 patients with CMA is shown in Figs. 9 and 10. A picture emerges that CMA is not a transient disease confined to the first months of life. Of the 39 children older than 2 years, over two-thirds have persistent CMA although a significant number of children developed tolerance to cow's milk subsequently. The immunological changes associated with remission of the disease are unclear. There is some evidence that patients with IgE-associated food allergy

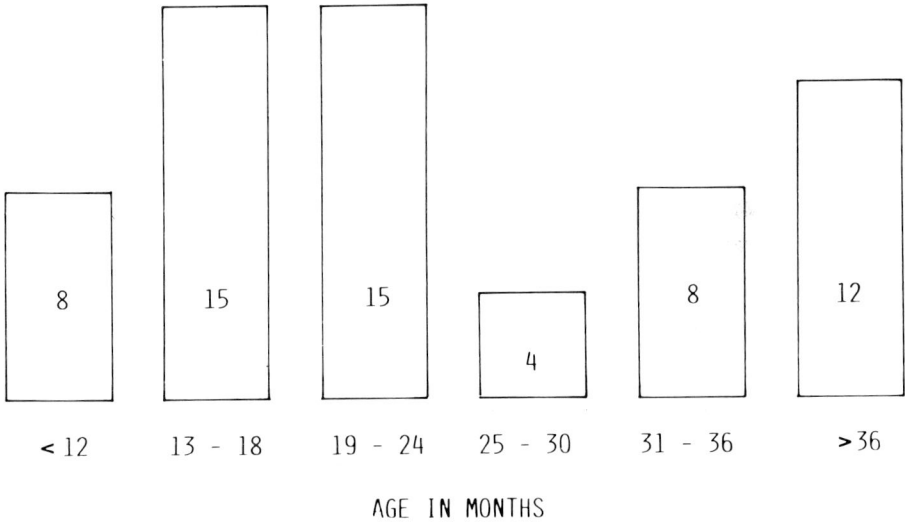

8   15   15   4   8   12

< 12   13 - 18   19 - 24   25 - 30   31 - 36   >36

AGE IN MONTHS

FIG. 9. Age of children with persistent cow's milk allergy (from initial cohort of 100 children).

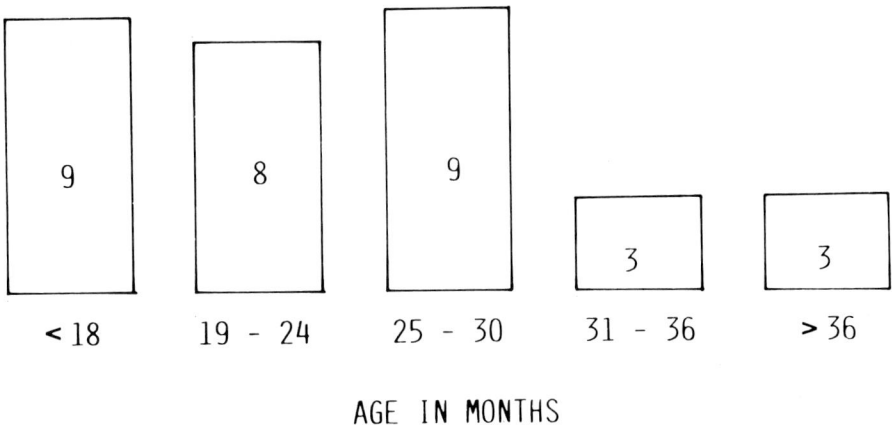

9   8   9   3   3

< 18   19 - 24   25 - 30   31 - 36   > 36

AGE IN MONTHS

FIG. 10. Age of 32 children tolerant to cow's milk (from initial cohort of 100 children).

develop tolerance to these foods despite the persistence of IgE hypersensitivity (21,22). It is unclear whether the pattern of clinical response to milk ingestion remains consistent throughout the duration of the disorder. Our preliminary findings suggest that most patients maintain a similar type of response while their disease persists although a few patients appear to show different patterns of disease when studied over several years. The clinical and immunologic outcome of hypersensitivity reactions to other foods in children with CMA is unknown.

ACKNOWLEDGMENT

The secretarial assistance of Mrs. Joan Sedmak is gratefully acknowledged.

REFERENCES

1. Heiner DC, Sears JW. Chronic respiratory diseases associated with multiple circulating precipitins to cow's milk. *Am J Dis Child* 1962;100:500.
2. Waldemann TA, Wochner RD, Laster L, et al. Allergic gastroenteropathy: a cause of excessive gastrointestinal protein loss. *N Engl J Med* 1967;276:761.
3. Wilson JF, Heiner DC, Lahey ME. Milk induced gastrointestinal bleeding in infants with hypochromic and microcytic anaemia. *JAMA* 1964;1989:122.
4. Whitfield MF, Barr DG. Cow's milk allergy in the syndrome of thrombocytopaenia with absent radius. *Arch Dis Child* 1976;51:337.
5. Jones RH. Congenital thrombocytopaenia and milk allergy. *Arch Dis Child* 1977;52:744.
6. Gryboski JD, Burkle F, Hillman R. Milk induced colitis in the infant. *Pediatrics* 1966;38:299.
7. Hill DJ, Ford RPK, Shelton MJ, Hosking CS. A study of 100 infants and young children with cow's milk allergy. *Clin Rev Allergy* 1984;2:125.
8. Hill DJ, Firer MA, Shelton MJ, Hosking CS. Manifestations of milk allergy in infancy: clinical and immunological findings. *J Pediatr* 1986;109:270.
9. Firer MA, Hosking CS, Hill DJ. Humoral immune response to cow's milk in children with cow's milk allergy. *Int Arch Allergy Appl Immunol* 1987;84:173.
10. Burgin-Woolf A, Signer E, Friess HM, Berger R, Burbalmer A, Just M. The diagnostic significance of antibodies to various cow's milk proteins (fluorescent immunosorbent test). *Eur J Pediatr* 1980;133:17.
11. Hill DJ, Ball G, Hosking CS. Clinical manifestations of cow's milk allergy in childhood. I. Associations with in-vitro cellular immune responses. *Clin Allergy* 1988 (*in press*).
12. Paganelli R, Levinsky RJ, Brostoff J, Wraith DG. Immune complexes containing food proteins in normal and atopic subjects after oral challenge and effect of sodium cromoglycate on antigen absorption. *Lancet* 1979;I:270.
13. Firer MA, Hosking CS, Hill DJ. The effect of antigen load on development of milk antibodies in infants allergic to milk. *Br Med J* 1981;283:693.
14. Jarrett EE. Activation of IgE regulatory mechanisms by transmucosal absorption of antigen. *Lancet* 1977;2:223.
15. Frick OL. Virus infections as triggers of allergy. *Clin Immunol Allergol* 1981;283.
16. Firer MA, Hosking CS, Hill DJ. Possible role for rotavirus in the development of cow's milk enteropathy in infants. *Clin Allergy* 1988;18:53.
17. Hill DJ, Duke AM, Hosking CS, Hudson IL. Clinical manifestation of cow's milk allergy in childhood. II. The diagnostic value of skin test and RAST. *Clin Allergy* 1988 (*in press*).
18. Hill DJ, Davidson GP, Cameron DJS, Barnes GL. The spectrum of cow's milk allergy in childhood. *Acta Paediatr Scand* 1979;68:847.
19. Townley RRW, Khaw KT, Schwachman H. Quantitative assay of disaccharidase activities of small intestinal mucosal biopsy specimens in infancy and childhood. *Pediatrics* 1965;36:911.
20. Ford RPK, Barnes GL, Hill DJ. Gastrointestinal hypersensitivity to cow's milk protein: the diagnostic value of gut function tests. *Aust Paediatr J* 1986;22:37.
21. Bock SA. The natural history of food sensitivity. *J Allergy Clin Immunol* 1982;69:173.
22. Sampson HA, McCaskill CM. Food hypersensitivity in atopic dermatitis. Evaluation of 113 children. *J Pediatr* 1985;107:669.

Food Intolerance in Infancy: Allergology, Immunology, and Gastroenterology, edited by Robert N. Hamburger. Carnation Nutrition Education Series, Vol. 1. The Carnation Co., Los Angeles/Raven Press, Ltd., New York © 1989.

Soy Protein Allergy

Edmund J. Eastham

Department of Child Health, Royal Victoria Infirmary, Newcastle upon Tyne, NE1 4LP, England

Following a brief historical review, this chapter examines the potential problems with soy protein isolate formulas, with particular reference to their antigenicity, allergenicity, and general impact on the immunological system. The clinical spectrum of soy allergy is described and its formula usage questioned with regard to prevention of allergy in susceptible individuals and in infants with colic.

The evidence suggests that in the healthy child soy is less allergenic than cow's milk, but when used as a substitute in cases where the small bowel is already damaged (postgastroenteritis, cow's milk allergy) the incidence of concomitant soy allergy may be substantial. Although the sales of these formulas are increasing, their use in selected instances is reviewed and, in many cases, contrary to the manufacturers' literature, have not withstood the rigors of good clinical trials.

SOY PROTEIN ALLERGY

For those being artificially fed, cow's milk has formed the basis for infant feeds for most of this century. With increasing scientific knowledge and improved manufacturing techniques, the present day array of formula choices are both safe and perfectly satisfactory for the vast majority of infants. For the small percentage that exhibit intolerance, an alternative is needed and the soybean would appear to be a satisfactory protein substitute. The sales of soy formulas have flourished particularly during the past 10 to 15 years. It is of interest that in the British Government's 1975 Department of Health and Social Security report on "Present-Day Practice in Infant Feeding" (1), there is no mention of all of these formulas. However, their current use has, in my opinion, tended to be indiscriminate and led to conflicting evidence and confusion among the medical and health-care professions. There are strong advocates for their use, backed by the high-powered sell of the manufacturers, but there are also those who feel that they should not be freely available without prescription and should only occasionally be prescribed (2). Like cow's milk formulas, however, they are in general safe, sustaining growth and development, although they are more expensive and they are without doubt the cause of allergic reactions.

HISTORICAL BACKGROUND

Economically and nutritionally, the main asset of the soybean is that it is rich in both protein (40%) and fat (20%). Like the lentil and pea, it belongs to the family, *Leguminosae,* and has been cultivated for centuries in Eastern Asia. The major producer today is the United States, which is responsible for over 60% of the world's total production.

The first description of its use as a substitute for cow's milk in infants was in 1909 by Ruhräh (3), and in 1929, Hill and Stuart (4) described a soybean powder formula for use in children with milk allergy. Several commercial formulas (first generation) then appeared which were based on fat-free soy flour, but various problems were soon encountered:

Presentation and taste. They had a caramel-like color and an unpleasant nutty flavor.

Carbohydrate intolerance. Because of various undigestible carbohydrates such as stachyose, increased flatulence and foul-smelling stools frequently occurred.

Vitamin deficiencies. Since organic solvents were used to extract the fat from the soy flour, the fat-soluble vitamins were lost. Deficiencies in vitamins A, K, and B_{12} were reported in the literature in the 1950s and 1960s (5–7).

Goitrogens. An unidentified component of soybean appears to have a goitrogenic effect in both animals and in a number of infants (8,9). However, iodine fortification counteracts this (10), and was therefore recommended as a precautionary measure (11).

Trypsin inhibitors. These antinutritional factors have received much attention, and, certainly in experimental animals, may cause growth retardation, pancreatic hypertrophy, and even adenocarcinoma (12). None of these, however, have been reported in infants, probably because the inhibitors are labile and 90% inactivated during preparation of the formulas. Their capacity to cause other problems is highlighted in a recent article (13) where the best known, the Kunitz soybean trypsin inhibitor, was reported to be the antigenic stimulant of an acute anaphylactic reaction in an adult female, whose symptoms developed "within minutes of tasting her infant's soy formula." Quite how important this compound is as an allergen remains to be seen.

Mineral deficiencies. Numerous studies have been conducted on the effect of soy protein on mineral availability and the interested reader is referred to a recent review (14). The main problem would appear to be phytic acid which chelates such ions as calcium, magnesium, zinc, copper, and iron (15). Most studies have focused on zinc and iron with conflicting results (16). From the practical point of view, any interference with mineral availability can readily be circumvented by fortification or addition of an enhancer (e.g., ascorbic acid in the case of iron).

In the mid-1960s a second generation soybean formula was developed based on a soy-protein isolate. The commercial production of this involves several steps, and results in an isolate of at least 90% protein. It is prepared from defatted soybean flakes obtained from high-quality, clean, dehulled soybeans. The flakes are extracted with water at neutral or slightly alkaline pH, to separate the soluble protein, carbohydrate, and mineral constituents from insoluble matter. The protein-containing extract is then separated from the residual flake material and acidified for precipitation. The resulting curd is then separated from the whey fraction, washed with water, and either spray-dried at its isoelectric point, or neutralized with sodium hydroxide and then spray-dried again.

SECOND GENERATION (SOY PROTEIN ISOLATE) FORMULAS

There are currently six of these formulas available in Britain, with little variation apart from the carbohydrate source. Their taste and palatability appear to be very acceptable. Potential problems with their use can be divided into four main headings: (a) growth; (b) mineral bioavailability; (c) carbohydrate intolerance; (d) immunological.

Growth

The biological quality of soy protein isolates, as determined by rat growth assay, has a range of 65 to 85% that of casein. When, however, the first limiting amino acid L-methionine is added, the quality of the protein improves to that of casein. In infant studies, a similar improvement in nitrogen balance was shown when a supplement of 20 mg/kg/day was added (16). This amino acid is now added to all modern formulas, which have been shown to sustain similar growth and serum chemical profiles when compared to breast milk and modified cow's milk formula (17–20). Differences in patient selection, types of soy feed given, and different methods of anthropometric data collection make it difficult to compare the large number of studies performed, but suffice it to say that there is fairly unanimous agreement that normal growth and development does occur.

Mineral Bioavailability

Studies using externally tagged zinc have shown that the highest absorption of zinc is from human milk and the lowest from soy isolate formulas (41% compared to 14%) (21). This low bioavailability in the presence of soy protein is probably caused by the 1% phytate content, and is thought to be a major factor in the symptom exacerbation of a child with acrodermatitis enteropathica (22).

A similarly decreased mineral bioavailability, or possibly a poor solubility, has been incriminated in a recent survey of 46 very low-birthweight infants who received one of three different feeds including a soy isolate, 60% of the latter developing radiological rickets and low serum phosphate levels and raised alkaline phosphatase (23). The study concluded that prolonged feeding with soy isolate formulas was to be avoided in infants less than 1,500 g birthweight.

Of equal concern, but as yet without any hard clinical data, is the high aluminum content of some of these formulas. Recent results were compared with those for fresh breast milk, cow's milk, and local tap water. Differences in concentration of greater than 150-fold were found, the soy isolate formulas all being more than 12 times the concentration of aluminum already implicated in cerebral toxicity (24).

Carbohydrate Intolerance

The marketability of all soy formulas is greatly enhanced by the absence of lactose, and one of the major sales indications for their use is following acute gastroenteritis which may be associated with a fall in enterocyte brush-border lactase levels and a secondary lactose intolerance. I advise caution, however, as not only may sucrase levels be depressed, but an occasional monosaccharide intolerance may also develop, making any of these formulas unsuitable.

Although rare, three other conditions would be exacerbated by the use of some of these formulas: congenital glucose/galactose malabsorption (all formulas), hereditary fructose intolerance, and sucrase-isomaltase deficiency (those containing sucrose).

Immunological

The basic assumption underlying the use of soy as a substitute for cow's milk is that it is less allergenic. It has frequently been used in the prophylaxis of allergic disease in newborns with a family history of atopic disease. It is equally advocated for the treatment of cow's milk protein intolerance. Trying to analyze the many studies done in the past few years is extremely difficult, if not impossible, because of difficulties in interpreting the results, the different diagnostic criteria used for selection, the varying lengths of the trials performed, some retrospective and some prospective, and the failure, in many, to perform double-blind crossover trials. The latter comment is particularly pertinent, because for the purist, nothing short of double-blind will suffice in order to obtain some idea of the placebo effect, which we all recognize as potentially large. Herein, in my opinion, lies a major and so far insurmountable problem: when comparing cow's milk with soy milk, most mothers will quickly spot the soy formula, no matter what it is packaged in. It is, therefore, impossible to have a true placebo.

Let us now examine the various, complicated, and still poorly understood immunological aspects involved with these formulas.

Protein Constituents

Most antigens are proteins and cow's milk contains at least 20. The globulin fraction of soybeans is the major protein component, comprising about 85%, and consists of four main subcomponents with approximate sedimentation constants of 15,

11, 7, and 2S (25). A comparison of the different protein bands in various formulas is shown in Fig. 1. There is evidence that the 2S-globulin has the highest allergenic potency, and that heat treatment at 80°C for 30 min enhances this potency (25). This is of interest, as we have shown that hemagglutination titer to soy, following intramuscular injection in rabbits, was higher when soy isolates were used compared to the crude soy powder extract (26). In contrast to cow's milk formulas, which become less antigenic after heat treatment (27), it is possible that the commercial preparation of soy isolates may actually enhance their antigenicity.

Antigenicity

The concept that the soybean is a weak antigen was fostered during the 1950s and 1960s, largely as a result of studies in guinea pigs. The factors involved in antigenicity alone are complex, and animal experiments are always difficult to extrapolate to human beings. In a study involving 25 normal infants fed casein hydrolysate, soy-based or milk-based formulas from birth (Table 1), we were able to demonstrate that the soy-based formula was at least as antigenic as the milk-based (28) (Figs. 2 and 3). Circulating antibodies developed in all infants with an initial rapid increase to 3 months and then little or no further rise thereafter.

High levels of hemagglutinating soy antibody have also been described in amniotic fluid, suggesting *in utero* sensitization (29), and secretory immunoglobulin A (IgA) antibodies against soy proteins are regularly found in the breast milk of mothers consuming such protein in their diets (30). These data all suggest that the soybean is not a weak antigen in humans.

Systemic Immunological Tolerance

Large molecular weight proteins are absorbed intact by the intestine in quantities which are nutritionally insignificant, but potentially important immunologically

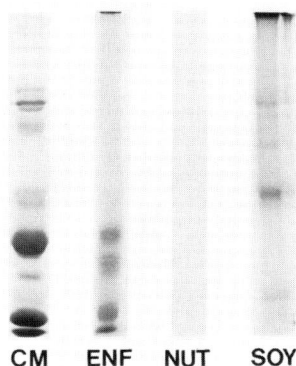

FIG. 1. Protein bands on sodium dodecyl sulfate-polyacrylamide gel electrophoresis of different formula feeds. Cow's milk (CM); modified cow's milk formula (ENF); protein hydrolysate formula (NUT); soy protein isolate formula (SOY).

CM ENF NUT SOY

TABLE 1. *Study groups*

Group	Formula	
	0–3 months	3–12 months
I	Milk base	Milk base
II	Milk base	Cow's base
III	Casein hydrolysate	Soy base
IV	Soy base	Soy base
V	Casein hydrolysate	Soy base

(31). In the majority of healthy people, the resulting immunological effects cause no apparent problems and, indeed, there is mounting evidence that the absorption of antigens after oral exposure leads to a simultaneous induction of specific systemic low-zone tolerance (32–34). The known factors controlling such reactions are complex (35), but involve IgA specific helper thymus-derived cells (T cells) and IgG and IgE suppressor cells in Peyer's patches (36). From the practical point of view, it is probably failure to develop this tolerance that somehow results in allergic reactions to food. The oral induction of tolerance has been achieved with a variety of substances both in animals and man, and, in the context of soy protein, we have shown that in rabbits, prior oral feeding with milk formula resulted in a state of partial systemic immunological tolerance, but that this was more profound and complete using soy-based formulas (26) (Figs. 4 and 5).

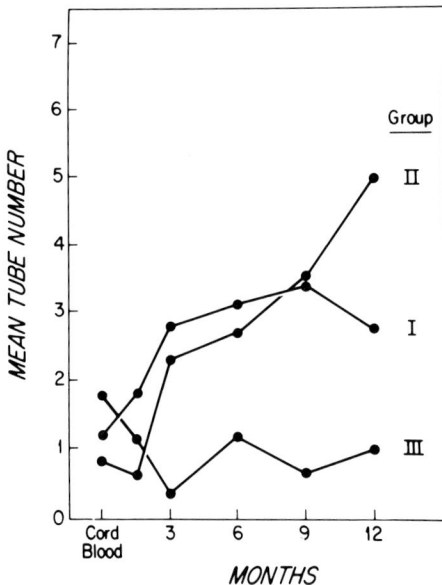

FIG. 2. Kinetics of production of hemagglutinins to cow's milk-based formula. (From Eastham et al., ref. 28, with permission.)

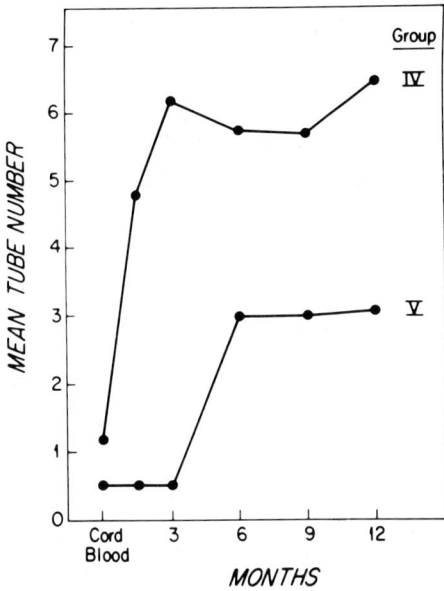

FIG. 3. Kinetics of production of hemagglutinins to soy-based formula. (From Eastham et al., ref. 28, with permission.)

The term, low zone, refers to the fact that the state of tolerance develops at a fairly critical small antigenic dose (i.e., that allowed by the healthy intestinal mucosa). Following acute gastroenteritis, however, the permeability of the mucosa increases as a result of tissue damage, and the amount of antigen reaching the Peyer's patch may be in excess of that necessary to maintain tolerance. This is probably very

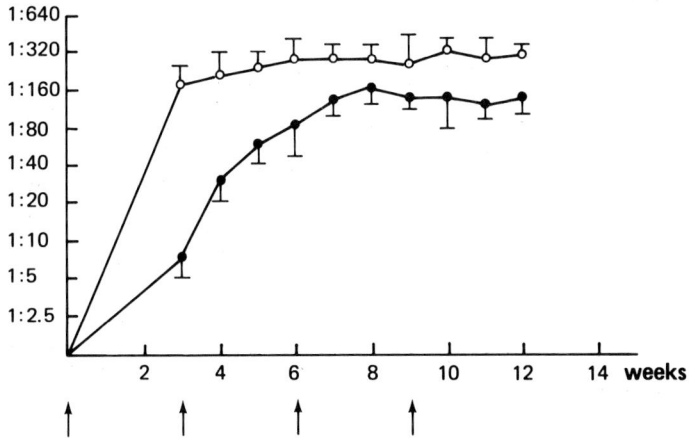

FIG. 4. Hemagglutinating anti-cow's milk antibody response after parenteral immunization with *(closed circle)* and without *(open circle)* prior oral feeding (mean ± SD). (From Eastham et al., ref. 26, with permission.)

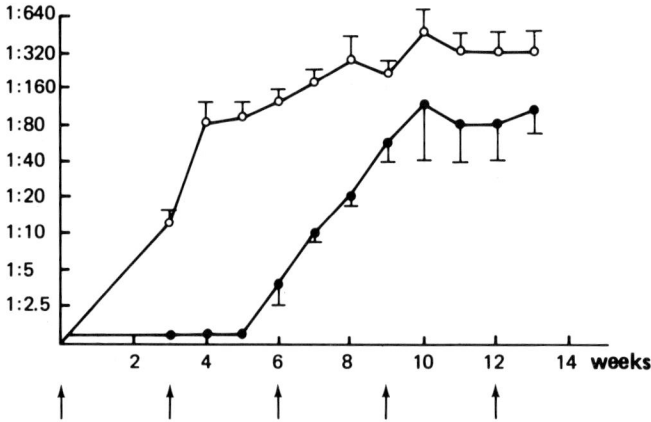

FIG. 5. Hemagglutinating antibody response after parenteral immunization with *(closed circle)* and without *(open circle)* prior oral feeding (mean ± SD). (From Eastham et al., ref. 26, with permission.)

relevant in clinical practice: in many cases, soy formulas are introduced at a time when the intestinal mucosa is damaged (e.g., gastroenteritis, cow's milk protein intolerance).

General Antibody Response

The body's response to any antigen may be influenced to some extent by the type of protein ingested (i.e., animal or vegetable, cow's milk or soy milk). A group in Veróna has published several reports since 1978, suggesting that healthy nonatopic infants fed high amounts of vegetable protein have lower immunoglobulin levels and more infections than do similar infants fed cow's milk (37,38). They have also recently published data (39) looking at antibody responses to polio virus, diphtheria, pertussis, and tetanus vaccine in a group of infants fed exclusively for 5 months on the breast or on one of four types of artificial feed varying in quality and quantity of protein. Antibody levels measured at 5 and 8 months showed a much lower response to all vaccines in those infants fed on the soy formula (Table 2) and the authors concluded that vegetable protein should not be given in infant feeds during the first months of life. Although this has been thought by some to be too dogmatic, the figures are nevertheless impressive and worrying. Further work in this area is awaited with interest.

Allergenicity

Antigenicity and allergenicity are not synonymous, and whatever the antigenic potency of a soy formula, it is a foreign protein and capable of producing an allergic reaction.

TABLE 2. *Mean antibody concentrations against polio type 2, diphtheria, and pertussis at 8 months of age in infants fed different types of formula*

Feed	Polio 2	Diphtheria	Pertussis
Human milk	1/316	1/1,507	1/380
Cow's milk formula	1/316	1/1,823	1/255
Soy formula	1/158	1/152	1/139

The first report of soy allergy was by Duke in 1934 (40), when he described an individual who was exquisitely sensitive and who lived and worked near a soybean mill. He also reported five cases of people working at this mill with asthma triggered by the same antigen, and he warned that the soybean might become a prominent source of allergy. During the next 20 years there was practically no evidence in the literature to support this prediction, but with its increasing usage, a variety of immunologically mediated intolerances to this protein have been reported.

Acute anaphylaxis is an immediate hypersensitivity reaction, occurring within a few minutes to hours of antigen challenge, and attributable to the IgE-mediated release of various chemical mediators. Although it seems to be rare, such a reaction following soy ingestion has been described (41,42). Three conditions must be met for anaphylaxis to occur: one initial exposure to a sensitizing agent, a latent period, and then a reexposure to the agent. Thus the increasing elimination of soy, followed by its reintroduction in children with allergic disease, can clearly create a potential for such a reaction and is considered a definite hazard by some (41).

Gastrointestinal symptoms, including diarrhea, vomiting, and failure to thrive, were some of the first recognized (43,44), and in 1972, Ament and Rubin (45) were the first to document a reversible flat jejunal lesion. This has subsequently been confirmed (46,47) and an immunological basis suggested by the finding of increased numbers of IgA- and IgM-containing cells in the lamina propria, and increases in serum IgA and IgG to soy at the time of the clinical reactions, together with changes in serum complement fractions three and four (46).

As well as the small intestine, the colon is the target organ in some cases of soy intolerance, and several reports of both enterocolitis in the low-birthweight infant and colitis in the older child have been published in the past few years (48–52). Rectal biopsies have shown an acute colitis with crypt abscesses, depletion of goblet cell mucus, and a polymorph leukocytosis within the lamina propria. Colonoscopic biopsies have shown, in addition, a noticeable increase in eosinophils and IgE-containing cells (52). Further evidence that this damage was immunologically mediated was a frequent family history of allergy, a blood eosinophilia, high concentrations of serum IgE, and positive IgE antibodies. In one study of enterocolitis, specific IgG and IgA antibodies were also significantly higher in those children with positive challenge responses (48).

Although skin testing and specific IgE measurements are neither consistently positive nor accurate in children with food allergies, there is a high incidence of soy sensitivity in older children with atopy on the basis of intracutaneous tests (53), and specific IgE antibodies to soy are often found in atopic children with severe eczema (54). Further evidence that clinical intolerance may be immunologically mediated comes from studies showing depressed neutrophil chemotaxis, enhanced random migration (55), and specific lymphocyte sensitization (56) to soy protein. Finally, a delayed and late turn-on of immunoglobulin has been postulated as a possible cause of gastrointestinal allergies, following a study of 98 infants with multiple allergies in whom this occurred in nearly a third (57).

The demonstration of all these immunological phenomena may just mean that the host is immunologically competent and has elaborated these biological molecules in the course of the normal immune response to a food. To attribute a pathogenic role to any of these protagonists, there are certain criteria which need to be fulfilled optimally, but these are beyond the scope of this paper.

At present we are only part of the way through these criteria with regard to soy allergy. The important question to ask is to what extent are soy formulas allergenic, particularly when compared to cow's milk? The estimated incidence of cow's milk allergy is variously reported as between 0.3 and 7.5% (58), reflecting differences in diagnostic criteria and patient referral patterns. The true incidence in Britain is thought to be around 1%. When soy is given to healthy infants there is evidence that the incidence of allergy is much less (59), although one study quoted 0.5%, which was still much lower than the 1.8% that was found for cow's milk (60). Relative to cow's milk, therefore, soy-based formulas are less allergenic when given to healthy infants, and this fact has helped to contribute to sales in the United States, where it is estimated that 10% of infants are receiving this type of formula. However, when used as a substitute for cow's milk in cases of cow's milk protein intolerance, allergy to soy develops in a far higher number of cases, figures varying from 15 to 50% (61–64). This is because the intestinal mucosa is more permeable and low-zone tolerance is probably broken. For this reason my personal practice is not to prescribe soy formulas in these circumstances, but to use one of the protein hydrolysate formulas.

Prevention of Allergy

The hypothesis to be analyzed is that soy protein formulas, when used exclusively from birth in infants at risk of developing allergic disease, have a delaying effect in preventing or postponing atopic manifestations. Such claims have been made for exclusive breast-feeding (65,66), although denied by others (67). There are two widely quoted studies from the 1950s and 1960s suggesting a beneficial effect of soy. Glaser and Johnstone (68) were the first to study the prophylactic potential, and they studied 96 infants from atopic families from birth to 6 months of age, and followed them until 6 years of age. The incidence of allergy was 15% in the soy group, 65% in control siblings, and 52% in nonrelated controls. In the later study, Johnstone and Dutton divided 240 children into two feeding groups and followed them prospectively until they were 10 years old. The incidence of asthma and rhinitis in the soy group was almost half (22.3%) that of the cow's milk group (42%) (69). More recently, breast-feeding supplemented with soy milk was found to exert a prophylactic effect on the development of atopic disease in at-risk infants (70), but it seems likely that it was the breast milk that was the more important factor. More recent, and in my opinion, better designed and conducted studies have shown that soy feeding produces no advantage over cow's milk in the prophylaxis of allergic disease (71–74).

Infant colic has been the subject of much recent speculation, and cow's milk has been suggested as a possible etiological cause (75,76). Not surprisingly, soy-based formulas were then tried as an alternative, but again there was no significant improvement in the colic (77).

I have attempted, in this paper, to balance the conflicting evidence that there are benefits in feeding soy formulas to infants, as a substitute for cow's milk formulas. Although it is true that the vast majority of infants would be able to tolerate them, show normal growth and development, and indeed have a lower incidence of protein intolerance, the numbers benefitting from this advantage, relative to cow's milk formulas, must be very small. This would not warrant the extra cost of mass changeover to these formulas. Their use in selected instances has been reviewed, and in many cases, contrary to the manufacturers' literature, has not withstood the rigors of good clinical trials. Cow's milk allergy is not common, but the concomitant occurrence of soy allergy (whichever figure you believe) is high enough to be cautious in recommending their use, particularly since protein hydrolysate formulas appear to be the most effective therapy and are virtually nonantigenic (78). Their use as prophylaxis against atopic disease in predisposed infants has also been examined. Since it has been estimated that only 10% of atopic diseases in childen under 6 years of age are caused by food (79), then it is not surprising that clinical trials have resulted in different conclusions. I personally find little in the literature to uphold the claim that soy formulas are protective. Their use in reducing infant colic has not been substantiated, and I remain concerned that the body's general antibody response may be depressed, resulting in more infections.

There is an urgent need for the studies from Verona, concerning responses to vaccines, to be repeated by other centers. Such studies should include soy protein isolate and protein hydrolysate formulas. Should they confirm these Italian studies with respect to soy, my own feeling is that these products should not be used at all in the first 6 months of life.

Finally, I have only concentrated on commercially available approved formulas. Many mothers obtain rather different forms of soy-based milks, usually from health food stores. These are unsuitable for babies as their composition lacks calcium, vitamins, and energy. How much allergy they cause is unknown!

REFERENCES

1. Department of Health and Social Security. *Present-day Practice in Infant Feeding*. London: Her Majesty's Stationery Office. 1975.
2. Taitz LS. Soy feeding in infancy. *Arch Dis Child* 1982;57:814–5.

3. Ruhräh J. The soybean in infant feeding. Preliminary report. *Arch Pediatr* 1909;26:496–501.
4. Hill LW, Stuart HC. A soybean preparation for feeding infants with milk allergy. *JAMA* 1929;93:986–90.
5. Cornfield D, Cooke RE. Vitamin deficiency: unusual manifestation in a 5½ month old baby. Case report. *Pediatrics* 1952;10:33–5.
6. Goldman HI, Desposito F. Hypoprothrombinemic bleeding in young infants: association with diarrhoea antibiotics and milk substitutes. *Am J Dis Child* 1966;111:430–2.
7. Davis RA, Wolf A. Infantile beriberi associated with Wernicke's encephalopathy. *Pediatrics* 1958;21:409–13.
8. Patton AR, Wilgus HS Jr, Harshfield GS. Goitrogenicity of soybean meal in chickens described for the first time. *Science* 1939;89:162–4.
9. Van Wyk JJ, Arnold MB, Wynn J, Pepper F. The effects of a soybean product on thyroid function in humans. *Pediatrics* 1959;24:752–60.
10. Block RJ, Mandle RH, Howard HW, Bauer CD, Anderson DW. The curative action of iodine on soybean goiter and the changes in the distribution of iodoamino acids in the serum and in thyroid gland digests. *Arch Biochem Biophys* 1961;93:15–24.
11. Sarret HP. Soy-based infant formulas. In: Hill LD, ed. *Proceedings of the World Soybean Research Conference*. Illinois: The Interstate Printers and Publishers. 1976.
12. McGuiness EE, Morgan RGH, Levison DA, Frape DL, Hopwood D, Wormsley KG. The effect of long-term feeding of soya flour on rat pancreas. *Scand J Gastroenterol* 1980;15:497–502.
13. Moroz LA, Yang WH. Kunitz soybean trypsin inhibitor: a specific allergen in food anaphylaxis. *N Engl J Med* 1980;302:1126–8.
14. Maga JA. Phytate; its chemistry, occurrence, food interaction, nutritional significance and methods of analysis. *J Agric Food Chem* 1982;30:1–9.
15. Liener IE. Naturally occurring toxicants in plant foods and milk. In: Freed DLJ, ed. *Health Hazards of Milk*. Eastbourne: Baillière Tindall, 1984;169–87.
16. Graham GG. Methionine or lysine fortification of dietary protein for infants and small children. In: Scrimshaw NS, Altshul AM, eds. *Amino Acid Fortification of Protein Foods*. Cambridge: MIT Press, 1971;222.
17. Fomon SJ. Requirements for protein and essential amino acids in early infancy. *Acta Paediatr Scand* 1973;62:33–45.
18. Sellars WA. Newgrowth charts: soy, cow and breast milk comparisons. *Ann Allergy* 1971;29:126–30.
19. Dean ME. A study of normal infants fed on soya protein isolate formula. *Med J Aus* 1973;1:1289–95.
20. Jung AL, Carr SL. A soy protein formula and a milk based formula. *Clin Pediatr* 1977;16:892–8.
21. Sandstrom B, Cererblad A, Lonnderdal B. Zinc absorption from human milk, cow's milk, and infant formula. *Am J Dis Child* 1983;137:726–9.
22. Glasgow JF, Elmes ME. Exacerbation of acrodermatitis enteropathica by soya-bean milk feeding. *Lancet* 1975;ii:769.
23. Kulkarni PB, Dorand RD, Bridger WM, Payne JH, Montiel DC, Hill JG. Rickets in premature infants fed different formulas. *South Med J* 1984;77:13–6.
24. Weintraub R, Hams G, Meerkin M, Rosenberg AR. High aluminium content of infant milk formulas. *Arch Dis Child* 1986;61:914–6.
25. Shibasaki M, Suzuki S, Tajima S, Hemoto H, Kuroume T. Allergenicity of major component proteins of soybean. *Int Arch Allergy Appl Immunol* 1980;61:441–8.
26. Eastham EJ, Lichauco T, Pang K, Walker WA. Antigenicity of infant formulas and the induction of systemic immunological tolerance by oral feeding: cow's milk versus soy milk. *J Pediatr Gastroenterol Nutr* 1982;1:23–8.
27. McLaughlin P, Anderson KJ, Widdowson E, Coombs RRA. The effect of heat on the anaphylactic-sensitizing capacity of cow's milk, goat's milk and various infant formulas fed to guinea pigs. *Clin Exp Immunol* 1979;35:454–62.
28. Eastham EJ, Lichauco T, Grady MI, Walker WA. Antigenicity of infant formulas: role of immature intestine on protein permeability. *J Pediatr* 1978;93:561–4.
29. Kuroume T, Oguri M, Matsumura T, Iwasaki I, Yuzuru K. Milk sensitivity and soybean sensitivity in the production of eczematous manifestations in breast-fed infants with particular reference to intrauterine sensitization. *Ann Allergy* 1976;37:41–6.
30. Hanson LA, Ahlstedt S, Anderson B, et al. The immune response of the mammary gland and its significance for the neonate. *Ann Allergy* 1984;53:576–82.

31. Walker WA, Isselbacher KJ. Uptake and transport of macromolecules by the intestine. Possible role in clinical disorders. *Gastroenterology* 1974;67:531–8.
32. Hanson DG, Nelson MV, Maia LCS, Hornbrook MM, Lynch JM, Roy CA. Inhibition of specific immune responses by feeding protein antigens. *Int Arch Allergy Appl Immunol* 1977;55:526–30.
33. Andre C, Heremans JF, Vaerman JP, Cambiasco CL. A mechanism for the induction of immunological tolerance by antigen feeding. Antigen-antibody complexes. *J Exp Med* 1975;142:1509–15.
34. Swarbrick ET, Stokes CR, Soothill JF. Absorption of antigens after oral immunization and the simultaneous induction of specific systemic tolerance. *Gut* 1979;20:121–5.
35. Anonymous. Oral encounters with antigen. *Lancet* 1981;i:702.
36. Ngan J, Kind LS. Suppressor T cells for IgE and IgG in Peyer's patches of mice made tolerant by administration of ovalbumin. *J Immunol* 1978;120:861–5.
37. Zoppi G. Gerosa F, Pezzini A, et al. Immunocompetence and dietary protein intake in early infancy. *J Pediatr Gastroenterol Nutr* 1982;1:175–82.
38. Zoppi G, Zamboni G, Bassani N, Vassoler G. Gammaglobulin level and soy protein intake in early infancy. *Eur J Pediatr* 1979;131:61–9.
39. Zoppi G, Gasparini R, Mantonvanelli F, Gobio-Casali L, Astolfi R, Crovari P. Diet and antibody response to vaccinations in healthy infants. *Lancet* 1983;ii:11–4.
40. Duke WW. Soy bean as a possible important source of allergy. *J Allergy* 1934;5:300–3.
41. David TJ. Anaphylactic shock during elimination diets for severe atopic eczema. *Arch Dis Child* 1984;59:983–6.
42. Mortimer EZ. Anaphylaxis following ingestion of soybean. *J Pediatr* 1961;58:90–2.
43. Cook CD. Probable gastrointestinal reaction to soybean. *N Engl J Med* 1960;262:1076–8.
44. Mendoz J, Meyers J, Snyder R. Soybean sensitivity: case report. *Pediatrics* 1970;46:774–6.
45. Ament ME, Rubin CE. Soy protein—another cause of the flat intestinal lesion. *Gastroenterology* 1972;62:227–34.
46. Perkkio M, Savilahti E, Kuitunen P. Morphometric and immunohistochemical study of jejunal biopsies from children with intestinal soy allergy. *Eur J Pediatr* 1981;137:63–9.
47. Poley JR, Kein AW. Scanning electron microscopy of soy protein-induced damage of small bowel mucosa in infants. *J Pediatr Gastroenterol Nutr* 1983;2:271–87.
48. McDonald PJ, Goldblum RM, Van-Sickle GJ, Powell GK. Food protein induced enterocolitis: altered antibody response to ingested antigen. *Pediatr Res* 1984;10:751–5.
49. Powell FK. Enterocolitis in low-birth-weight infants associated with milk and soy protein intolerance. *J Pediatr* 1976;93:553–60.
50. Halpin TC, Byrne WJ, Ament ME. Colitis, persistent diarrhoea, and soy protein intolerance. *J Pediatr* 1977;91:404–7.
51. Powell GK. Milk and soy-induced enterocolitis of infancy. *J Pediatr* 1978;93:553–60.
52. Jenkins HR, Pincott JR, Soothill JF, Milla PJ, Harries JT. Food allergy: the major cause of infantile colitis. *Arch Dis Child* 1984;59:326–9.
53. Fries JH. Studies on the allergenicity of soybean. *Ann Allergy* 1971;29:1–7.
54. David TJ. The investigation and treatment of severe eczema in childhood. *Int Med* 1983;Suppl 6:17–25.
55. Butler HL, Byrne WJ, Marmer DJ, Euler AR, Steele RW. Depressed neutrophil chemotaxis in infants with cow's milk and/or soy protein intolerance. *Pediatrics* 1981;67:264–8.
56. Van Sickle GJ, Powell GK, McDonald PJ, Goldblum RM. Milk and soy protein induced enterocolitis: evidence for lymphocyte sensitization to specific food proteins. *Gastroenterology* 1985; 88:1915–21.
57. Gryboski JD, Kocoshis S. Immunoglobulin deficiency in gastrointestinal allergies. *J Clin Gastroenterol* 1980;2:71–6.
58. Bahna SL, Heiner DC. *Allergies to Milk*. New York: Grune and Stratton, 1980.
59. American Academy of Pediatrics' Committee on Nutrition. Soy protein formulas: recommendations for use in infant feeding. *Pediatrics* 1983;72:359.
60. Halpern SR, Sellars WA, Johnson RB, Anderson DW, Saperstein S, Reisch JS. Development of childhood allergy in infants fed breast, soy or cow's milk. *J Allergy Clin Immunol* 1973;51:139–51.
61. Walker-Smith JA. Gastrointestinal allergy. *Practitioner* 1978;220:562–9.
62. Gerrard JW, MacKenzie JWA, Goluboff N, Garson JZ, Maningas CS. Cow's milk allergy: prevalence and manifestations in an unselected series of newborns. *Acta Paediatr Scand* 1973;234:1–21.
63. Jakobsson I, Lindberg T. A prospective study of cow's milk protein intolerance in Swedish infants. *Acta Paediatr Scand* 1979;68:853–9.

64. Visakorpi JK, Immonen P. Intolerance to cow's milk and wheat gluten in the primary malabsorption syndrome in infancy. *Acta Paediatr Scand* 1967;56:49–55.
65. Matthew DJ, Taylor B, Norman AP, Turner MW, Soothill JF. Prevention of eczema. *Lancet* 1977;i:321–4.
66. Saarinen UM, Kajosaari M, Backman A, Siimes MA. Prolonged breast-feeding as prophylaxis for atopic disease. *Lancet* 1979;ii:163–6.
67. Kramer MS, Moroz B. Do breast-feeding and delayed introduction of solid foods protect against subsequent atopic eczema. *J Pediatr* 1981;98:546–50.
68. Glaser J, Johnstone DE. Prophylaxis of allergic disease in the newborn. *JAMA* 1953;153:620–2.
69. Johnstone DE, Dutton AM. Dietary prophylaxis of allergic disease in children. *N Engl J Med* 1966;274:715–7.
70. Businco L, Marchetti F, Pellegrini G, Cantini A, Perlini R. Prevention of atopic disease in 'at-risk new borns' by prolonged breast feeding. *Ann Allergy* 1983;51:296–9.
71. Brown EB. A prospective study of allergy in a pediatric population. *Am J Dis Child* 1969;117: 693–8.
72. Kjellman N-IM, Johansson SGO. Soy versus cow's milk in infants with a biparental history of atopic disease, development of atopic disease and immunoglobulins from birth to four years of age. *Clin Allergy* 1979;9:347–58.
73. Gruskay FL. Comparison of breast, cow and soy feedings in the prevention of onset of allergic disease: a 15 year prospective study. *Clin Pediatr* 1982;21:486–91.
74. Moore WJ, Midwinter RE, Morris AF, Colley JRT, Soothill JF. Infant feeding and subsequent risk of atopic eczema. *Arch Dis Child* 1985;60:722–6.
75. Jakobsson I, Lindberg T. Cow's milk as a cause of infantile colic in breast-fed infants. *Lancet* 1978;ii:437–9.
76. Evans RW, Ferguson DM, Allardyce RA, Taylor B. Maternal diet and infantile colic in breast-fed infants. *Lancet* 1981;i:1340–2.
77. Lothe L, Lindberg T, Jakobsson I. Cow's milk formula as a cause of infantile colic. A double-blind study. *Pediatrics* 1982;70:7–10.
78. Eastham EJ, Walker WA. Adverse effects of milk formula ingestion on the gastrointestinal tract. *Gastroenterology* 1979;76:365–74.
79. Bleumink E. Food allergy and the gastrointestinal tract. In: Asquith P, ed. *Immunology of the Gastrointestinal Tract*. Edinburgh: Churchill Livingstone, 1979;195.

Food Intolerance in Infancy: Allergology, Immunology, and Gastroenterology, edited by Robert N. Hamburger. Carnation Nutrition Education Series, Vol. 1. The Carnation Co., Los Angeles/Raven Press, Ltd., New York © 1989.

Maternal Diet During Pregnancy and Lactation

Ranjit Kumar Chandra

Pediatric Research, Medicine, and Biochemistry, Memorial University of Newfoundland, St. John's, Newfoundland, Canada

The spectrum of atopic disease includes eczema, asthma, rhinitis, and a variety of other disorders. Allergic diseases are common causes of childhood illness. An interaction of genetic and environmental factors is considered to underlie the pathogenesis of atopic illness. A family history of allergy is elicited in about 70% of all patients with atopy. Biparental history is a stronger predisposing factor than uniparental history. Of the allergens considered responsible for precipitating symptoms, inhalants are more important for reactive bronchopulmonary disease whereas foods are more often contributors to eczema and other skin manifestations. The range of severity of symptoms varies widely, from mild to life-threatening. The heavy burden of atopic illness in terms of physical and emotional costs has led to attempts at prevention. It is clear that exclusive breast-feeding affords partial protection. However, the undoubted occurrence of serious atopic disease even among the exclusively breast-fed has prompted us to postulate that sensitization to food antigens may occur *in utero* as well as via breast milk after birth (1). In view of these considerations, we have conducted several studies to evaluate the role of maternal diet during pregnancy and lactation.

IDENTIFICATION OF HIGH-RISK INFANTS

For successful implementation of a preventive program, it is essential to identify a relatively small group of subjects who are at high risk of developing the disease. In the case of atopic disease, three lines of investigations have been pursued. The initial enthusiasm for using macromolecular uptake in the intestine has been dampened by subsequent careful work. The two promising indices of risk for atopy are cord blood immunoglobulin E (IgE) levels and thymus-derived cell (T-cell) subsets.

Immunoregulatory Thymus-Derived Cells

IgE underlies the genesis of many of the manifestations of atopic disease. The production of IgE is regulated by the balance of helper and suppressor T cells. Thus it is logical to consider using the number and function of T-cell subsets as an index of high risk.

There is considerable experimental evidence to indicate that suppressor T cells inhibit synthesis of reaginic IgE antibodies and deficiency of these cells enhances the risk of IgE-mediated immunopathology (2). Removal of suppressor cells by adherence or selective irradiation alters IgE levels. Similarly, cyclophosphamide selectively enhances IgE production. This effect of immunoregulatory T cells on IgE production is largely antigen-nonspecific. These animal observations are lent support from studies in human subjects. Strannegard et al. (3) found reduced proportion of rosette-forming T lymphocytes in 233 atopic children compared with 59 controls. The discrepancy between results in later studies may be caused in part by methodologic differences. For instance, techniques that do not permit detection of low avidity binding of sheep red blood cells may not show differences between atopic and control patients.

With our ability to identify T-cell subsets using monoclonal antibodies, studies have shown a higher ratio of T4/T8 cells largely owing to reduction of suppressor T8 cells (4) and abnormal suppressor cell function often using concanavalin A-stimulated cell cultures (5). The degree of abnormality in suppressor cell assay correlated with the duration of disease.

The interpretation of the results of studies on T-cell subsets in atopic disease, reviewed recently by Björkstén (6) and by Chandra (1), should be done with caution. It is possible that changes in immunoregulatory cells are the result rather than a cause of allergic disorders. The potent effects of histamine and other chemical mediators released during allergic reactions on inflammatory cells and lymphocytes are well documented. However, in recent prospective studies of infants 4 to 6 weeks old without any symptoms or signs of allergy the reduction in the number of suppressor T8 cells preceded the development of atopic eczema (Table 1) (7), thereby making it possible to attribute a primary rather than a secondary role to these changes. Confirmatory data were published recently (8).

Cord Blood Immunoglobulin E Levels

An increase in serum IgE levels has been observed in over 80% of patients with atopic disease. Thus, elevated IgE concentration is a strong indication of the presence of allergy in children. The synthesis and release of IgE are regulated by many factors, both genetic and environmental. There is a strong influence of age on serum IgE levels. Very small amounts of antigen, in picogram concentrations, are adequate for sensitization and formation of IgE antibodies (9). Large doses of antigen result in production of antibodies of other immunoglobulin isotypes. The regulation

TABLE 1. *Thymus-derived cell (T-cell) subpopulations in infants with and without family history of atopy*

Group	Percentage of cells		
	T4-Positive	T8-Positive	T4-T8
Negative history			
Healthy	51 ± 3.2	28 ± 4^a	1.9 ± 0.21^c
Symptomatic	47 ± 3.7	20 ± 1.9^b	2.6 ± 0.33^d
Positive history			
Healthy	45 ± 4.1	25 ± 2.0^a	2.0 ± 0.25^c
Symptomatic	49 ± 3.5	17 ± 2.5^b	2.8 ± 0.51^d

The results are expressed as mean ± SEM.
Values with different subscript letters are significantly different.

of reaginic antibodies by maternal influences and age of exposure has been extensively studied. The fetus is capable of synthesizing IgE from the 11th week of gestation (10) and it is attractive to suggest that newborn infants who subsequently become symptomatic may already show a tendency to produce IgE in greater amounts than nonatopic subjects. Thus, one might find higher cord blood IgE in infants who subsequently become atopic. Indeed this possibility has been investigated and the data indicate that high and low IgE response is already coded at birth (11). For example, Croner et al. (12) found that 70% of infants with positive family history for atopy and high cord blood IgE showed evidence of atopy by 24 months of age. However, many studies have methodological flaws (1) in that they do not mention the type of feeding (breast or artificial), and the type and time of weaning food introduced. Moreover, careful period assessment of a prospective basis was not included. Our data show that cord blood IgE is a strong predictor of atopic eczema in young infants, irrespective of family history (13). However, there is a significant influence of infant feeding.

The predictive value of cord blood IgE in the development of atopic disease was evaluated in a prospective study of two groups of infants (13). Elevated cord blood IgE greater than 0.7 U/ml was associated with a high risk of development of atopic disease in the first 2 years of life (52.8 and 58.8% in the groups with or without family history of atopy, respectively), whereas levels less than 0.7 U/ml carried a low risk (13.4 and 1.1%, respectively, in the groups with or without family history). Of 120 infants in Group 1 with positive family history of atopic disease, 53 showed cord blood IgE 0.7 U/ml or greater. Among these 53 infants, 31 were breast-fed exclusively for a minimum of 3 months (mean duration 5.7 months) and only 9 (29.0%) showed evidence of atopic disease (eczema, recurrent wheezing, or both). Among the 22 who were formula-fed, 19 (86.3%) became symptomatic. These differences are statistically significant ($p<0.01$, Chi-square analysis). Sixty-seven infants had cord blood IgE less than 0.7 U/ml; 41 were breast-fed of whom 3 (7.3%) developed atopic disease, whereas of the 26 who were formula-fed, 6 (23%) became symptomatic. These figures also are statistically significant ($p < 0.05$, Chi-square test). Of 106 infants in Group 2 with negative family history, 17 showed elevated cord blood IgE higher than 0.7 U/ml. Of these 17 infants, 8 were breast-fed and 3 (37.5%) developed eczema and/or recurrent wheezing, whereas 9 were formula-fed and 7 (77.7%) became symptomatic. Eighty-nine had cord blood IgE < 0.7 U/ml; 43 were breast-fed, and none showed symptoms of allergic disease until 2 years of age, whereas only 1 (2.17%) of the 46 on the formula developed eczema.

SENSITIZATION OF THE FETUS AND YOUNG INFANT

There is much indirect information and some definite observations to indicate that sensitizing amounts of food antigens can reach the fetus during intrauterine life and via breast milk after birth (Chandra, *manuscript in preparation,* and refs. 14–18). These data have been reviewed by Saarinen (16) and by Chandra (1). Intrauterine sensitization against foreign antigens has been shown and food ingested by the mother can be found in breast milk and cause symptoms in the baby. It is logical to suggest that the protective effect of breast-feeding on the development of atopic disease may be enhanced by modifying the mother's diet during pregnancy and during the time the infant is being breast-fed. The modification of the mother's diet may therefore be expected to influence the incidence of atopic disease.

INFANT FEEDING AND ECZEMA

Atopic eczema may be precipitated or aggravated by foods to which the infant is sensitized. In our prospective studies, we observed a significant beneficial effect of exclusive breast-feeding for at least 3 to 4 months on subsequent occurrence of eczema (13,19). This protective effect of breast-feeding against atopic disease has been seen in a number of prospective studies (20). Businco et al. (21) used a carefully designed protocol employing breast-feeding or soya milk and only selected weaning after 6 months and a controlled diet for the mother during lactation. Comparing the study groups with the control group in which infants were fed cow's milk, they demonstrated a protective effect of breast-feeding on the development of allergy. Some investigations, largely retrospective, were unable to demonstrate any beneficial effect of breast-feeding on incidence of atopic disease (22). For example, one report concluded that breast-feeding and delayed introduction of solid foods do not protect against subsequent atopic eczema (23). An important drawback of this study, however, is the fact that it was a retrospective investigation in which the parents of children aged 1 month to 20 years were interviewed regarding feeding history, family history, and demographic data. Obviously the reliability of such a history long after the events had taken place would be questionable. Furthermore, many of the negative studies examined general population samples rather than children from atopic families.

The possible mechanisms for the protective effect of human milk include reduced exposure to sensitizing food proteins such as β-lactoglobulins, anti-infective properties that reduce the incidence of infections, and increased maturation of intestinal barrier (24–26).

MATERNAL FOOD ANTIGEN AVOIDANCE DURING PREGNANCY AND LACTATION

The possibility of acquiring food desensitization during fetal life and the demonstration of food antigens in breast milk have led to the logical suggestion that maternal antigen avoidance during pregnancy and lactation would reduce the risk of atopic eczema during infancy.

We have recently reported the results of a prospective study of maternal antigen avoidance during pregnancy and lactation on the incidence and severity of atopic eczema in infants at high risk of developing the disorder (15). One hundred twenty-one women with a history of a previous child with atopic disease were randomly allocated during the next pregnancy to antigen avoidance or control groups. Dietary advice consisted of almost complete exclusion of milk and dairy products, egg, fish, beef, and peanut throughout pregnancy and lactation. A total of 109 completed the study. Maternal antigen avoidance was associated with reduced occurrence of atopic eczema and the skin involvement was less extensive and milder.

The maternal antigen avoidance and control groups were found to be matched for several confounding variables (Table 2) that may influence compliance, choice of the mode of infant feeding, the development of atopic eczema, and follow-up. Ma-

TABLE 2. *Confounding variables*

	Group 1 Antigen avoidance advice (*N* = 55)	Group 2 Control (*N* = 54)
Family income ($)	36,242 ± 5,160[a]	32,499 ± 6,388
Maternal education		
University	23	25
High school	19	18
Less than high school	13	11
Family history of atopy		
Biparental	12	15
Uniparental	21	23
Birthweight (kg)	3.36 ± 0.26	3.51 ± 0.33
Low birthweight (< 2,500 g)	3	3
Duration of breast-feeding (months)	5.3 ± 0.6	6.1 ± 1.1
Age of introduction of solids (months)	6.2 ± 0.9	6.5 ± 1.2
Pets	21	18
Parental smoking	12	15

[a]Mean ± SD.
Differences between the two groups are statistically not significant.

TABLE 3. *Influence of maternal antigen avoidance and mode of feeding on incidence of atopic eczema in infants*

Groups	N	Eczema present	No eczema	Statistical analysis (Fisher's exact probability test)
Group 1 (Maternal food antigen avoidance)	55	17	38	
Breast-fed	35	5	30	$p = 0.0046$
Formula-fed	20	12	8	
				$p = 0.0503$
Group 2 (Control)	54	24	30	$p = 0.7864$
Breast-fed	36	11	25	$p = 0.0509$
Formula-fed	18	13	5	
				$p = 0.6933$

ternal antigen avoidance was associated with reduced occurrence of atopic eczema (Table 3). Among the 55 in Group 1 who completed the trial of antigen avoidance, 17 infants developed atopic eczema, 5 of 35 were breast-fed, and 12 out of 20 who were formula-fed. Among the offspring of 54 control mothers in Group 2 given no dietary restrictions, eczema was observed in 24 infants, 11 of 36 breast-fed and 13 of 18 formula-fed. The incidence of atopic eczema was significantly reduced in Group 1, mainly among the breast-fed group. Fewer exclusively breast-fed infants developed eczema compared with formula-fed infants both in Groups 1 and 2. For the entire group of breast-fed infants, the incidence of eczema was significantly less compared with the formula-fed group. The beneficial preventive effect of breast-feeding was more marked when combined with maternal antigen avoidance. The extent of atopic eczema as estimated by an objective scoring system was significantly less in the antigen avoidance group (Table 4). The breast-fed infants had a lower score compared with formula-fed babies both in Groups 1 and 2. One or more of the food antigens were detected in breast milk samples obtained from 3 of 20 mothers

TABLE 4. *Influence of maternal antigen avoidance and mode of feeding on severity and extent of atopic eczema in high-risk infants*

Groups	Breast-fed	Formula-fed
Group 1 (Maternal antigen avoidance)	20 ± 3^a	32 ± 3^b
($N = 55$)	($N = 35$)	($N = 20$)
Group 2 (Control)	29 ± 4^b	46 ± 5^c
($N = 54$)	($N = 36$)	($N = 18$)

The results are expressed as mean ± SEM of eczema score (see Methods). Values designated with a different subscript letter differed significantly from one another on Student's t test analysis, a versus c, $p < 0.01$; b versus c, $p < 0.05$.

TABLE 5. *Presence of dietary antigens in breast milk*

	Mothers tested (N)	β-Lactoglobulin	Casein	Ovalbumin	Any antigen
Group 1 (Antigen avoidance advice)	20	3	2	1	3[a]
Group 2 (Control)	16	12	7	10	15[a]

[a]Chi square, $\chi^2 = 22.0$; $p < 0.01$.

in Group 2 controls (Table 5). These differences are significant statistically. Thus, avoidance of common dietary allergens during pregnancy and lactation enhanced the preventive beneficial effect of exclusive breast-feeding on the incidence of atopic eczema among infants at high risk.

ENVIRONMENTAL ENGINEERING FOR THE PREVENTION OF ATOPIC DISEASE

The potential contribution of food allergy to the development of atopic disease (eczema, asthma, others) has stimulated studies on prevention, employing exclusive breast-feeding, hypoallergenic formulas, and maternal dietary restrictions during pregnancy and lactation. Many studies have found a reduction, but not elimination, of atopic eczema among high-risk infants fed exclusively on the breast. Study design differences, particularly disregard of confounding variables (Table 6), may be

TABLE 6. *Confounding variables influencing the scientific validity of studies of the association between breast-feeding and atopic disease*

Prospective versus retrospective
Duration and exclusive nature of breast-feeding
Definition of disease
Time of introduction of solids
Small number of subjects
Dropout rate
Social demographic characteristics
Attendance at day-care facility
Environmental control (smoking, dust, pets)
Compliance
Blinding
Lack of supportive immunology data
Statistical analysis

TABLE 7. *Maternal antigen avoidance*

Gestational period during which potential allergens are excluded
Range of food antigens excluded
Compliance
Number of subjects and dropouts

responsible for differences in the results of various studies (27–29). The apparent failure of even exclusive breast-feeding to entirely prevent atopic symptoms may be attributed to several factors (21–36). One, sensitization may have occurred *in utero* so that it is already too late at birth to entirely prevent atopic disease. Two, food antigens may be passed into human milk and cause allergic symptoms among the breast-fed group. The latter possibility has been suggested by the detection of such antigens in human milk and by the amelioration of colic-like symptoms and of eczema in infants by antigen avoidance by mothers during lactation (30–36).

Some of the variables that may influence the outcome of trials of maternal food avoidance in prevention of allergic disease are listed in Table 7. This may explain the discrepancy between the results of our studies (15) and those observed by Kjellman *(unpublished observations)*. The Swedish study began dietary precautions in the third trimester of pregnancy, long after the fetus is capable of becoming sensitized (19). Secondly, only two foods, egg and milk, were avoided. Finally, a casein hydrolysate was fed to the mothers and it is possible that this preparation may contain sensitizing molecules (see Hill, *this volume*).

In order to reduce the risk of sensitization and thereby that of atopic disease, a plan of environmental engineering should be followed (Table 8) (1,37). It would be prudent to begin preventive measures during pregnancy and continue them after birth for the first 4 to 6 months of life. Thus, the maximum benefit may be expected to accrue from antigen avoidance during the antenatal period, followed by breast-feeding (with continuing precautions related to mother's diet) or a protein hydrolysate formula.

TABLE 8. *Environmental engineering*

Pregnancy	Avoid allergenic foods
Infancy	Prolong breast-feeding
	Delay solid foods
	Reduce exposure to inhalants
	Reduce risk of infection
	Eliminate parental smoking

REFERENCES

1. Chandra RK. Prevention of atopic disease. Environmental engineering utilizing antenatal antigen avoidance and breast feeding. In: Goldman A, Hanson LA, Atkinson SA, eds. *Effect of Human Milk Upon the Recipient Infant*. New York: Plenum *(in press)*.
2. Kishimoto T. IgE class-specific suppressor T cells and regulation of IgE response. *Prog Allergy* 1982;32:265–317.
3. Strannegard IL, Lindholm L, Strannegard O. Studies of T lymphocytes in atopic children. *Int Arch Allergy Appl Immunol* 1976;50:684–91.
4. Butler M, Atherton D, Levinsky RJ. Quantitative and functional deficit of suppressor T cells in children with atopic eczema. *Clin Exp Immunol* 1982;50:92–8.
5. Rola-Pleszczynski M, Blanchard R. Abnormal suppressor cell function in asthmatic children. *Clin Allergy* 1981;12:323–30.
6. Björkstén B. Atopy allergy in relation to cell-mediated immunity. *Clin Rev Allergy* 1984;2:95–106.
7. Chandra RK, Baker M. Numerical and functional deficiency of suppressor T cells precedes the development of atopic eczema. *Lancet* 1983;ii:1393–4.
8. Tanio V-M. Lymphocyte subsets in infants; relationship to feeding, atopy, atopic heredity, and infections. *Int Arch Allergy Appl Immunol* 1985;78:305–10.
9. Jarrett EEE. Activation of IgE regulatory mechanisms by mucosal absorption of antigen. *Lancet* 1977;ii:223–6.
10. Miller DL, Hirovnen T, Gitlin D. Synthesis of IgE by the human conceptus. *J Allergy Clin Immunol* 1973;52:182.
11. Orgel HA, Hamburger RN, Bazaral M, Gorrin H. Development of IgE and allergy in infancy. *J Allergy Clin Immunol* 1975;56:296–304.
12. Croner S, Kjellman N-IM, Eriksson B, Roth A. IgE screening in 1701 newborn infants and the development of atopic diseases during infancy. *Arch Dis Child* 1982;57:364–8.
13. Chandra RK, Puri S, Cheema PS. Predictive value of cord blood IgE in the development of atopic disease and role of breast-feeding in its prevention. *Clin Allergy* 1985;15:517–22.
14. Jakobsson I, Lindberg T, Benediktsson B, Hansson BG. Dietary bovine beta-globulin is transferred to human milk. *Acta Paediatr Scand* 1985;74:341–5.
15. Chandra RK, Puri S, Suraiya C, Cheema PS. Influence of maternal food antigen avoidance during pregnancy and lactation on incidence of atopic eczema in infants. *Clin Allergy* 1986;16:565–9.
16. Saarinen UM. Prophylaxis for atopic disease. Role of infant feeding. *Clin Rev Allergy* 1984;1:151–67.
17. Kuroume T, Oguri M, Matsumara T, Iwadaki I, Knabe Y, Kawahe S, Negishi K. Milk sensitivity and soybean sensitivity in the production of the eczematous manifestations in breast-fed infants with particular reference to intrauterine sensitization. *Ann Allergy* 1976;37:41.
18. Cant AJ, Bailes JA, Marsden RA, Hewitt D. Effect of maternal dietary exclusion on breast-fed infants with eczema: two controlled studies. *Br Med J* 1986;293:231–3.
19. Chandra RK. Prospective studies of the effect of breast feeding on the incidence of infection and allergy. *Acta Paediatr Scand* 1979;68:691–4.
20. Mathew DJ, Taylor B, Normal AP, Turner MW, Soothill JF. Prevention of eczema. *Lancet* 1988;i:321–24.
21. Businco L, Marchetti F, Pelligrini G, Cantani A, Perlinin R. Prevention of atopy disease in "at risk newborns" by prolonged breast-feeding. *Ann Allergy* 1983;51:296.
22. Fälth-Magnusson K, Oman H, Kjellman N-IM. Maternal abstention from cow's milk and egg in allergy risk pregnancies; effect on antibody production in the mother and the newborn. *Allergy* 1987 *(in press)*.
23. Kramer MS, Moroz B. Does breast feeding and delayed introduction of solid food protect against subsequent eczema? *J Pediatr* 1981;98:546–58.
24. Chandra RK. Immunological aspects of human milk. *Nutr Rev* 1978;36:265–72.
25. Soothill JK, Stokes CR, Turner MW, Norman AP, Taylor B. Predisposing factors and the development of reaginic allergy in infancy. *Clin Allergy* 1976;6:305–19.
26. Chandra RK. Physical growth of exclusively breast-fed infants. *Nutr Res* 1982;2:275.
27. Saarinen JM, Kajosaari M, Backman A, Siimes MA. Prolonged breast feeding as prophylaxis for atopic disease. *Lancet* 1979;ii:163–6.

28. Hide DW, Guyer BM. Clinical manifestations of allergy related to breast and cow's milk feeding. *Ann Allergy* 1981;56:172.
29. Fergusson DM, Horwood LJ, Beautrais AL, Shannon FT, Taylor B. Eczema and infant diet. *Allergy* 1981;11:325–9.
30. Gerrard JW. Allergies in breast-fed babies to foods ingested by mothers. *Clin Rev Allergy* 1984;2:143–9.
31. Jakobsson I, Lindberg T. Cow's milk as a cause of infantile colic in breast-fed infants. *Lancet* 1978;ii:437–9.
32. Warner JO. Food allergy in fully breast-fed infants. *Clin Allergy* 1980;10:133–6.
33. Van Asperen PP, Kemp AS, Mellis CM. Immediate food hypersensitivity reactions on the first known exposure to the foods. *Arch Dis Child* 1983;58:253.
34. Shannon WR. Demonstration of food proteins in human breast milk by anaphylactic experiments on guinea pigs. *Am J Dis Child* 1921;223–7.
35. Matsumura T, Kuroume T, Oguri M, Iwasaki I. Egg sensitivity and eczematous manifestations in breast-fed newborns with particular reference to intrauterine sensitization. *Ann Allergy* 1975; 35:221–9.
36. Chandra RK, ed. *Food Intolerance*. New York: Elsevier, 1984;103–17.
37. Chandra RK. Environmental engineering in the prevention of atopic disease: how early is early enough? In: Chandra RK, ed. *Food Allergy*. St. John's: Nutrition Research Education Foundation, 1987;373–87.

Food Intolerance in Infancy: Allergology, Immunology, and Gastroenterology, edited by Robert N. Hamburger. Carnation Nutrition Education Series, Vol. 1. The Carnation Co., Los Angeles/Raven Press, Ltd., New York © 1989.

General Discussion for Section IV

Ranjit Kumar Chandra, Cecil Collins-Williams, Edmund J. Eastham, Samuel Fomon, and David Hill

Dr. Fomon: I've asked Dr. Cecil Collins-Williams to present some preliminary data, which he is presently analyzing, on a study of the incidence of allergy in Oriental patients compared to Caucasian patients.

THE INCIDENCE OF MILK ALLERGY IN ORIENTAL AND CAUCASIAN INFANTS A PRELIMINARY REPORT

Cecil Collins-Williams

University of Toronto, Toronto, Ontario, Canada M5P IN5

The following results were obtained from a survey questionnaire response from: Group 1, nine experienced pediatric allergists (former fellows), and Group 2, nine less experienced physicians with many Oriental patients.

The interpretation of Table 1 is somewhat difficult because the more experienced and highly trained allergy specialist physicians reported no difference in true immu-

TABLE 1. *The incidence of true immunoglobulin E (IgE)-mediated milk allergy and other adverse reactions to milk*

Group	Incident	Oriental	Caucasian
1	Allergy	3.2%	3.4%
	Adverse reactions	7.1%	8.5%
2	Allergy	9.1%	2.9%
	Adverse reactions	12.8%	5.6%

TABLE 2. *The incidence and duration of breast-feeding*

Group	Incidence/Duration	Oriental	Caucasian
1	Incidence	57%	52%
	Duration	3.7 months	3.8 months
2	Incidence	39%	62.5%
	Duration	4.9 months	4.25 months

noglobulin (IgE)-mediated allergy to milk in Oriental or Caucasian infants; whereas the general pediatricians (Group 2), with larger numbers of Oriental families in their practices, believe the incidence of true milk allergy is over three times higher in the Oriental infants. Could this be due to a large difference in the number of mothers who breast-fed their infants? Table 2 provides some data on this point.

Among the experienced allergists (Group 1), they report no difference in the incidence or the duration of breast-feeding between the Oriental and the Caucasian mothers. The general pediatricians noted a 50% higher incidence of breast-feeding in their Caucasian mothers compared to the Oriental mothers.

No significant difference in symptoms of milk allergy was observed or reported in the two groups.

As I stated, this is an exploratory study which is still under way. Perhaps the results will be clearer when a larger number of families has been screened and the data subjected to statistical analysis. I searched the literature and could find no data on this topic and would therefore appreciate hearing from anyone with relevant information.

Dr. Fomon: Thank you, Dr. Collins-Williams. We are now ready for questions.

Dr. Guesry: Pierre Guesry from Vevey, Switzerland. Dr. Hill, I was very impressed by the high number of patients with casein hydrolysate intolerance that you showed in one of your slides. Could you tell us how you did the diagnosis? Was it by *in vitro* test, was it by challenge test, and how do you interpret this high rate of allergy to casein hydrolysate?

Dr. Hill: I think you've got to bear in mind firstly that our patients are a highly selected group and they only come to us if they have major gastrointestinal problems and gross eczema. They really do represent the very severe end of the spectrum of food hypersensitivity. Diagnosis, as I indicated, was not as critically evaluated as was cow's milk allergy. The diagnosis is based clinically on the development of symptoms when the child ingests the casein hydrolysate formula. The range of symptoms in patients with casein hydrolysate hypersensitivity is similar to those for cow's milk allergy. Symptoms remit when the casein hydrolysate is excluded. There are no other laboratory tests done with them.

Dr. Guesry: Dr. Chandra, in your study when you try to assess the importance of removing allergen during pregnancy you also remove allergen during the lactation period in the same mother. So how are you able to differentiate the effect of removing allergen during pregnancy and during lactation alone?

Dr. Chandra: Initially, I showed a study in which maternal antigen avoidance was started only at birth, and in that group, the incidence of atopic eczema was roughly 18%, whereas in the group where the food avoidance was started in early pregnancy the incidence was 11%. Thus, there appears to be an additive effect of such dietary precautions during pregnancy and lactation.

Dr. Guesry: You don't think then to have a group of avoidance during pregnancy and no avoidance during lactation?

Dr. Chandra: We had very few women in that group, and therefore I cannot be sure if dietary precautions during pregnancy alone would be helpful, although the trends are suggestive. In the formula-fed group, if their mothers had taken dietary precautions during pregnancy, there was a significantly lower total eczema score, even though the incidence of eczema was no different from that in formula-fed infants whose mothers had not taken any dietary precautions during pregnancy.

Dr. Guesry: Dr. Eastham, you showed a gel electrophoresis of different types of food, and in soya there were less bands of so-called allergen than in cow's milk. I think you have to take into account that in order to migrate in the gel the protein has to be soluble, and part of the soy proteins are insoluble. Thus, they could not migrate and you would not see them.

Dr. Eastham: I would agree, yes.

Dr. Walker-Smith: I am Walker-Smith, London, England. Dr. Hill, I was very interested in your observations about rotavirus. Group 2 is the one in which I would have anticipated you would get a positive answer. I wasn't clear whether you retrospectively analyzed those children and there was a clear-cut history of gastroenteritis or, in fact, whether some that had no history of a preceding gastroenteritis but presumably had had a subclinical illness. Could you clarify that?

Dr. Hill: Yes, it was a retrospective study. We didn't really answer the question as to whether the rotavirus was acquired because the children had underlying gut disease or because the rotavirus infection precipitated the enteropathy.

Dr. Walker-Smith: It's very difficult, the chicken and the egg, isn't it, and which comes first.

Dr. Fomon: Let me make a nutritional comment about soy formulas. I think that it has been well demonstrated that babies who react to cow's milk can in many cases probably react to soy formula if you give them a long enough time, maybe even half of them or most of them. So what I suspect is that the 15 or 20% of infants in the United States who are being fed soy formulas are being fed soy formulas for reasons that are not very sound. On the other hand, soy-based formulas as currently marketed are, in my opinion, of equivalent nutritional quality to milk-based formulas. I have only one slight reservation, and that relates to skeletal mineralization. Most of the skeletal mineralization problems have concerned the small preterm infants and they have been reported with the use of a formula in which the minerals were not well suspended. It is uncertain whether the minerals ever reached the babies, and that would surely explain a lack of mineralization. Presently marketed formulas appear to have much better mineral stability and it may be that, even from the point of view of mineralization of the skeleton, milk-based and isolated soy protein-based formulas are equivalent. Do any of the panelists want to comment?

Dr. Eastham: Dr. Fomon, we have spoken today about soy formulas and we have both alluded to soy protein isolate formulas. I think someone should point out that there are also substantial numbers of soy formula and products sold by health food manufacturers and health food stores that are potentially dangerous for small babies, since most of these do not contain vitamin D and their calcium/phosphate ratios are certainly not what we would regard as nutritionally optimal. A lot of mothers do buy soy milk from health food stores believing that because it is a ''health'' food store, they are nutritionally adequate. I think someone should go down on record as saying that these are not healthy products and should not be fed to infants at all.

Food Intolerance in Infancy: Allergology, Immunology, and Gastroenterology, edited by Robert N. Hamburger. Carnation Nutrition Education Series, Vol. 1. The Carnation Co., Los Angeles/Raven Press, Ltd., New York © 1989.

Introduction to Section V

Lewis A. Barness

Department of Pediatrics, University of South Florida, College of Medicine, Tampa, FL 33162

The most common food allergy of infants consuming only cow's milk is cow's milk. The frequency of occurrence of cow's milk allergy is not certain and has been variously estimated as 3/1,000 or 7/100. Although the discrepancy in these numbers is large, either number represents only a fraction of those infants placed on substitute formulas for food allergy. Diagnosis is frequently made without testing because, when a mother complains that her infant hasn't the disposition or the activity that she expects of her infant, it is easier to change the type of feeding than to do extensive tests. That the child may then be considered a vulnerable child is frequently overlooked. That the feeding regimen may be inadequate for that child is sometimes not considered.

For the rare infant who does not tolerate milk, several approaches are possible. The most easily accomplished is the elimination of lactose in those lactase-deficient or galactosemic children. For those infants intolerant to cow's milk protein, hydrolysis of the protein has been somewhat successful but cost and other considerations limit its usefulness. Pure amino acid formulas, even if possible to use for prolonged periods, suffer from nutritional deficits, hence the need for peptides. Other starting proteins or different hydrolytic processes may result in more acceptable products.

No one challenges the lower incidence of allergic manifestations in the breast-fed infant compared with the bottle-fed infant, although the precise incidence in either type of feeding is unknown. Nonetheless, certain phenomena appear reasonable at this time which may help explain the differences and which may provide direction for prevention.

It appears that the breast-fed infant receives multiple antigens, generally in small quantities. Secretory immunoglobulin A (sIgA) limits absorption of these and directs the body to produce antibodies. Repeated exposure produces tolerance.

In contrast, the solely formula-fed infant is exposed early to relatively few antigens in relatively high amounts. Because the dosage is high, allergic reaction rather than tolerance occurs. Offering a hypoallergenic formula to such infants with allergic manifestations already present should alleviate those manifestations. However, to start infants at birth on hypoallergenic formulas may indeed produce a result opposite to that desired. Infants who are asymptomatic and who in the normal course of feeding presumably rapidly develop tolerance of dietary proteins, not exposed to any allergens early, might well develop severe manifestations on exposure later.

If this scheme is correct then, in addition to developing hypoallergenic foods for the symptomatic infants, efforts might be extended to find substances for either the breast- or bottle-fed infant which make the gut less permeable, perhaps by accelerating gut maturing.

If a scale is made of the severity of allergic reactions, death, anaphylaxis, respiratory and central nervous systems, gastrointestinal system, and dermatological system may be the deciding order of importance. Although the most obvious symptoms in the newborn are related to gastrointestinal and dermatological systems, hope is that correction or mitigation of these may prevent other disease states later. Even though it is not clear that food allergies are the cause of respiratory allergies later, availability of hypoallergenic foods may help clarify these issues.

Food Intolerance in Infancy: Allergology,
Immunology, and Gastroenterology, edited by
Robert N. Hamburger. Carnation Nutrition
Education Series, Vol. 1. The Carnation Co., Los
Angeles/Raven Press, Ltd., New York © 1989.

Hypoallergenic Formulas

P. R. Guesry, M. C. Secretin, R. Jost, J. J. Pahud, and J. C. Monti

Nestlé Technical Assistance Company, CH-1800 Vevey, Switzerland

In spite of a long-standing interest in cow's milk allergy, it is surprising to observe the difference in opinion about the true frequency of the disease, which ranges from 1 to 7% (1). One of the reasons for this seems to be that in many cases the real rate is underestimated because the condition is difficult to diagnose, but also because few practitioners were interested in diagnosing a disease for which there was no therapy.

For a while in the 1950s and 1960s, soy formulas were considered suitable for the management of babies suffering from food allergy, and cow's milk allergy in particular, and for ensuring prophylaxis in cases involving high-risk infants (2). Glaser and Johnstone (2) at that time and many publications since then, demonstrating the very high rate of sensitization to soy (3–5), made it clear that soy is not hypoallergenic, and interest in the problem dropped again.

Now that truly hypoallergenic formulas are available and prevention can be proposed in high-risk infants (6), interest in food allergy has been renewed. This interest is even greater now that it is agreed that "early exposure to cow's milk increases the risk not only of adverse reactions to this milk but also of developing allergies to other foods" (7).

Two new prospective studies (8,9), very well monitored including challenge test, give the same rate of 5% of true cow's milk allergy in an unselected population of infants.

When discussing hypoallergenic formulas for prevention of cow's milk allergy, the problem is to define what we mean by hypoallergenic formula, and to be sure that we do not replace one allergen by another. We must also make sure that we keep the nutritional level of the formula optimal. We must prove the efficacy of the formula and be able to guarantee its hypoallergenicity, batch after batch. Last but not least, the taste of the formula should be good enough to be used exclusively over a lengthy period (at least 4 to 6 months) and the price should not prevent prolonged usage.

WHAT IS A HYPOALLERGENIC FORMULA?

Any protein or large peptide repetitively introduced parenterally could induce secretion of immunoglobulin E (IgE) and, after a period of sensitization, a further introduction could trigger the chain of immunological events leading up, through secretion of IgE or IgG and mediators (10), to the clinical manifestations of allergy. If we would discuss the allergenicity of parenteral food, only free amino acids or di- and maybe tripeptides would be suitable.

When discussing formulas we have to take into account the digestion that takes place in a baby's digestive tract and the filtration through the mucous layer and the intestinal cell wall. Of course intact protein could escape through this physiological mechanism, as is shown by the presence of foreign intact protein in the plasma of babies (11), but by and large this process is efficient and dramatically reduces the amount of foreign protein introduced into the immunological system.

For these reasons the classical animal model (12), consisting of repeated parenteral injections of the allergen added to Freund's adjuvant followed by an intravenous challenge, is interesting for measuring the reduction in allergenicity obtained by a certain process and for comparing different formulas, but it is not a suitable model for trying to predict the clinical efficiency of a given formula.

We could be tempted to test hypoallergenic formulas *in vitro* using serums from patients who are already polysensitized, or *in vivo* by doing skin tests on patients suffering from food allergy. Again, these tests are interesting but could be misleading as they do not take into account the physiological processing of the small quantity of allergens which possibly remain in the human intestine, nor the unknown quantity of allergen which can be tolerated or even become tolerogenic (13).

These tests may also be too specific and, for example, an intact soy protein will give no reaction if the patient is specifically sensitized to cow's milk, which does not guarantee of course that he would not become sensitized if submitted to repeated contacts.

Research during recent years was aimed therefore at developing animal models more representative of the clinical situation, i.e., studying oral sensitization of animals (14,15) which is not completely satisfactory because the way mice, rats, and guinea pigs react to allergens differs from what happens in humans.

Attempts were also made to define hypoallergenicity on the basis of peptide size. A threshold of 5,000 daltons has been proposed by some authors (16). We do not think that such a rigid limit is of great value. It is well known that peptides, such as calcitonin (mol wt 3,600) and gastrin (mol wt 2,100), could become allergenic (17). Elsayed and Ajold (18) have shown that a synthetic peptide made of 16 amino acids could find IgE antibodies from allergic patients, and Dailey (19) produced peptone shock or anaphylaxis in sensitized animals with peptones whose molecular weight was largely under 5,000 daltons. However, it is not clear that they were able to sensitize virgin animals with such a product even by parenteral route and less still by oral route, demonstrating the clear distinction that should be made between a product aimed at being prophylactic and a therapeutic product for patients who are already sensitized.

On the other hand MacLaughlan et al.'s (20) experiments showed that by heating the protein one can reduce allergenicity to a large extent without altering the molecular weight of the protein by changing its tertiary structure.

The conclusion to be drawn from this is that only *in vivo* studies on animal models or human beings can give more precise information on the reduction in allergenicity of a given protein after processing. *In vitro* tests should only be used to monitor the process when the results have been confirmed by *in vivo* studies, and for checking each and every batch of commercial products.

We believe that an infant formula should only be labeled as hypoallergenic when the quantity of potentially allergenic material has been drastically reduced (at least 100 times) but, more importantly, when animal studies resembling clinical conditions show that virgin animals could not be sensitized orally and when clinical trials also show no oral sensitization of at-risk newborns.

ALLERGEN REPLACEMENT

The whole history of dietary management of food allergy up to very recent years has been based on allergen replacement. The Greeks and Romans recognized cow's milk allergy and proposed replacement by goat's milk. This practice was still common at the turn of the century and a few practitioners still believe that goat's milk can be given to patients allergic to cow's milk. Goat's milk is usually collected under conditions of poor hygiene. It is excessively rich in mineral salts and deficient in certain vitamins, especially D, C, B_6, B_{12}, and folic acid, which makes it unsuitable, without modification, for feeding human infants (21). More important still is the fact that goat's and cow's milk protein share common allergens, making unmodified goat's milk as allergenic as cow's milk.

Utilization of meat-based formulas gives similar results owing to the cross-reactivity of beef and even lamb protein and cow's milk proteins.

The belief that casein is less allergenic than whey is very controversial.

The idea that a soy-based formulation might be beneficial in cases of cow's milk allergy, or even for prevention, started in the early 1950s (2). Even then Glaser and Johnstone warned their readers about the risk of inducing soy protein allergy, but their warning has gone unheeded and soy-based formulas are heavily promoted by manufacturers as hypoallergenic. This has led to a 20% range of consumption for soy-based formulas in certain countries, and the publication of many articles describing soy protein allergy (3–5,22–24).

The only possibility of obtaining truly hypoallergenic formulas without using free amino acids, which have their specific nutritional disadvantage, is to modify the structure of the native protein sufficiently in such a way that the antigenic sites are not close enough to link two receptors (Fig. 1). This could be achieved in two ways, by heat treatment which changes the ternary structure of the protein, and by hydrolysis.

HEAT TREATMENT

Heat treatment alone (25) is capable of reducing the allergenicity of native protein. The sensitivity of protein to heat varies according to the structure of the protein itself. For example, whey proteins, and particularly β-lactoglobulin, are more sensi-

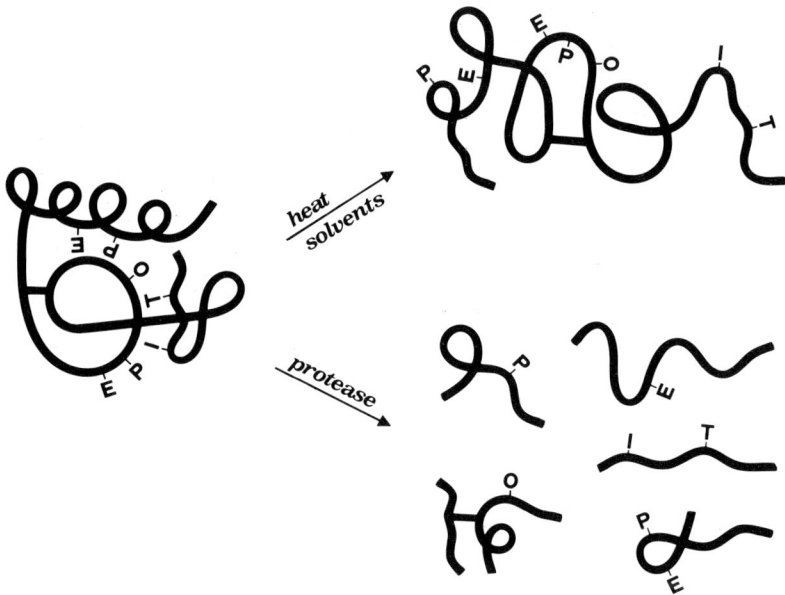

FIG. 1. Modification of the structure of a native protein. Heat or solvents change the ternary structure. Enzymatic proteolysis splits the amino acid sequence. (R. Jost, with permission.)

tive to heat than casein. However, even for whey protein the heat denaturation necessary to reduce significantly the allergenicity would induce such a Maillard reaction that the nutritional value would be reduced to an unacceptable extent (26). Another drawback of heat treatment is the risk of inducing, by change of ternary structure, the formation of new epitopes which were not present in the native proteins, or more probably the demasking of hidden epitopes. Heat treatment alone is unable to produce good quality hypoallergenic formulas. However, within certain pH limits, by monitoring Ca^{++} concentration and with precise timing, heat treatment will complete hydrolysis without diminishing the nutritional value of the protein.

PROTEIN HYDROLYSIS

A better way of breaking the epitopes down is to split the protein molecule into peptides. Acid hydrolysis induces severe amino acid degradation, decreasing its nutritional value. Enzymatic proteolysis by endopeptidase, such as trypsin and chymotrypsin (27), is more gentle and preserves the quality of the amino acids and peptides produced. The extent of the hydrolysis can be modulated by its duration. Prolonged hydrolysis over many hours increases the number of cleaved sites and improves hypoallergenicity (28).

One disadvantage is that the number of sites which could react with glucose or galactose is increased and the risk of lysine blockage is greater. Another is the bad taste which develops in the product when a large quantity of free amino acids or of di- and tripeptide is produced. Another disadvantage of prolonged hydrolysis is the increase in the osmolarity of the product. The American Academy of Pediatrics recommends (29) that the osmolarity of infant formulas should remain under 400 milliosmols.

This price to pay when increasing hydrolysis to decrease allergenicity of a protein underlines the necessity to choose between extreme solutions in agreement with a given program. It is always possible to further decrease allergenicity of a protein down to a mixture of amino acids, but the bad taste, the high price, and more importantly, the lower nutritional value will prevent its prolonged usage or will make it unsuitable for infants' growth.

The sensitivity to endopeptidase hydrolysis is also dependent on the type of protein. α-Caseins, β-caseins, β-lactoglobulins, and α-lactalbumin are highly sensitive to trypsin hydrolysis (30). On the other hand, κ-caseins, bovine serum albumin, and immunoglobulins are quite resistant to hydrolysis in their native state. Faced with such resistance, a combination of hydrolysis and heat treatment could become necessary.

NUTRITIONAL ADEQUACY

As already mentioned, when designing a hypoallergenic formula there is a risk of having a protein of poor nutritional quality. Besides their strong allergenicity, soy formulas also present various nutritional problems. The amino acid imbalance of soy protein could easily be corrected by the addition of methionine, although free amino acids increase the osmolarity of the formula and are less well absorbed than peptides (31). A more serious problem is the impairment of iron absorption (32) owing either to phytic acid present in soy formulas or to the protein itself. Impairment in calcium absorption is probably caused by the lack of lactose (33) in these formulas, but the defect in bone densification observed with soy formulas (34) is either caused by a phosphorus or a zinc absorption defect for which the phytic acid is responsible.

When using a heat-treated, enzymatically hydrolyzed protein there is a risk of impaired nutritional adequacy, which could be related to the poor amino acid pattern of the native protein being hydrolyzed or to the heat treatment, especially when this takes place after hydrolysis as this increases the number of chemically reactive sites.

With regard to the quality of the raw material used, no pediatrician would use standard infant formulas composed of gelatin and soy. After hydrolysis the amino acid pattern of such a mixture could not be improved. In the 1960s, the introduction of starter formulas enriched with whey was regarded as a considerable improvement over the old formulations, containing 80% of casein and only 20% of whey, owing to the poor amino acid pattern of the casein. This amino acid pattern is even worse when the formula is made of 100% casein. Such a poor amino acid pattern makes the addition of free amino acids necessary and has the drawback mentioned above.

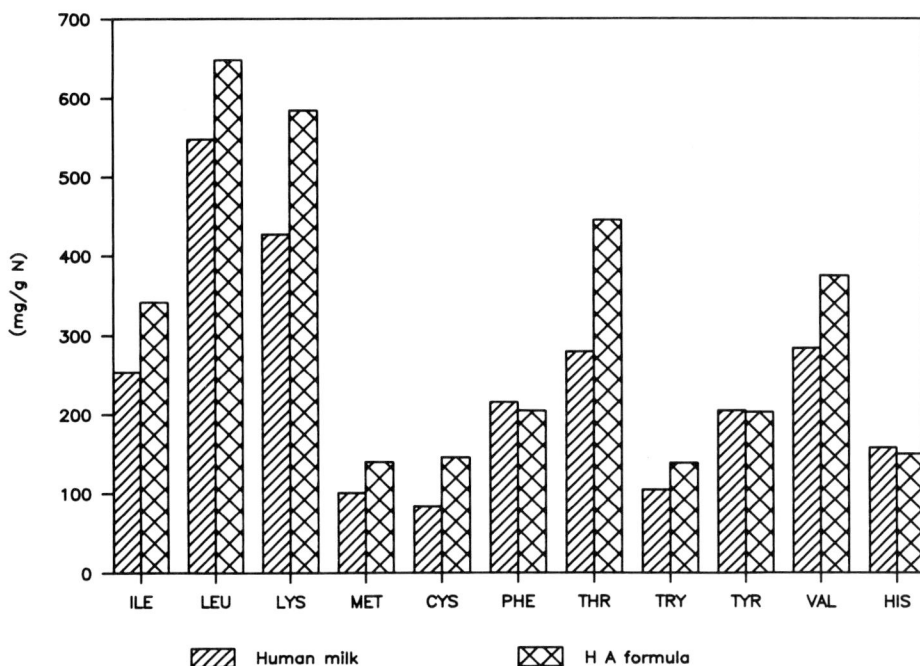

FIG. 2. Comparison of amino acid pattern of human milk and hypoallergenic formula (Carnation Good Start H.A.).

The amino acid pattern of a formulation made with whey protein hydrolysate (HA) is very close to the standard pattern of human milk (Fig. 2).

Lactose, which is the only sugar in human milk, should be used whenever possible for newborns who are at risk of developing allergy but are not sick because lactose enhances calcium absorption (33).

TABLE 1. *Protein efficiency ratio, biological value, and net protein utilization of hydrolyzed whey protein (LHA) compared with casein*

	Hydrolyzed formula HA, %	Casein reference, %
Protein efficiency ratio		
Absolute value	3.5	2.5
Casein	140.0	100.0
Biological value	88.4	69.8
Net protein utilization	68.4	56.8

Note: Carnation Good Start H.A. and the European formula with HA in the name are essentially the same formulation.

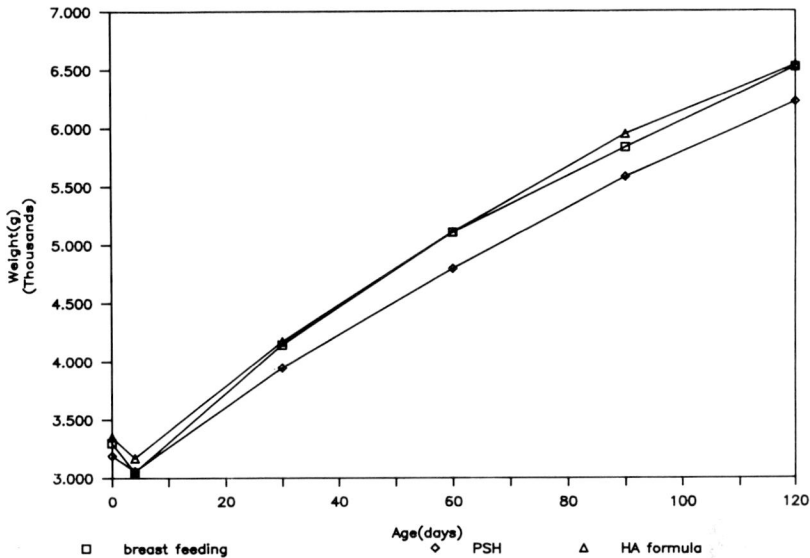

FIG. 3. Growth pattern of breast-fed babies, babies fed with whey protein hydrolysate (HA), and fed with a formula containing 50% of casein. (Clinical study by Dr. Alain, with permission.)

Heat treatment should also be monitored carefully in order not to block the lysine nor to induce the production of lysinoalanine which could impair the bioavailability of zinc (35). The fact that we have chosen whey protein rather than casein as raw material drastically reduces the risk of producing lysinoalanine.

Finally, protein quality must be tested in animals before starting clinical trials on the formula.

Protein efficiency ratio, biological value, and net protein utilization have been measured in the HA formula and found good (Table 1).

Growth monitoring of the first babies receiving the formula is mandatory, and those receiving HA exclusively showed a growth pattern similar to that for breast-fed babies (Fig. 3) (Alain, *personal communication*), which confirms the perfect nutritional value of the product.

TESTS OF HYPOALLERGENICITY

In Vivo

Tests during the early period of development were chosen so as to be able to check the progress of the hydrolysis and of heat treatment on a suitable animal model in which sensitization would be checked orally (14,15), to be more representative of clinical reality. Specially bred guinea pigs were fed for 6 weeks with either a control product or the product to be tested and subsequently they were challenged

ORAL SENSITIZATION CAPACITY
PCA Titrations

Standard
Formula

Hydrolys.
Formula

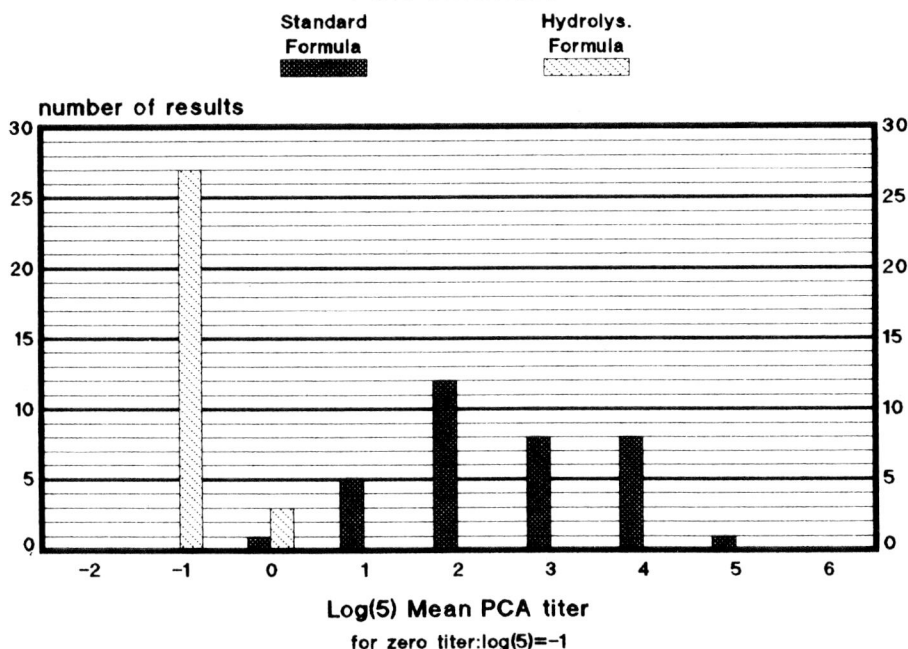

FIG. 4. Passive cutaneous anaphylaxis titers of guinea pigs fed with whey protein hydrolysate (HA) or a standard formula. Passive cutaneous anaphylaxis (PCA).

by intravenous injection of the intact protein or of the hydrolyzed protein. Results were judged according to the presence or absence and the severity of the clinical manifestations of allergy. The serum of the animals was drawn and used for inducing passive cutaneous anaphylaxis in virgin animals.

The interest of this test, besides the fact that it resembles the true clinical situation, is that it allows two different properties of the product to be tested.

When the guinea pig is fed for 6 weeks with HA and then challenged with intact protein, the prophylactic properties of the product can be measured.

When the guinea pig is fed with untreated cow's milk protein and then challenged with hydrolyzed protein one can evaluate the potential therapeutic effect of the product. This test has confirmed the high allergenicity of skim milk and whey protein (94 to 100% reaction) and the validity of the model. It has also confirmed the allergenicity of soy proteins.

These tests have shown that, when sensitized with whey protein or whole milk, guinea pigs do not react to intravenous injection of the hydrolyzed protein used as raw material for HA. Only 1 animal out of 51 fed with HA reacted to an intravenous challenge with whey protein. It is not easy to interpret this unique reaction, and one cannot completely exclude the fact that this guinea pig may have received intact milk protein.

Passive cutaneous anaphylaxis has confirmed the clear difference between the plasma of animals fed with intact protein and those fed with HA (Fig. 4).

In Vitro

During the development period, radioimmunoassay for remaining traces of β-lactoglobulin and peptides carrying monovalent epitopes was used to follow up the progress of the hydrolysis (Fig. 5). Radioimmunoassay is particularly useful under these conditions as it is quantitative and shows that a reduction of more than 100 times could be achieved for β-lactoglobulin (27).

Immunoblotting was also used to identify the remaining traces of proteins in the final product. This is very important since the hydrolysis of the protein was satisfactory for certain products of competitors, but significant quantities of intact protein were found in the final product through addition of lactose (Fig. 6) or lecithin. This points out the importance of hydrolyzing the protein in the presence of lactose, which should not be added after hydrolysis, and to check the final commercial product and not only the hydrolyzed protein.

The two tests are very sensitive but have the disadvantage of being difficult to

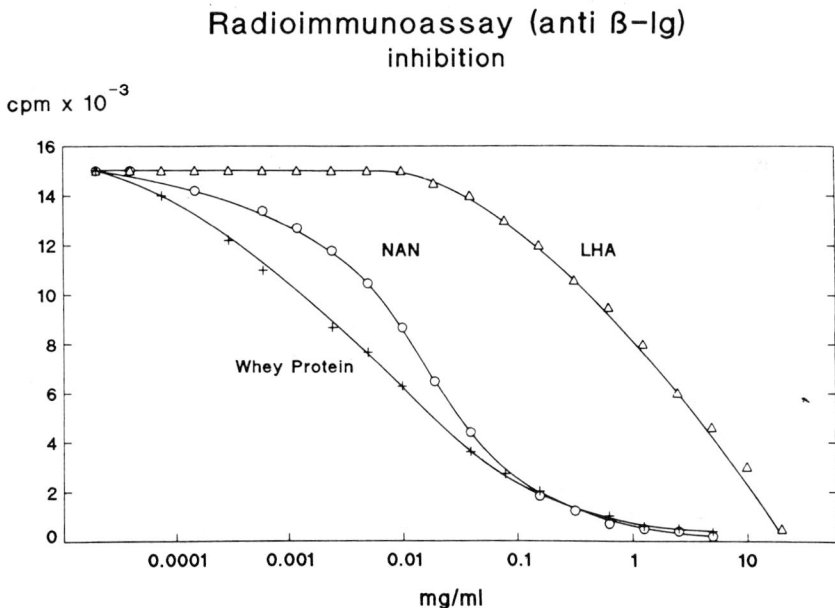

FIG. 5. Radioimmunoassay for β-lactoglobulin of whey protein, starter nonhydrolyzed formula (NAN), and hydrolyzed formula HA (LHA).

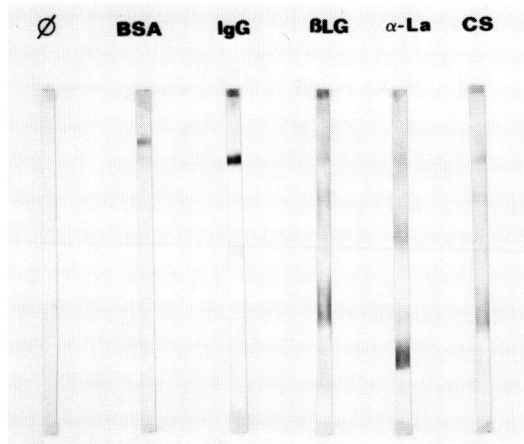

FIG. 6. Immunoblotting of edible lactose. Ø is the blank performed with normal rabbit serum.

carry out in a factory when each batch must be tested, and they are also too specific to serve as a screening test aimed at spotting any kind of contamination which could take place in a factory.

For practical purposes we have chosen to combine a broad screening test (sodium dodecyl sulfate-polyacrylamide gel electrophoresis) (Fig. 7) and a specific test for

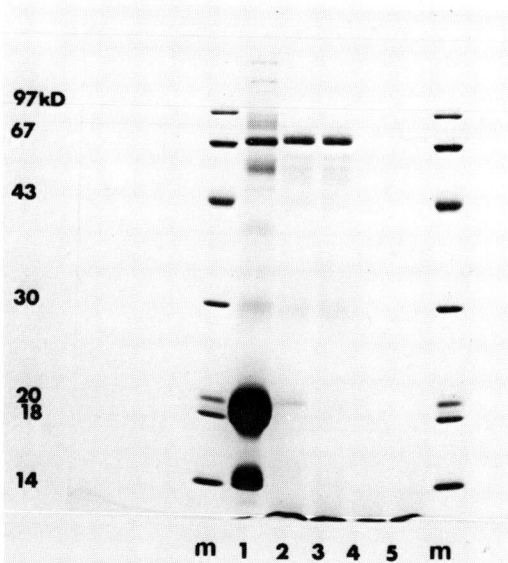

FIG. 7. Sodium dodecyl sulfate-polyacrylamide gel electrophoresis of whey protein hydrolysate (HA). Markers (M), substrate (whey proteins) (1), different stages of hydrolysis (2 and 3), HA end-product before and after heat treatment (4 and 5).

LHA7-IV   LHA7-A-V

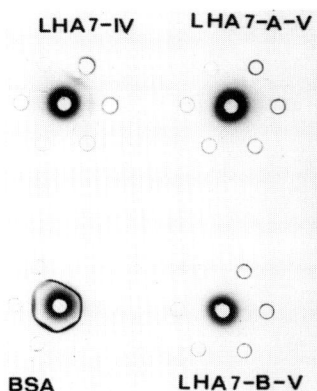

FIG. 8. Double immunodiffusion test. Bovine serum albumin (BSA) reference; two finished products; and product, whey protein hydrolysate (HA).

BSA   LHA7-B-V

the most frequently encountered allergen in our raw material (β-lactoglobulin) and the most resistant (bovine serum albumin) sought out with radial immuno-diffusion (Fig. 8).

CLINICAL TRIALS

All these *in vitro* and *in vivo* studies confirmed that HA is hypoallergenic and it could then be submitted to clinical trials, which is the only way to be certain of the hypoallergenicity of the product.

The first one (36) was designed to check that it would not be possible to sensitize atopic babies to HA. In order to be conclusive, the study was designed to involve the maximum statistical risk. Only babies with a family history of atopic disease were selected, and the way HA was administered, during the 1st week of life only followed by a period of 4 months with exclusive breast-feeding, was intended to maximize the risk (37). When HA was reintroduced at 4 months, none of the 45 at-risk babies manifested symptoms of allergy.

Since then many studies have been, or are being, conducted which demonstrate the prophylactic efficacy of HA in at-risk babies (6). In some indications, such as eczema and sleep disorders (38), HA has been proven effective as a therapeutic agent. However, the usage of HA for therapeutic purposes should be handled carefully, and it is not recommended for babies suffering from chronic diarrhea or when the symptoms of allergy of type I with anaphylactic shock are present.

REFERENCES

1. Gerrard JW, MacKenzie JWA, Goluboff N, Garson JZ, Maningas CS. Cow's milk allergy: prevalence and manifestations in unselected series of newborns. *Acta Paediatr Scand [Suppl 234]* 1973;1–21.
2. Glaser J, Johnstone DE. Prophylaxis of allergic disease in the newborn. *JAMA* 1953;153:620–2.
3. Eastham EJ, Lichauco T, Grady MI, Walker WA. Antigenicity of infant formulas: role of immature intestine on protein permeability. *J Pediatr* 1978;93:561–4.

4. Kjellman NIM, Johansson SGO. Soy versus cow's milk in infants with a biparental history of atopic disease: development of atopic disease and immunoglobulins from birth to 4 years of age. *Clin Allergy* 1979;9:347–58.

5. Gruskay FL. Comparison of breast, cow, and soy feedings in the prevention of onset of allergic disease. *Clin Pediatr* 1982;21:486–91.

6. Vandenplas Y, Deneyer M, Sacre L, Loeb H. Influence of feeding breast milk, adapted milk formulas and a new hypoallergenic formula on allergic manifestations in infants. In: Reinhardt D, Schmidt E, eds. *Food Allergy*. Nestlé Nutrition Workshop Series, New York: Raven Press, 1988;17:257–64.

7. Foucard T. Development of food allergies with special reference to cow's milk allergy. *Pediatrics* 1985;(Suppl.):177–81.

8. Bock SA. Prospective appraisal of complaints of adverse reactions to foods in children during the first three years of life. *Pediatrics* 1987;79:683–8.

9. Forget P, Leclercq-Foucart J, d'Hondt C, et al. Intolérance au lait chez le nourrisson. *Rev Méd Liège* 1988;42:257–60.

10. Bellanti JA, El-Rafei A, Peters SM, Harris N. Comparative studies of specific IgG4 and anti IgE antibody in patients with food allergy. In: Reinhardt D, Schmidt E. eds. *Food Allergy*. Nestlé Nutrition Workshop Series. New York: Raven Press, 1988;17:51–61.

11. Jakobsson I. Gut absorption of macromolecules: a short communication. In: Reinhardt D, Schmidt E, eds. *Food Allergy*. Nestlé Nutrition Workshop Series. New York: Raven Press, 1988;17:243–4.

12. Ratner B, Dworetzky M, Oguri S, Aschheim L. Effect of heat treatment on the allergenicity of milk and protein fractions from milk as tested in guinea-pigs by parenteral sensitization and challenge. *Pediatrics* 1958;648–52.

13. Jarrett EE. Activation of IgE regulatory mechanisms by transmucosal absorption of antigen. *Lancet* 1977;ii:223–5.

14. McLaughlan P, Anderson KJ, Coombs RRA. An oral screening procedure to determine the sensitizing capacity of infant feeding formulae. *Clin Allergy* 1981;11:311–18.

15. Pahud JJ, Schwarz K, Granato D. Control of hypoallergenicity by animal models. In: Reinhardt D, Schmidt E, eds. *Food Allergy*. Nestlé Nutrition Workshop Series, New York: Raven Press, 1988;17:199–207.

16. Crumpton MJ. Protein antigens: the molecular bases of antigenicity. In: Sela M, ed. *The Antigens*. New York: Academic Press, 1974;II:1–78.

17. De Weck AL. Low molecular weight antigens. In: Sela M, ed. *The Antigens*. New York: Academic Press, 1974;II:141–247.

18. Elsayed S, Ajold J. Immunochemical analysis of cod fish allergen M. Locations of the immunoglobulin binding sites as demonstrated by the native and synthetic peptides. *Allergy* 1983;38:449–59.

19. Dailey R. Peptones. US Department of Commerce. National Technical Information Service. *Bulletin PB.284* 1978:882.

20. MacLaughlan P, Anderson KJ, Widdowson EM, Coombs RRA. Effect of heat on the anaphylactic-sensitizing capacity of cow's milk, goat's milk, and various infant formulae fed to guinea-pigs. *Arch Dis Child* 1981;56:165–71.

21. Coveney J, Darnton-Hill I. Goat's milk and infant feeding. *Med J Aust* 1985;143:508–10.

22. Mortimer ER. Anaphylaxis following ingestion of soy bean. *J Pediatr* 1961;58:90–4.

23. Halpin TC, Byrne WJ, Ament ME. Colitis, persistent diarrhea, and soy protein intolerance. *J Pediatr* 1977;91:404–7.

24. Van Sickle GJ, Powell KG, McDonald P, Goldblum RM. Milk- and soy protein-induced enterocolitis: evidence for lymphocyte sensitisation to specific food proteins. *Gastroenterology* 1985;88:1915–21.

25. Heppel LMJ, Cant AJ, Kilshaw PJ. Reduction in the antigenicity of whey proteins by heat treatment: a possible strategy for producing a hypoallergenic infant milk formula. *Br J Nutr* 1984;51:29–36.

26. Kilshaw PJ, Heppell LMJ, Ford JE. Effects of heat treatment of cow's milk and whey on the nutritional quality and antigenic properties. *Arch Dis Child* 1982;57:842–7.

27. Pahud JJ, Monti JC, Jost R. Allergenicity of whey protein: its modification by tryptic in vitro hydrolysis of the protein. *J Pediatr Gastroenterol Nutr* 1985;4:408–13.

28. Jost R, Monti JC, Pahud JJ. Whey protein allergenicity and its reduction by technological means. *Food Tech* 1987;41:118–21.

29. American Academy of Pediatrics, Committee on Nutrition. Commentary on breast feeding and infant formulas, including proposed standards for formulas. *Pediatrics* 1976;57:278–85.

30. Jost R. Physicochemical treatment of food allergens: application to cow's milk protein. In: Reinhardt D, Schmidt E, eds. *Food Allergy*. Nestlé Nutrition Workshop Series. New York: Raven Press, 1988;17:187–97.
31. Silk DBA, Clark ML, Marrs TC, et al. Jejunal absorption of an amino acid mixture simulating casein and an enzymatic hydrolysate of casein prepared for oral administration to normal adults. *Br J Nutr* 1975;33:95–100.
32. D'Souza SW, Lakhani P, Waters HM, Boardman KM, Cinkotai KI. Iron deficiency in ethnic minorities: association with dietary fibre and phytate. *Early Hum Dev* 1987;15:103–11.
33. Ziegler EE, Fomon SJ. Lactose enhances mineral absorption in infancy. *J Pediatr Gastroenterol Nutr* 1983;2:288–94.
34. Steichen JJ, Tsang RC. Bone mineralization and growth in term infants fed soy-based or cow's milk-based formula. *J Pediatr* 1987;110:687–92.
35. Furniss DE, Hurrell RF, Finot PA. Modification of urinary zinc excretion in the rat associated with the feeding of Maillard reaction products. *Acta Pharmacol Toxicol (Copenh)* 1986;59 [Supp 7]:188–90.
36. Gerke R, Reinhardt D, Schmidt E. Hypoallergenic formula: a feeding trial in newborn infants from atopic families. In: Reinhardt D, Schmidt E, eds. *Food Allergy*. Nestlé Nutrition Workshop Series. New York: Raven Press, 1988;17:209–13.
37. Strobel S, Ferguson A. Immune responses to fed antigen in mice: systemic tolerance or priming is related to age at which antigen is first encountered. *Pediatr Res* 1984;18:588–94.
38. Kahn A, François G, Sathoux M, et al. Sleep characteristics in milk intolerant infants. *Sleep* 1988;11:291–7.

Food Intolerance in Infancy: Allergology, Immunology, and Gastroenterology, edited by Robert N. Hamburger. Carnation Nutrition Education Series, Vol. 1. The Carnation Co., Los Angeles/Raven Press, Ltd., New York © 1989.

Introduction to the New Carnation Good Start H.A. Formula

Ernie Strapazon

Carnation Company, Los Angeles, CA 90036

In 1988 the Carnation Company introduced in the United States the new hypoallergenic formula named Carnation Good Start H.A. It is a product of Nestlé research and it is based on the ingredients presented in Table 1.

Complete nutritional information on Carnation Good Start H.A. is provided in Table 2. Five fluid ounces, when the product is reconstituted as directed, provides 100 calories with 9.8% protein, 46% fat, and 44.2% carbohydrate.

In Table 3 is a nutrient comparison of breast milk to Carnation Good Start H.A. and three other commercially available infant formulas.

Clinical studies have shown that Good Start H.A. will provide significant benefits for American babies and their parents and also for American physicians. The chapters following this one provide data based upon clinical studies using the Carnation Good Start H.A. formula by clinical investigators from Europe, Canada, and the United States. This is followed by a chapter containing a general discussion of infant formulas, hypoallergenicity, and Carnation's Good Start H.A. formula. Re-

---

TABLE 1. *Ingredients in Carnation Good Start H.A.*

42% Enzymatically hydrolyzed reduced minerals whey and whey protein concentrate (from cow's milk)
24% Vegetable oils (palm olein, high-oleic safflower, and coconut)
17% Maltodextrin
14% Lactose[a]
1% Lecithin
Less than 1% of each of the following:
    Calcium chloride, potassium chloride, potassium citrate, calcium phosphate, choline bitartrate, sodium ascorbate (vitamin C), salt, magnesium chloride, taurine, ferrous sulfate (iron), inositol, zinc sulfate, L-carnitine α-tocopherol acetate (vitamin E), niacinamide, calcium pantothenate, copper sulfate, riboflavin, vitamin A acetate, pyridoxine hydrochloride (vitamin B_6), thiamine mononitrate, folic acid, phylloquinone (vitamin K), potassium iodide, vitamin D_3, manganese sulfate, biotin, and vitamin B_{12}

---

[a]Note that 70% of the carbohydrate in Good Start H.A. is lactose.

sponses to questions on the formulation, rationale of the constituents, and comparison with other infant formulas are included in the discussion.

The Carnation Company reminds the physicians, nutritionists, and allied health workers, as well as the Carnation marketing team, of its absolute and unswerving commitment to the promotion of breast-feeding as the uncontested best way to feed human newborn infants. Carnation Good Start H.A. will be a valued complement to breast-feeding when needed, will provide a highly digestible hypoallergenic alternative to soy-based formulas, and will be the formula of choice when mother elects to wean her infant, especially in allergy-prone families.

TABLE 2. *Complete nutritional information on Carnation Good Start H.A.*

Contents	Amount	
Protein	2.4	g
Fat	5.1	g
Carbohydrate	11	g
Water	135	g
Linoleic acid	450	mg
Vitamins:		
Vitamin A	300	IU
Vitamin D	60	IU
Vitamin E	1.2	IU
Vitamin K	8.2	μg
Thiamin (vitamin B_1)	60	μg
Riboflavin (vitamin B_2)	135	μg
Vitamin B_6	75	μg
Vitamin B_{12}	0.22	μg
Niacin	750	μg
Folic acid (folacin)	9	μg
Pantothenic acid	450	μg
Biotin	2.2	μg
Vitamin C (ascorbic acid)	8	mg
Choline	12	mg
Inositol	6.1	mg
Minerals:		
Calcium	64	mg
Phosphorus	36	mg
Magnesium	6.7	mg
Iron	1.5	mg
Zinc	0.75	mg
Manganese	7	μg
Copper	80	μg
Iodine	8	μg
Sodium	24	mg
Potassium	98	mg
Chloride	59	mg
Others:		
L-Carnitine	10	mg/qt
Taurine	50	mg/qt

TABLE 3. *Comparison—infant formulas per 100 calories*

Nutrient	Units	Breast milk	Good Start H.A.	Similac	Prosobee	Nutramigen
Protein	g	1.5	2.4	2.22	3.0	2.8
Fat	g	5.4	5.1	5.37	5.3	3.9
Carbohydrate	g	10.0	11.0	10.7	10.0	13.4
Linoleic acid	mg	540	450.0	1,300.0	1,000.0	2,000.0
Calories/liter		710.0	670.0	676.0	670.0	670.0
Vitamins:						
A	IU	310.0	300.0	300.0	310.0	310.0
D	IU	3.0	60.0	60.0	62.0	62.0
E	IU	0.32 mg	1.2	3.0	3.1	3.1
K	μg	0.29	8.2	8.0	15.0	15.6
B_1	μg	29.1	60.0	100.0	78.0	78.0
B_2	μg	48.6	135.0	150.0	94.0	94.0
B_6	μg	28.5	75.0	60.0	62.0	62.0
B_{12}	μg	0.07	0.22	0.25	0.31	0.31
C	mg	5.6	8.0	9.0	8.1	8.1
Niacin	μg	208.0	750.0	1,050.0	1,250.0	1,250.0
Folic acid	μg	6.9	9.0	15.0	15.6	15.6
Pantothenic acid	μg	250.0	450.0	450.0	470.0	470.0
Biotin	μg	0.6	2.2	4.4	7.8	7.8
Choline	mg	12.5	12.0	16.0	7.8	13.3
Inositol	mg	—	6.1	4.7	4.7	4.7
Calcium	mg	38.9	64.0	75.0	94.0	94.0
Phosphorus	mg	19.4	36.0	58.0	74.0	62.0
Magnesium	mg	4.9	6.7	6.0	10.9	10.9
Iron	mg	0.04	1.5	1.8	1.88	1.88
Zinc	mg	0.17	0.75	0.75	0.78	0.78
Manganese	μg	0.08	7.0	5.0	25.0	31.0
Copper	μg	35.0	80.0	90.0	94.0	94.0
Iodine	μg	15.3	8.0	15.0	10.0	7.0
Sodium	mg	25.0	24.0	28.0	36.0	47.0
Potassium	mg	73.0	98.0	108.0	122.0	109.0
Chloride	mg	58.0	59.0	66.0	83.0	86.0
Taurine	mg	5.6	8.0	6.7	6.0	6.0
Carnitine	mg	—	1.6	1.6	—	—

From Tsang RC and Nichols BL, eds. *Nutrition During Infancy*. Philadelphia: CV Mosby, 1988.

Food Intolerance in Infancy: Allergology, Immunology, and Gastroenterology, edited by Robert N. Hamburger. Carnation Nutrition Education Series, Vol. 1. The Carnation Co., Los Angeles/Raven Press, Ltd., New York © 1989.

Experience with the Carnation Hypoallergenic Formula, Good Start H.A.

Robert N. Hamburger

University of California San Diego, Pediatric Immunology and Allergy Division M-009-D, La Jolla, CA 92093

As mentioned in my introduction, there may be a significant difference between the findings in the laboratory of cross-reactivity between immunoglobulin E (IgE) antibody to cow's milk proteins and their enzymatic hydrolysate. Some years ago we demonstrated that some infants' IgG and/or IgE antibody to cow's milk recognized epitopes (peptides) in a casein hydrolysate (Nutramigen). Nevertheless, many infants with true allergy to cow's milk were fed Nutramigen without developing any clinical problem (1). More recently, an infant of 4 months of age was described (2) who was breast-fed, yet developed laboratory proven radioallergosorbent test (RAST) IgE antibody to cow's milk 4 +, soy protein 3 +, egg 4 +, and corn 4 +, and had serious anaphylactic allergic reactions to milk (in mother's diet), soy (Isomil), intravenous Intralipid, Nutramigen, and lamb-based formula. His total serum IgE level was reported to be 1,022 IU/dl. This remarkable baby tolerated only Vivonex, a chemically defined, free amino acid-based, completely elemental diet. Although the mother of this infant reported never having fed cow's milk-based formula to her baby, our studies of diet restriction compliance (3) revealed that infants were frequently fed milk, egg, or wheat despite denial by the parents and often without the parents' awareness.

In a manner similar to our earlier studies with Nutramigen, we examined, in the laboratory, the new Carnation hypoallergenic formula, Good Start H.A. With serums from known milk-allergic individuals we looked for cross-reactivity with both IgG (precipitins) and IgE (enzyme immunoassay) antibody to the new H.A. formula. As expected, we found an occasional individual whose antimilk antibody recognized an epitope on the partially digested cow's milk whey protein in H.A. formula. Thus, we were led to caution our co-workers to utilize this new formula as a prophylactic or preventive feeding in families with bilateral allergic diseases or with prior histories of milk intolerance; not to treat known milk-allergic or milk-intolerant individuals. Nevertheless, a physician in my Division at the University of California San Diego, with informed consent, tried the Carnation H.A. formula in an infant with anemia, colic, and bloody diarrhea from cow's milk formula (4), with remarkable success. In collaboration with our Pediatric Gastroenterology service (Doctors Self and Katz) we are studying a group of severely milk-intolerant infants and children (5) with regard to the usefulness of Carnation's Good Start H.A. in improving nutrition and growth and development.

With the support of the Carnation Company, we have begun an open clinical trial of their Good Start H.A. formula in families with prior histories of milk intolerance in parents and/or siblings. In the first few families enrolled, there has been good acceptance by both infants and older children (1 to 8 years old) and by two breast-feeding mothers; confirming the Company's claim of remarkable good taste despite the enzymatic digestion and heat treatment of this nutritionally complete formula. Within the next 18 months we should begin to see some data on the incidence of sensitivity or intolerance to this formula. To date we are able to confirm the clinical impression gained in Europe of an excellent addition to the pediatrician's arsenal of weapons against the development of cow's milk allergy; and contrary to expectations, Good Start H.A. has been useful in already milk-sensitized infants and children when used under direct supervision.

We are pleased to see that the Carnation Company is including the concept that "Breast is Best" (6) in all its advertising and marketing materials and is not promoting this new formula as a substitute for breast milk. We pediatricians should avoid using guilt or scare tactics (7) to increase breast-feeding; we must improve our educational and guidance efforts, especially with new mothers, to assure the resurgence of almost universal breast-feeding (8).

ACKNOWLEDGMENTS

This work was partially supported by grants from the Carnation Company, the Elizabeth and Carroll Boutell Fund, and the University of California San Diego Pediatric Immunology and Allergy Foundation. The assistance of Janice R. Turner, Linda Galbreath, Jill Gilbert, and Maria Ware is very much appreciated.

REFERENCES

1. Hamburger RN, Heller S, Mellon MH, O'Connor RD, Zeiger RS. Current status of the clinical and immunological consequences of a prototype allergic disease prevention program. *Ann Allergy* 1983;51:281–9.
2. Habib FK, Fishman HJ, Bellanti JA. Severe anaphylaxis, eczema, food allergy and hypergammaglobulinemia E in an infant. Case report. *Ann Allergy (in press)*.
3. Hamburger RN, Casillas R, Johnson R, Mellon M, O'Connor RD, Zeiger R. Long-term studies in prevention of food allergy: Patterns of IgG anti-cow's milk antibody responses. *Ann Allergy* 1987;59:175–8.
4. Wilson NW, Self TW, Hamburger RN. Severe cow's milk induced colitis in a four day old exclusively breast-fed neonate. *Ann Allergy* (Abstr.) *(in press)*.
5. Bahna SL, Heiner DC. *Allergies to Milk*. New York: Grune & Stratton, 1980.
6. Stanway P, Stanway A. *Breast Is Best*. London: Pan Books, Ltd, 1983.
7. Davis MK, Savitz DA, Graubard BI. Infant feeding and childhood cancer. *Lancet* 1988;2,8607, 65–8.
8. Wilson NW, Hamburger RN. Allergy to cow's milk in the first year of life and its prevention. Continuing Medical Education Review. *Ann Allergy* 1988;61:323–8.

Food Intolerance in Infancy: Allergology,
Immunology, and Gastroenterology, edited by
Robert N. Hamburger. Carnation Nutrition
Education Series, Vol. 1. The Carnation Co., Los
Angeles/Raven Press, Ltd., New York © 1989.

In Vitro Testing of Cow's Milk Allergens and Hypoallergenic Formulas

Ulrich Wahn

*Children's Hospital, Free University of Berlin, Fachbereich 3,
Heubnerweg 6, D-1000 Berlin 19, Federal Republic of Germany*

This chapter presents some data on *in vitro* testing of cow's milk allergens and hypoallergenic formulas. We were interested in finding an appropriate model to test the hypoallergenicity of modified cow's milk proteins, and of course one possibility was to test those products for their ability to bind to human immunoglobulin E (IgE) antibodies from the serums of allergic patients. The way we did it, in cooperation with the group of Dr. H. Lowenstein in Copenhagen, was to do two-dimensional electrophoresis of protein mixtures and see, after incubation with serums of allergic patients, whether those fractions and those molecules were still able to bind human IgE, which can be detected by binding to radiolabeled anti-IgE, which in turn can be detected by autoradiography (1).

Figure 1 shows just the whey proteins of cow's milk. This can also be done in a similar way with the casein fraction. The whey consists of a number of different proteins and if they bind to human IgE from a patient's serum, statistical measurements can be made on which proteins are more likely to bind IgE and which ones are not. It appears from the two examples with hydrolyzed casein that some hydrolysates are not at all able to bind to these IgE antibodies, but that should not lead to the conclusion that cow's milk protein hydrolysates are really completely nonallergenic. It has been shown from other models that cellular tests are more sensitive compared to studies utilizing crossed radioimmunoelectrophoresis (CRIE).

If one changes to a cellular test, are washed leukocytes containing basophils a useful tool for the determination of the allergenic potency of food proteins? And if so, how much is the mediator releasing activity of the cow's milk proteins reduced after enzymatic digestion and heat treatment, as is the case in hypoallergenic formulas? We tested a number of cow's milk proteins, purified proteins, in serial dilutions and incubated them with basophils of sensitized infants and children and measured the histamine which was released into the supernatants (2,3).

Figure 2 shows an example, an unusual example, because this is a patient who reacts only to casein. Usually, as milk consists of many proteins, we observe IgE-

273

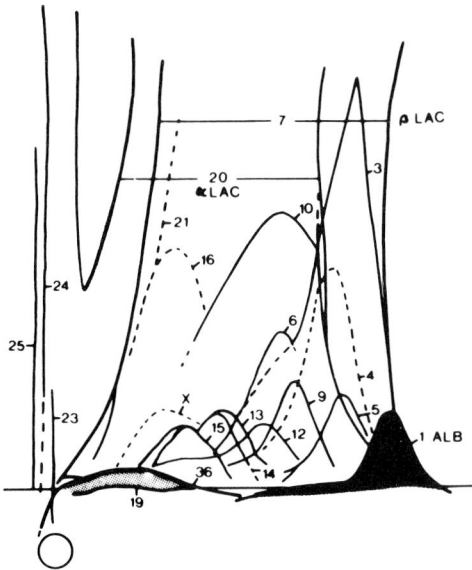

FIG. 1. Crossed immunoelectrophoretic pattern of bovine whey. (From Gjesing et al., ref. 1, with permission.)

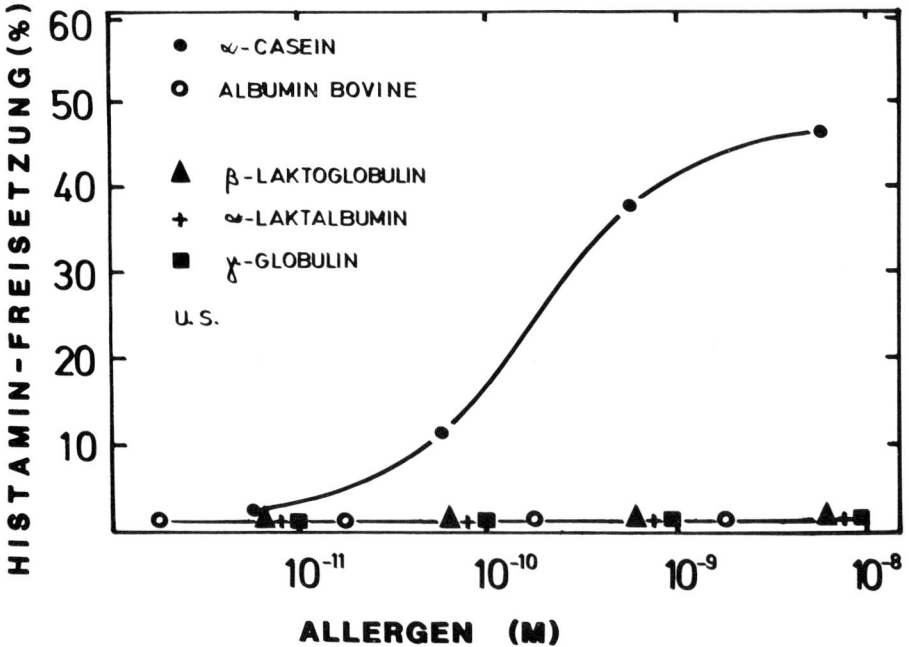

FIG. 2. Histamine release from washed leukocytes of a patient with sensitivity to casein and not to any of the whey proteins.

mediated cellular responses (histamine release) with three, four, or five protein fractions. However, in this case just casein induced histamine release.

From these experiments you can calculate the sensitivity to a specific protein, which can be defined by the antigen concentration from the ascending part of the dose-response curve necessary to induce a certain percent of mediator release, for example, 30 or 20% histamine release. This is the parameter which is presented in Fig. 3. It demonstrates that casein and β-lactoglobulin are allergens in the majority of cases.

We recently performed a study with 64 children, aged 3 months up to 12 years, and we tested their serums for specific IgE to cow's milk and to individual cow's milk proteins. In addition we did histamine release studies with their cells utilizing five different hydrolyzed formulas. Patients had a variety of different allergic symptoms which will not be presented. Out of these 64 patients, 29 (45%) had serum IgE to cow's milk which was radioallergosorbent test (RAST) 2 + or higher, whereas 35 had RAST test 0, so they served as controls. In order to test the sensitivity and specificity of our cellular tests, we compared these data with histamine release. In this highly sensitized group, positive histamine release to at least one of the proteins was found in 15 of the 29 RAST-positive patients (52%), whereas histamine release was negative in 14 out of these 29 patients. This was up to a concentration of 10 μg/ml for each protein. In the control group (negative RAST for milk proteins) there was positive histamine release to one of the milk proteins in only 4 cases out of 35 (11%), whereas in 31 cases it was negative. Those were judged to be nonspecific histamine releases.

Different hypoallergenic formulas have been tested at up to concentrations of 10 μg/ml, because at higher concentrations, pilot experiments have shown nonspecific

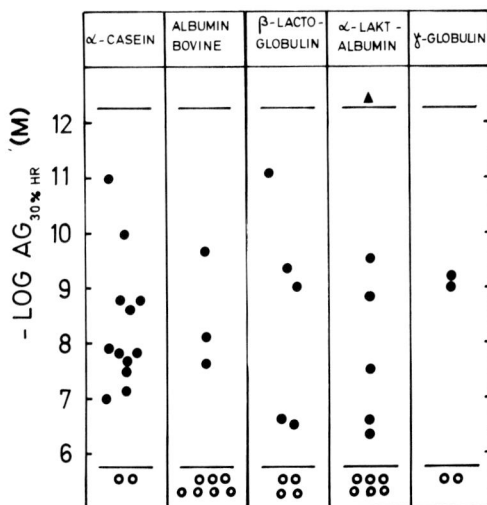

FIG. 3. Basophil sensitivity to cow's milk proteins determined by *in vitro* histamine release from washed leukocytes of allergic donors.

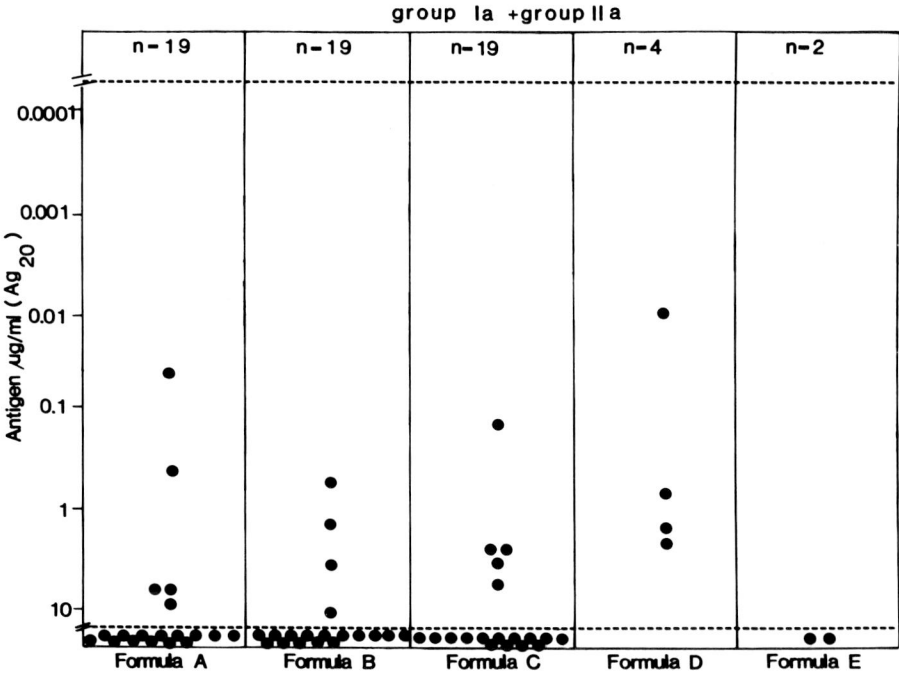

FIG. 4. Histamine releasing activity of five different hydrolysates prepared from various protein sources. Leukocyte donors were all sensitive to cow's milk proteins. Ag_{20} indicates the concentration of the hydrolysate necessary to induce 20% of the histamine release.

histamine release, histamine release which is calcium-dependent, and which does not occur in non-allergic controls. Figure 4 provides preliminary data on several hypoallergenic formulas, and shows that some of them are still releasing histamine at higher concentrations in very sensitive patients, although most of them are completely negative in the histamine release test. Formula E is the hypoallergenic formula which we are discussing in this symposium. So far we have tested 9 patients with clear evidence of cow's milk allergy by positive *in vitro* tests and 8 out of these 9 patients were negative by means of the histamine-release test.

We believe that histamine release from basophils is a useful tool to test for allergenic activity and for the hypoallergenicity of cow's milk protein formulas. More studies are necessary to determine whether an optimum of hypoallergenicity has been reached or whether this can be still further improved.

ACKNOWLEDGMENTS

This work was partially supported by grants from the Carnation Company and the Deutsche Forschingsgemeinschaft (DFG Wa 409/5-1). The assistance of Dr. Susanne Lan and Mrs. Iris Wertmann is very much appreciated.

REFERENCES

1. Gjesing B, Osterballe O, Schwartz B, Wahn U, Lowenstein H. Allergen-specific IgE antibodies against antigenic components in cow milk and milk substitutes. *Allergy* 1986;41:51–6.
2. Wahn U, Ganster G. Kuhmilchproteine als allergene. In: Wahn U, ed. *Aktuelle probleme der pad. Allergologie*. FDR: Gustav Fischer Verlag, 1983;121–6.
3. Wahn U, Thiemeier M, Ganster G. Kuhmilchallergie bei sauglingen und kleinkindern. *Allergologie* 1984;7:361–3.

Food Intolerance in Infancy: Allergology, Immunology, and Gastroenterology, edited by Robert N. Hamburger. Carnation Nutrition Education Series, Vol. 1. The Carnation Co., Los Angeles/Raven Press, Ltd., New York © 1989.

International Experience with a New Hypoallergenic Formula, Federal Republic of Germany

Eberhard Schmidt and J. Eden-Köhler

Children's Hospital of the University of Düsseldorf, Düsseldorf, Federal Republic of Germany

There have been a number of studies on the acceptance of a new hypoallergenic formula in Germany (HA), one of which has been published (1). One study in Düsseldorf (2) was carried out on a rather small number of infants from families with high risk for atopic disease in order to test the immunologic safety of HA formula when used as a prefeeding formula before full lactation sets in.

After using HA formula initially, the infants were fully breast-fed for 4 to 6 months. When mothers wished to wean, their infants were again given HA formula over a whole month before cow's milk-formula was introduced, thus using a most aggressive sensitizing mechanism to test the product. The different feeding steps were accompanied by laboratory investigations for immunoglobulin E (IgE) basophil release test, and eosinophil count. In this group of 45 infants, no signs of sensitization against HA formula were encountered. However, two infants were sensitized against cow's milk protein during the breast-feeding period (Fig. 1).

At present, a prospective feeding trial is going on to test the hypotheses that HA formula should be able to postpone or prevent the manifestation of atopy in infants at risk from their family history. Some characteristics of the study are shown in Table 1. For the purpose of this Symposium, a first check into the data is undertaken without the attempt at this stage to apply statistical analysis. The yet small size of the groups stands against it (see Table 2).

Table 2 gives the present figures for the incidence of atopic reactions in the various feeding groups. There is a considerable problem about how to classify skin alterations not representing classical atopic dermatitis below 3 months of age. They are presently described as "dry scaly skin." Only a clinical recheck will clarify how many infants with this manifestation will later on get atopic dermatitis.

All that can be said at the present stage of the trial is that these preliminary data show a trend which seems to point to a certain protective effect, or whatever it is, of HA formula toward manifestations of atopic disease in infants at risk. Further evidence will be presented when groups are large enough for statistical analysis.

279

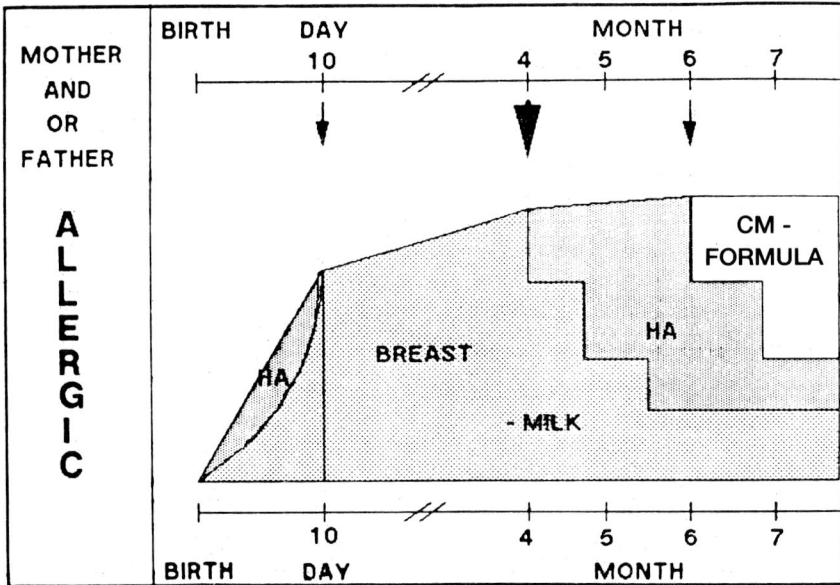

FIG. 1. Study design to evaluate the immunological safety of hypoallergenic (HA) formula when used as prefeeding formula before lactation sets in. *Arrows* indicate laboratory tests: IgE, basophil release test, and eosinophil count.

TABLE 1. *Characteristics of ongoing prospective feeding trial on hypoallergenic formula*

Basic population: approximately 10,000 newborns
Newborns at risk: approximately 1,000
Risk factors evaluated:
　Parental history for atopy
　Cord blood IgE
Hospital based:
　10 obstetric units
　in Düsseldorf, Cologne, and Neuss
Start: January 1988
Duration of observation: until the infants' age of 2 years.

TABLE 2. *Preliminary results on 146 infants between 4 and 6 months of age for the incidence of atopic reactions[a]*

Feeding-groups[b]	No atopy	Dry scaly skin	Atopic eczema	Rhinitis	N	Skin lesions, %	Atopies, %
1 Human milk, maternal diet	14	2	—	—	16	12.5	0.0
2 Human milk, no maternal diet	41	5	3	—	49	16.3	6.1
3 Human milk, 3 mo then HA formula	12	—	2	—	15	13.3	13.0
4 Human milk, 3 mo then cow's milk formula	7	2	2	—	11	36.4	18.2
5 HA, from birth	24	5	1	—	30	20.0	3.3
6 Cow's milk formula, from birth	11	6	1	1	19	42.0	10.5

[a]Intermediate data.
[b]Feeding-groups are as follows: Group 1: Breast milk only, mothers on restriction for milk, egg, and fish. Group 2: Breast milk only, no dietary restrictions for the mother. Group 3: Breast milk for 4 to 12 weeks, then hypoallergenic (HA) formula. Group 4: Breast milk for 4 to 12 weeks, then cow's milk-based formula. Group 5: HA formula from birth. Group 6: Cow's milk-based formula from birth.

REFERENCES

1. Zabransky S, Zabransky M. Preliminary clinical experience with a hypoallergenic infant formula. *Extracta Pediatr* 1987;11:10–2.
2. Schmidt E, Reinhardt D, Gerke R. The use of a hypoallergenic milk formula in newborns. *Der Kinderarzt* 1987, No. 5;627.

Food Intolerance in Infancy: Allergology,
Immunology, and Gastroenterology, edited by
Robert N. Hamburger. Carnation Nutrition
Education Series, Vol. 1. The Carnation Co., Los
Angeles/Raven Press, Ltd., New York © 1989.

A Clinical Trial with a New Hypoallergenic Formula

Yvan Vandenplas and Helmuth Loeb

Academic Children's Hospital, Free University of Brussels, 1090 Brussels, Belgium

Food allergies, and particularly cow's milk allergy, often appear to be familial, possibly owing to a genetic hyperreactivity to respond with increased immunoglobulin E (IgE) production in general, rather than to inheritance of sensitivity to specific food allergens. Milk allergy in these infants is common because cow's milk formula is usually the first and most prevalent food in the infant's diet (1). Cow's milk contains more than 25 distinct proteins that may act as antigens in man. The antigenicity differs from protein to protein and seems to depend on host factors as well as on a combination of genetic, environmental, and adjuvant factors. The most important allergens are β-lactoglobulin, casein, lactalbumin, and bovine serum albumin. Efforts to reduce the incidence of food allergy are expected to be most rewarding when used in young children. Infants are considered at high risk for food allergy, probably because of the increased intestinal mucosal permeability to incompletely digested macromolecules and the lack of an adequate protection by secretory IgA at the mucosal membrane surface. The risk is especially high in atopic infants (i.e., those from families with atopy (2)).

MATERIAL AND METHODS

Infants at risk for allergy because of a family history of atopy were studied. At least one of the parents or brothers/sisters of the infant had to present atopic disease (Table 1), sustained by a positive radioallergosorbent test (RAST) or skin prick test, and symptoms had to disappear if treated. Among other general information, history of the nearest family for allergic manifestations (e.g., eczema, urticaria, hay fever, asthma, etc.) was available, and consent of the parents was obtained by a questionnaire during the prenatal consultation at 34 weeks of gestation. Parents were informed that their infants were going to be included in a trial with a new formula, but were not informed about the hypoallergenic properties of the formula.

Five groups of babies were studied (Table 2). It was decided to include the number of infants necessary to end up with five groups of 15 infants each, because a

TABLE 1. *Number of atopic relatives (father/mother/brothers/sisters) in each different group*

Group	No. of atopic relatives		
	1	2	3
1	7	7	1
2	9	4	2
3	9	6	0
4	8	6	1
5	7	8	0

large number of drop-outs in some groups (i.e., stopping breast-feeding before 4 months) had to be expected (Table 2). Trying to exclude as much as possible the influence of, for example, climatologic factors, inclusion was chronological (first infant: group 1, second infant: group 2, etc.).

All babies were followed during a 4-month period. This short period of follow-up was chosen because it permitted a strict separation in a breast-fed and a formula-fed group, and the avoidance of other food allergens (e.g., orange juice). All babies stayed at home during those 4 months.

A screening test for atopy (Phadebas IgE paper radioimmunosorbent test [PRIST] dosage method) was performed in all infants on the 5th day of life. At 4 months, an IgE level was repeated, a RAST (cow's milk, casein, lactalbumin, lactoglobulin; Pharmacia Diagnostics, Uppsala, Sweden) and a skin prick test (Bencard, Brentford, England) for cow's milk were performed in asymptomatic infants. In symptomatic infants, laboratory investigations were performed when symptoms were at their worst, before administration of the hypoallergenic formula. A Student's *t* test was used for the statistical evaluation.

Cow's milk allergy was suspected if the infant had symptoms involving the gas-

TABLE 2. *Groups of infants studied, and drop-outs*

Group (N = 15)	Group description
1	HA[a] exclusively from birth on during 4 months. No drop-outs.
2	HA from birth on during 2 months; an adapted formula from 2 to 4 months. Four drop-outs (parents who refused changing to an adapted formula).
3	Adapted formula from birth on during 2 months; HA from 2 to 4 months. Two drop-outs.
4	Exclusively breast-fed during 4 months. Six drop-outs.
5	Adapted formula during 4 months. One drop-out.

[a]HA, hypoallergenic formula.

trointestinal and/or respiratory tract and/or the skin. Diagnosis was suspected if urticaria or asthma (if an infectious origin was excluded) appeared; or when vomiting, diarrhea, colics, or eczema lasted for more than 1 week in the absence of any organic disease such as infantile pyloric stenosis, infectious gastroenteritis, or cystic fibrosis.

Laboratory investigations (e.g., culture, sedimentation rate, white blood cell count) were performed in symptomatic infants.

Confirmation of the diagnosis was made by demonstrating relief of the symptoms for 3 to 4 weeks with the avoidance of cow's milk, and the reappearance of symptoms at its reintroduction (3). Although central nervous system manifestations (e.g., irritability, restlessness, insomnia [4]) have been demonstrated to be related to cow's milk allergy, these were not taken into account (none of our patients did present one of these symptoms).

The adapted formula administered was identical in all infants (casein/whey ratio, 40/60%; protein, 1.65 g/100 ml; fat, 3.4 g/100 ml, carbohydrates [lactose 100%], 7.4 g/100 ml). The hypoallergenic formula (HA) had the following composition: the fat consists essentially of vegetable oils (palm, safflower, and coconut oil). The carbohydrates are lactose (70%) and dextrin-maltose (30%). The proteins are a whey protein, hydrolyzed by trypsin under specific conditions. Hypoallergenic tests (radioimmunoassay, immunoallergens, and *in vivo* animal tests) were performed before administration (5). This hydrolysate contains <0.1 μg/mg β-lactoglobulin or $<0.04\%$ of the initial concentration; it contains almost no casein (5).

RESULTS

Results are shown in Table 3. Mean IgE levels on day 5 (0.8 to 1.2 U/ml) were distributed rather similarly in all groups. IgE levels had a significantly lessened increase during the first 4 months of life in the infants on HA compared with the other groups, except for the breast-feeding group, where the difference was not significant. The mean IgE level at 4 months (for all 15 infants in each group) of group 1 (1.9 U/ml) was not significantly different from mean IgE of the breast-fed group (group 4:2.7 U/ml); but both were significantly lower ($p<0.01$) as mean IgE levels in the other groups (group 2 HA-adapted formula [AdFo], 10.1 U/ml; group 3 AdFo-HA, 8.5 U/ml; group 5 AdFo, 15.7 U/ml). Differences between groups 2, 3, and 5 were not significant. The evolution of the IgE level in infants with a positive screening test is shown in Fig. 1. It has to be noticed that in a number of infants of all groups ($N=13$) IgE levels were identical at the 5th day of life and at 4 months (<0.2 U/ml). In none of the infants, the IgE at 4 months was lower than on the 5th day of life.

Weight gain was not significantly different in the groups on HA ($+105\%$) (group 1), on exclusive breast-feeding ($+96\%$) (group 4), and on adapted formula ($+103\%$) (group 5). This may be related to the great individual weight variation in each group (birthweight: 2,495 to 4,420 g). Individual weight gain was smaller, although not significantly, in the breast-fed group.

TABLE 3. *Evolution of laboratory investigations and symptoms of atopy in all infants*

Test	Group 1 HA[a]	Group 2 HA–AdFo	Group 3 AdFo–HA	Group 4 BF	Group 5 AdFo
IgE > 1.3 U/ml day 5 (N)	5	6	5	5	6
IgE > 4.0 U/ml 4 months[b] (N)	2	8	7	2	8
RAST positive (N)	0	1	1	0	1
Skin prick test positive (N)	0	3	2	0	2

Symptoms of atopy (N = total)		2 months	4 months	2 months	4 months		
	0	0	6	4	0	1	8
IgE > 1.3 U/ml day 5 (N)	0	0	3	2	0	1	5
IgE > 4.0 U/ml 4 months (N)	0	0	5	3	0	1	5
Dermatological symptoms	0	0	3	3	0	1	6
Gastrointestinal symptoms	0	0	3	2	0	0	6
Respiratory symptoms	0	0	1	0	0	0	1

[a]HA, hypoallergenic formula; AdFo, adapted formula; BF, breast-feeding.
[b]Laboratory investigations were performed at 4 months or when manifestations were at their worst.

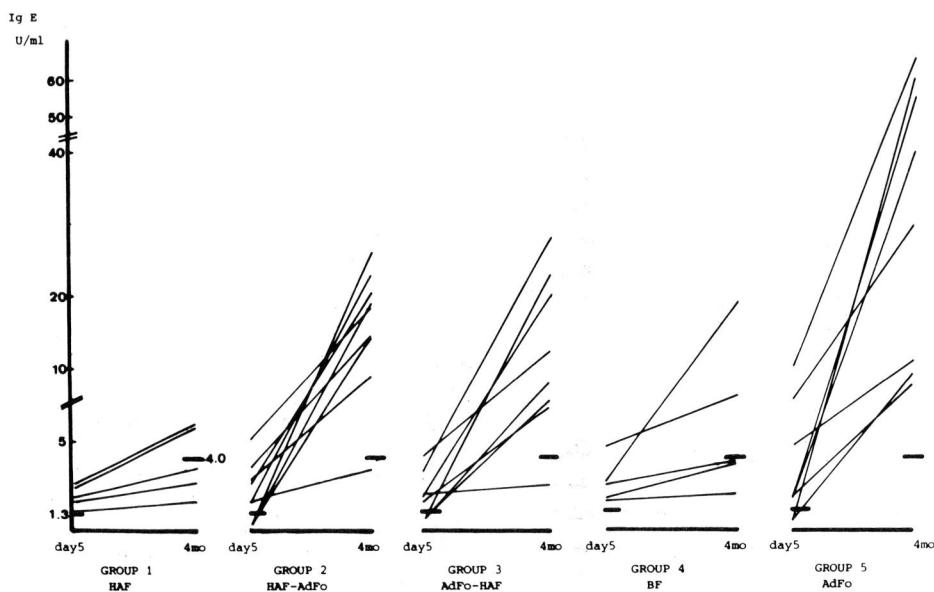

FIG. 1. Evolution of immunoglobulin E (IgE) levels in infants with a positive screening test: IgE levels on day 5 > 1.3 U/ml.

Group 1

Fifteen infants with a positive family history were fed with HA exclusively during 4 months. In five of them the IgE level on the 5th day of life was >1.3 U/ml (Table 3). After 4 months, none of these infants had developed symptoms of atopy (Table 3). All infants tolerated HA very well. The skin prick test was negative in all infants.

Group 2

Fifteen infants (six of them had an IgE level >1.3 U/ml) were fed during 2 months with HA, and then changed to an adapted formula. All infants were free of symptoms at 2 months, but before 4 months, six infants of this group had presented allergic manifestations that disappeared on HA and reappeared on the previous cow's milk formula (IgE level on day 5 was >1.3 U/ml in three of these infants, and >4.0 U/ml at 4 months in five infants). In one infant more than one system was involved. The RAST was positive in one infant for β-lactoglobulin. Three infants had a positive skin prick test.

Group 3

Fifteen infants received an adapted formula from birth (5 infants had an IgE level >1.3 U/ml on day 5). Four infants had developed allergic manifestations before the age of 2 months. The symptoms disappeared on HA, and reappeared with the initial cow's milk formula. No infant on HA presented symptoms at 4 months. One infant had a positive RAST for β-lactoglobulin. The IgE level on day 5 was >1.3 U/ml in five infants and >4.0 U/ml at 4 months in seven infants. Only three of the latter had developed symptoms of atopy. The skin prick test was positive in two infants.

Group 4

IgE level on the 5th day of life was >1.3 U/ml in five infants, and >4 U/ml at 4 months in two infants. One infant in the breast-fed group suffered from eczema before he was 1 month old. The mother appeared to eat more cow's milk products since lactation. Symptoms disappeared when the mother received a cow's milk-free diet. No infant had a positive skin test.

Group 5

In six infants, IgE level on day 5 was >1.3 U/ml. Eight of the infants with a positive family history and an adapted formula from birth had developed atopic symptoms before the age of 4 months. Symptoms disappeared on HA in all eight infants, and reappeared on cow's milk. In five infants more than one system were involved. One RAST was positive for cow's milk and casein. Skin prick tests were positive in two infants. Symptoms appeared in three infants before 2 months of age, in five infants between 2 and 4 months.

DISCUSSION

Atopic disease was documented in 18/45 (40%) of the infants with a positive family history and receiving a cow's milk formula (regardless of the IgE level on the 5th day of life), compared with a 40% incidence in a retrospective study we performed (2). In the infants receiving an adapted formula and with a positive neonatal screening test for allergy ($N = 17/45$; 38%) (compared to 39% in the retrospective study) atopy was detected in 8/17 (47%) compared to 49% in a previous study, performed in a group of 275 infants with a positive family history. So, although the number of infants in each group was small ($N = 15$), the incidence of atopy in the groups with an adapted formula (groups 2, 3, and 5) was very similar to the incidence we reported before in much larger groups (2). The number of infants with IgE level >1.3 U/ml on day 5 was rather evenly distributed in the five groups studied. Distribution of positive family history was identical in the five groups.

The frequency of atopic manifestations in our population was smaller as compared to the results in other studies, in whom the incidence varied from 44.4 to 88.9% (6–10). The high number of infants with more than one atopic relative ($N = 35/75$) increased risk of atopy for the infant (11). The consideration that the study was not double-blind (although parents were not informed about the hypoallergic properties) contributed to an overestimation of allergic manifestations. Gastrointestinal symptoms seem to be most common, which may be explained because the gastrointestinal tract is the first target of the food antigens.

Hypersensitivity phenomena in infants are rare in the 1st month of life. Their peak time of onset is at 4 to 6 weeks in formula-fed infants.

The cornerstone of diagnosis in food allergy is a complete history and unequivocal clinical reaction to elimination of the offending food and to subsequent challenge under defined conditions (3,12). Laboratory tests may be useful, but are not contributory in most cases. There is a lack of correlation between skin tests and oral food provocation. A better correlation exists between family history and food challenge.

Postnatally, breast-feeding should be the mode of choice with the mother avoiding indulgence of milk, eggs, and nuts. Supplementation with other foods should be very gradual and not begin before 6 months of age (13), which is very hard to obtain in modern Western societies with out-of-the-house working mothers. Breast milk can contain foreign proteins that are able to elicit symptoms of food allergy in the breast-fed infant (14). The fact that only nanogram quantities of foreign antigens are present does not detract from this potential allergenic effect. On the contrary, Jarrett (15) has shown in animals that small doses are more potent in producing immediate-type hypersensitivity than are large doses. Societal and cultural educational programs about allergy and exposure to food antigens could possibly improve the results obtained with breast-feeding. In a recent review article on breast-feeding, protection by breast-feeding for atopic eczema was claimed in only 10 of 22 analyzed studies; for asthma, protection rate was 7/12 studies (16).

When breast-feeding cannot be provided, a number of formulas can be considered. Soybean formulas have been recommended because they had a lower incidence of allergy (17). However, a concern has been expressed regarding a possible increase in the incidence of sensitivity to soy protein (up to 30%) with the increase in its use (18).

Other potentially hypoallergenic formulas such as meat-based formula and heat-treated cow's milk are available, but their usefulness for long-term prophylaxis against food allergy has not been adequately studied. Casein- and lactalbumin-hydrolysate formulas are a potent dietary therapy for the treatment of cow's milk allergy, but their preventive use is limited because of high cost. Therefore, the concept of the new formula we studied is very interesting, and deserves further study, as well as for therapy (in mild cases) as for prevention.

The effect of exclusive breast-feeding during the first months of life upon prevention of cow's milk allergy has been suggested, although the possibility exists of intrauterine sensitization (19). It is justified, however, to strongly recommend exclusive breast-feeding for at least the first 4 months in newborns from a family with a history of atopy. If breast-feeding is impossible, a formula like HAF maybe provides an alternative worthwhile to study more rigorously. Whether a practice like this may be able to not only prevent or postpone the development of food allergy, but also of allergy in general, remains an open question. The latter remains also unproved for prolonged breast-feeding (16). The long-term prophylaxis of atopy by breast-feeding seems at least a "golden jubilee of controversy" (16). In a recent study, prolonged breast-feeding was concluded to not contribute to the prevention of infantile atopy and respiratory tract infections (20). One of the main reasons for this could be the heterogenicity of breast milk with regard to its protective capacity: inadequate quantities of maternal IgA antibodies to food allergens appear to play a permissive role in the development of infantile allergic disease in breast-fed infants (21). HA exclusively for 2 months certainly seems only to postpone the appearance of atopy.

ACKNOWLEDGMENTS

This work was partially supported by grants from Nestlé. The assistance of Mrs. M.J. Mozin and Dr. P. Guesry was very much appreciated.

REFERENCES

1. Bahna SL, Furukawa CT. Food allergy: diagnosis and treatment. *Ann Allergy* 1983;51:574–80.
2. Vandenplas Y, Sacre L. Influences of neonatal serum IgE concentration, family history and diet on the incidence of cow's milk allergy. *Eur J Pediatr* 1986;145:493–6.

3. Gerrard J W, Shenessa M. Food allergy: two common types as seen in breast and formula fed babies. *Ann Allergy* 1983;50:375–9.
4. Kahn A, Mozin MJ, Casimir G, Montauk L, Blum D. Insomnia and cow's milk allergy in infants. *Pediatrics* 1985;76:880–4.
5. Pahud JJ, Monti JC, Jost R. Allergenicity of whey protein: its modification by tryptic in vitro hydrolysis of the protein. *J Pediatr Gastroenterol Nutr* 1985;4:408–13.
6. Croner S, Kjellman N-IM, Eriksson B, Roth A. IgE screening in 1701 newborn infants and the development of atopic disease during infancy. *Arch Dis Child* 1982;57:364–8.
7. Duchâteau J, Casimir G. Neonatal serum IgE concentrations as a predictor of atopy. *Lancet* 1983;i,413–4.
8. Katz DH. New concepts concerning the clinical control of IgE synthesis. *Clin Allergy* 1979;9:609–24.
9. Michel FB, Bousquet J, Grellier P. Comparison of cord blood immunoglobulin E concentrations and maternal allergy for the prediction of atopic diseases in infancy. *J Allergy Clin Immunol* 1980;65:422–30.
10. Michel FB, Bousquet J, Coulomb V. Prediction of the high allergic risk newborn. In: Johansson SGO, ed. *Diagnosis and Treatment of IgE Mediated Diseases,* Amsterdam-Oxford, Princeton: Excerpta Medica, 35–7.
11. Kjellman N-IM. Development and production of atopic allergy in childhood. In: Baström H, Ljungstedt N, eds. Skandia International Symposia. *Theoretical and Clinical Aspects of Allergic Diseases,* Stockholm (1983): Almqvist and Wicksell, 1982;57-73.
12. Stern M, Walker W A. Food allergy and intolerance. *Pediatr Clin North Am* 1985;32:471–92.
13. American Academy of Pediatrics. Committee on Nutrition: Breast-Feeding. *Pediatrics* 1978; 62:591–601.
14. Kilshaw PJ, Cant AJ. The passage of maternal dietary protein into human breast milk. *Int Arch Allergy Appl Immunol* 1984;75:8–15.
15. Jarrett E. Stimuli for the production and control of IgE in rats. *Immunol Rev* 1978;41:52–76.
16. Kramer MS. Does breast-feeding help protect against atopic disease? Biology, methodology, and a golden jubilee of controversy. *J Pediatr* 1988;112:181–90.
17. Johnston DE, Dutton AM. Dietary prophylaxis of allergic diseases in children. *N Engl J Med* 1966;274:712–9.
18. Kjellman N-IM, Johansson SGO. Soy versus cow's milk in infants with a biparental history of atopic disease: development of atopic disease and immunoglobulins from birth to four years of age. *Clin Allergy* 1979;9:347–51.
19. van Asperen PP, Kemp A S, Mellis CM. Immediate food hypersensitivity reactions on the first known exposure to the food. *Arch Dis Child* 1983;58:253–6.
20. Savilahti E, Tainio VM, Salmenpera L, Siimes MA, Perheentupa J. Prolonged exclusive breast-feeding and heredity as determinant in infantile atopy. *Arch Dis Child* 1987;62:269–73.
21. Machtinger S, Moss R. Cow's milk allergy in breast-fed infants: the role of allergens and maternal secretory IgA antibodies. *J Allergy Clin Immunol* 1986;77:341–7.

Food Intolerance in Infancy: Allergology, Immunology, and Gastroenterology, edited by Robert N. Hamburger. Carnation Nutrition Education Series, Vol. 1. The Carnation Co., Los Angeles/Raven Press, Ltd., New York © 1989.

General Discussion for Section V

Sami L. Bahna, Lewis A. Barness, Ranjit Kumar Chandra, Pierre R. Guesry, Robert N. Hamburger, David J. Hill, Russell J. Merritt, Eberhard Schmidt, Ernie Strapazon, Yvan Vandenplas, and Ulrich Wahn

Dr. Dolovich: Dolovich, Hamilton. Does trypsin remain in the Carnation Good Start H.A. preparation?

Dr. Guesry: The quantity of trypsin which remains in the product is the object of release procedures and we check that there is less than 1 part per million (ppm). There is an autodigestion of the trypsin at the end of the process.

Dr. Dolovich: Insofar as there seems to be lactose present, is there not a problem in giving it to children who have had milk protein intolerance where there might be lactose intolerance present?

Dr. Guesry: This product is a prophylactic product which is going to be given to infants at risk of developing symptoms of allergy and who so far are normal. So I don't see why normal infants, even at risk, would not receive lactose. That is one part of the answer. The other part of the answer is that you are probably aware that there are more and more studies coming from developing countries sponsored by the World Health Organization showing that in acute diarrhea, removing lactose from the diet is no longer recommended.

Dr. Dolovich: It's just that one of Dr. Hamburger's examples of cow's milk intolerance was where the lactose might have been the problem. Another question is, in those situations where there is milk allergy, if one were going to propose its use, should one do a skin test with the new formula preparation before giving it?

Dr. Guesry: Again, I think we have to make a clear distinction between a therapeutic and the prophylactic usage, and in this latter case I do not think it is necessary at all to make any test. If you would like to use the product for therapy, which is not recommended by us, and I have to be very clear on that, then you should take all precautions. In other words, if the baby is suffering from insomnia, I think, as Dr. Kahn has shown, it's a good indication there is very little risk and you could go ahead and use the product. If the baby is suffering from eczema, I think you may be able to use the product. On the other hand, if there are manifestations of anaphylaxis or chronic prolonged diarrhea—severe diarrhea—you should not use the product, or if you do so because you have nothing else, then you have to do a cow's milk radioallergosorbent test (RAST), or skin test, and you should take the responsibility for the additional risk.

Dr. Dolovich: Is there any information on whether or not people who are milk-allergic or have eczema or have any of these conditions, whether insomnia or otherwise, in fact have any *in vivo* reactivity to the material such as, do they have a positive skin test to the hypoallergenic formula?

Dr. Guesry: Well, I think Robert Hamburger answered that question earlier.

Dr. Dolovich: With *in vitro* tests, I think.

Dr. Guesry: Have you done skin tests, Dr. Hamburger?

Dr. Hamburger: No, only *in vitro* tests with RAST.

Dr. Wahn: I could just comment that there are few case reports, and I don't think they have been published, that in highly sensitive cow's milk-allergic babies there may be a residual skin test activity.

Dr. Schmidt: I would like to add a warning about the therapeutic use of the H.A. formula in our area where HA formula is already highly used in many infants. We have seen an infant who was cow's milk-allergic who went into a severe reaction when fed by the parents with HA formula in the hope to treat milk allergy.

Dr. Hamburger: That is a critical kind of incident which should alert us to a rare but serious hazard.

Dr. Kjellman: We tested this HA product *in vivo* with skin tests, and 7 out of 15 or 47% showed a skin prick test reaction which was about 50% the size of the skin prick test with cow's milk. So, in known cow's milk-allergic patients you should really take care and make a test before you try feeding the HA formula to the patients. We have also done RAST tests with blood from the same patients, and the RAST reactions are there. They are much weaker than with cow's milk, but it's really not nonallergenic, it is correctly labeled HA, for *hypoallergenic*.

Dr. Bahna: We are planning in our prospective study to test any infant who might develop allergic reactions on that formula. This is a prophylactic study. I don't anticipate a major problem because of the immunochemical studies that were done by Jean-Jacques Pahud and his colleagues in Vevey that were presented by Dr. Guesry. The hydrolysis reduced the quantity of the intact protein to a tremendous degree. It's almost trace quantities, and the guinea pig studies that were presented also showed that allergenicity of the hydrolyzed whey is remarkably low or almost nil.

Dr. Hamburger: I want to second the statements made by Doctors Kjellman and Bahna, that with those rare true IgE-mediated anaphylactic infants, please be extremely cautious. I have never seen any product to which some baby wouldn't react and react violently, and those babies who know how to make a true anaphylactic reaction, those are the ones to watch out for.

Dr. Devries: Jeffery Devries from Detroit, Michigan. Food allergies are fairly uncommon. Therefore, even if this formula were to be used universally as a prophylactic measure, the number of cases of food allergy that it would prevent would be relatively small. Other manifestations of atopic disease are much more common. Is there any experimental evidence that preventing food allergies in this way might lead to a decrease of other manifestations of atopic disease?

Dr. Hamburger: The data from the studies by Doctors Zeiger, Mellon, et al., and we collaborated with them, suggest very strongly that the prevention of food allergy in early infancy results in a marked decrease in asthma in the first few years of life in young children. So I think we are expecting to see some decrease in the other major allergic diseases in those babies in whom we successfully delay or prevent the onset of atopic sensitization in early infancy.

Dr. Barness: I think that is very important. A speaker indicated increasing allergic manifestations in this country. If prevention of food allergy in infancy is going to prevent asthma later, I believe this will be a real advance.

Dr. Zimmerman: Zimmerman, Toronto, Canada. I would like to reiterate something the other speakers have commented on. At this meeting there has been a tendency to use what we could call the European definition of food allergy, and it confuses IgE and non-IgE mechanisms so that when everything is lumped together, it's possible to talk about allergy in large groups of patients. But then in the two cases that Dr. Hamburger presented, he talked about a group that I am particularly interested in, the highly atopic, infants who have an IgE of 1,000 IU/ml or more. When you examine those infants immunologically, they are very turned-on in the IgE pathway. If you put their bone marrow-derived cells (B cells) in culture, they spontaneously make IgE. They make IgE to a wide range of food proteins in the first year and they convert very early to inhalants. Now, that child is at risk of anaphylaxis versus the case which was used as another example of allergy, which was a protein-losing enteropathy, and which is non-IgE-mediated. The other point with which I want to take issue is that it's impossible for me to conceive of being able to trypsinize a protein and not have residual undigested intact protein. In the data that have been shown today, I've really not gotten a feeling for the amount of undigested residual there is in the formula. These infants are going to produce IgE both to the undigested and possibly even to the epitopes showing up on the peptides from the digested proteins. So I think it's wrong to lump together all these illnesses so that you may get the mistaken notion that we are influencing necessarily atopic diseases in atopic infants. The other thing is, in our evaluation of infants presenting with asthma, many of them present with an IgE that is essentially normal; I don't see that there is necessarily a contribution from it. In summary, the point I'm trying to make is to talk about food allergy in relationship to a group that may or may not be atopic, in which the symptoms are due primarily to viral infections at day-care settings that are triggering the asthma. This lumps together and expands and perhaps even confuses what we are looking at clinically.

So after that long commentary, is there any evidence or are there any data on what the lower limit of intact protein or peptide large enough to cross-react is in the new H.A. formula? I should see some kind of inhibition data, RAST inhibition, something that gives me an idea of the lower limit of the intact protein so I can get a feeling for whether we really have something that will not present a problem.

Dr. Barness: Are you asking for the size of the protein, the size of the peptides, or the amount of each in the formula?

Dr. Zimmerman: Well, there have been a number of things commented upon, even the question of colic, for example. If in breast milk you have the transfer of cow's milk protein at a level of 40 ng/ml, then the question is, when you give 8 ounces of this H.A. formula, is the residual protein that is intact still going to represent something like 40 ng/ml, or are we way down below that level? Also, what is the lower limit of level permitted in a production run, especially when it's batch-produced for general consumption?

Dr. Guesry: It's quite difficult to answer that precisely. We know that the reduction of the quantity of β-lactoglobulin, for example, to take the most abundant type of protein in the formula, is reduced by about 250 times.

Dr. Zimmerman: So give me a calculation then in milligrams per milliliter, what does that amount to?

Dr. Guesry: I do not have that information available at the moment.

Dr. Hamburger: Your question, Dr. Zimmerman, seems a reasonable one, but our preliminary data using both direct RAST and RAST-inhibition with the Carnation Good Start H.A. formula, suggest that it is more complex than how significant the trace amounts of undigested proteins and/or large peptides are. Some infants' serums with high titer IgE anti-cow's milk-antibody react to a slight extent with the H.A formula and others do not. Similarly, blocking a milk-antimilk RAST with H.A. formula varies from 0% to a maximum of 17% thus far in the first few serums tested. Obviously, the smaller the whey protein digested peptides remaining in the formula, the better, if the good taste, good nutrition, and reasonable price can all be maintained.

Dr. Corder: Fred Corder of Mitchellville, Maryland. Even though the recommendation is that this is a hypoallergenic formula that is to be used primarily as a prophylactic agent, it is going to be put on the grocer's shelf for the general public to use. My concern is the parents who have children who have presented with problems of eczema, problems of asthma are going to be picking this up without recommendations and seeing hypoallergenic on the formula, they are going to be using this as a treatment instead of as a prophylactic, even without the recommendations of their physician. Do you have any data that there may be some advantage to these patients, or that they are at greater risk in terms of the formula being used, and it is my opinion it will be used, as a therapeutic without physician recommendation because it will be on the grocer's shelf.

Dr. Barness: Dr. Schmidt, what is happening at this time in Europe?

Dr. Schmidt: Well, what you said is very familiar to us because Good Start H.A. was introduced in my country before we had any results about the preventive effects, and of course it is used by parents in the good hope that they can prevent disease. This is a problem that we try now to find the indications, the true indications, for prevention. That's all I can say at this moment. This is what we are working on now.

Dr. Barness: Dr. Strapazon or Dr. Guesry, are there any precautions to prevent this type of activity in a drug store or in a supermarket?

Dr. Guesry: I could understand any concern, but I wonder why our colleague is concerned by the fact that the family could in certain circumstances choose to give the Good Start H.A. instead of a soy formula. Apparently he is not concerned that the baby is receiving a soy formulation without a good indication, which can be purchased in many types of stores without physicians' guidance. We know that Carnation Good Start H.A. is safe and nutritious. We know that this product is effective in certain applications. So I do not really share his concern.

Dr. Corder: The concern is only raised in my mind because the panel is specific to say that our recommendation is that this is to be primarily used as a preventive formula. I have not heard that this is a formula that may be used without any particular limitation. It has been said at least twice in this last discussion that it is a prophylactic formula. That is why I raised the question that if your recommendation for this formula is that it is a prophylactic formula, then is there any reason or reservation for just saying it's a formula that can be used such as soy formulas are put on the market, but they are not put on the market as a recommendation from the company saying it's a prophylactic formula.

Dr. Hamburger: Could Dr. Schmidt tell us if there have been any problems as a general rule with the formula being available in the stores in Germany?

Dr. Schmidt: No, there have been no problems as far as I know, and it has been widely used. Of course the medical profession was looking for indications because we were afraid that something could happen, but I must admit that it seems to be safe and nothing has happened in the population that I know of. We would, however, prefer indications for us from the medical profession. That's clear. But on the whole, it seems to be a safe formula for use by everybody.

Dr. Zucker: Preston Zucker of New Jersey. Just some practical questions. I didn't hear the fat source identified in this formula. What preparation will be available and will it only be in powder or in ready-to-feed or concentrated liquid, and when is it expected to be available in the local communities?

Dr. Guesry: For the time being the only formulation will be in powder form, as has been shown by Dr. Strapazon. About the fat composition of the product? It is 100% vegetable oils including palm olein, high-oleic safflower, and coconut oils. We have tested the fat absorption of this mixture in human newborns, because as you know, it's the only way to be sure that the fat absorption is good, and we obtained a fat absorption of 90%, which is as good as or even better than any other infant formula. The date of availability in the United States will be in October 1988.

Dr. Zucker: What would be your recommendation if you were using this H.A. formula prophylactically on an infant who then developed a rotavirus infection?

Dr. Guesry: I would continue the formula since we know that rotavirus increases the risk of penetration of the intestinal mucosa by intact protein. I think post-acute diarrhea is a very good indication for the use of such a formula. Perhaps Dr. Walker-Smith would also like to comment on that.

Dr. Walker-Smith: I agree. I mean, I would agree that if you got rotavirus gastroenteritis when you were on this formula it would be a decided advantage because you would be having less chance of sensitization with whole protein. But just one point for clarification. Just as if you were on an ordinary adapted formula of course it contains lactose. So you might develop lactose intolerance during rotavirus, but that of itself wouldn't be particularly important and it wouldn't be particularly a drawback in that situation. But obviously if you had cow's milk-sensitive enteropathy, I would support the view that you would not be using this formula if a child had postenteritis syndrome. Again, it would be of value as a prophylaxis if you acquired rotavirus while you were on this formula. So I would support that view.

Dr. Dolovich: Someone mentioned that at least to some extent there are marketing issues and ways in which promotion will take place, and I wonder if the panel would comment on an advertisement in a recent medical journal advising Good Start H.A. I don't know what message will go to the public, but this is an item that will go to physicians, and the first indication for Good Start H.A. is "For formula intolerance instead of soy." Another statement is: "Resolves symptoms of milk allergy or intolerance such as spitting up, skin rash, runny nose, and colic." That, to me, is a therapeutic intervention that is being described in an advertisement, and I wonder if you would comment.

Dr. Strapazon: The issue is really the severity of the symptom that is being presented. I think in cases of mild symptoms, the data indicate that the product is effective. In cases of severe symptoms it might not be appropriate, and even other hydrolysate products such as Alfare or Nutramigen or one of the other ones out there might not be effective. As we have heard, in life-threatening anaphylaxis only an elemental amino acid formula might be safe. So it's really a decision that has to be made by the physician. Our intention was that this decision would be made under the supervision of a physician and a physician would be adequately informed to give the correct advice.

Dr. Guesry: Dr. Dolovich asked what type of information would go to the public. We are clear on that. All promotional and all medical information is aimed at the doctors and nothing will be given to the general public about this new formula, which is an adjunct to breast milk in normal babies and in babies in families with allergy.

Dr. Strapazon: The only information that will be directed at the public, and clearly without any mention of the Carnation Company or the product at all, is that in cases of formula intolerance, where there are problems with a nursing infant, the public are advised to see their physician. Our message is that the physician is the individual best informed to make that type of determination and he or she should be consulted.

Dr. Zimmerman: Dr. Eastham reminded us in his lecture on soy intolerance of all the problems that happened when soy formula was first developed, such as the vitamin deficiencies that occurred and the chloride problem and things like that. Has this product been tested over a period of time, let's say a year or so, in normal newborns to know that it promotes bone density, that it promotes growth, that it promotes no vitamin deficiencies and no hyperchloredemia or anything like that?

Dr. Guesry: As you have heard from Dr. Schmidt, the product has been on the market for almost two years now. We (Nestlé) have sold about 700 tons of the product and more than 100,000 babies have been fed with this product, and some for many, many months.

Dr. Zimmerman: But what I meant was has it been tested? I mean, have you done the studies that show that nothing happened? You think how long it took us to figure out that soy had a lot of deficiencies, and just feeding it to a bunch of infants for a year without testing those specific things like bone mineralization doesn't answer the question. For example, the soy formula on prematures is a good example.

Dr. Guesry: Specifically we have not yet studied bone mineralization of premature infants fed this formula.

Question: So you are not recommending it, I take it then, for prematures?

Dr. Guesry: We are presently doing a study feeding this formula to premature infants.

*Food Intolerance in Infancy: Allergology,
Immunology, and Gastroenterology,* edited by
Robert N. Hamburger. Carnation Nutrition
Education Series, Vol. 1. The Carnation Co., Los
Angeles/Raven Press, Ltd., New York © 1989.

Prophylaxis of Allergy in Infants and Conclusions on Food Intolerance

Robert N. Hamburger

*University of California San Diego, Pediatric Immunology and Allergy Division M-009-D,
La Jolla, CA 92093*

The diagnosis and management of food allergy today cannot be practiced with the available hard data and the known facts (1,2). To help our patients we use everything clinically available: diet, support, challenge (3), trial and error, placebo, laboratory (4) and skin tests (5), reassurance and medication (6). The art of medicine was never more challenged than in the care of the possibly food allergic, food intolerant patient.

The introduction to the United States of a new infant formula that has the potential for good nourishment with hypoallergenicity is certainly welcomed. The experience in Europe (7,8) is reassuring, but the extent of usefulness has not been adequately explored. For example, is it useful and acceptable as a food for older children following an acute gastroenteritis until the gastrointestinal lining has healed? Could a nursing mother drink it herself to protect her potentially allergic infant from cow's milk sensitization via her breast milk? How long is the optimum length of use of this hypoallergenic milk in normal infants and in infants with bilateral family histories of allergy? In fact, the most important question of them all still needs to be answered: Just how hypoallergenic is this new infant formula?

Some years ago we were studying a casein hydrolysate formula in my laboratory in preparation for our second prophylaxis of allergy study. I informed the manufacturer that serums from some highly cow's milk-allergic infants reacted with milk protein peptides in the formula. In fact, we found some rather large peptides in the casein hydrolysate formula and in addition, traces of other milk proteins besides the known casein. Nevertheless, when used in our clinical prophylaxis study as a supplement to breast-feeding, not one allergic reaction occurred in over 100 infants from highly allergic families, although allergic reactions to Nutramigen have been reported in the literature. Our analysis of the new whey milk protein hydrolysate confirms reports from Italy (9) that some highly atopic infants have IgE–anti-cow's milk-protein antibody that cross-reacts with peptides in the whey protein hydrolysate as well as to the casein hydrolysate formulas. Thus we would predict that this new infant hypoallergenic formula will be most useful in preventing sensitization to cow's milk proteins rather than therapeutically for infants already sensitized to cow's milk. The term hypoallergenic is a relative term, since some infants, some people, will react to almost anything which man creates.

Before concluding, I would like to present some thoughts on the value of a prophylaxis regimen in the prevention, postponement, or amelioration of atopic allergic diseases of childhood. Ever since the massive study of 20,000 infants by Grulee and Sanford (10) in 1936 proved beyond any doubt that exclusive breast-feeding reduced the incidence of eczema more than sevenfold compared to cow's milk feeding, dozens of more recent studies have served to confuse the issue. The interpretation of the results of our own recently completed double-blind, randomized, controlled study (11) has been influenced by the differing views of the two senior members of the research team (RNH and RSZ). Looking at the data, I concluded that despite the fact that both the study and the control mothers breast-fed and the level of compliance (12) was low in the study group, the cumulative and period prevalence was lower in five out of six allergic diseases (eczema, hives, asthma, and gastrointestinal symptoms: but not in allergic rhinitis) in the prophylaxis patients. That, to me, is a highly significant result implying a much greater value of the prophylaxis regimen than is immediately evident. If adherence to the regimen could be improved, I believe the statistical significance would be markedly improved.

Despite the difference in interpretation of the data, we both agree, as do all those who participated in this rigorous study, that in order to reduce the incidence of allergic disease in infants from highly allergic families, we recommend:

(a) Maternal avoidance of milk, egg, and peanut products during lactation (with calcium supplementation).
(b) Infants being weaned from the breast or supplemented should be fed a hydrolyzed hypoallergenic formula (peptides preferably smaller than 1,500 daltons) instead of cow's milk or soy formula until 12 months of age.
(c) Infant avoidance of solid foods for 6 months, cow's milk for 12 months, and egg, peanut, and fish for at least 24 months.
(d) Parental smoking to be discontinued; furry pets, molds, mites, and dust to be removed from the home (with special emphasis in the infant's room).

In conclusion, this is the first of an ongoing series of symposia on food intolerance with special reference to infants and children. The Carnation Company has made the strongest possible commitment to the promotion and encouragement of breast-feeding as the optimum way to feed almost all human infants (13). They, in collaboration with Nestlé SA, have vowed to search for and improve supplementary and complementary infant foods in order to provide ideal nourishment in the most hypoallergenic infant diet possible. In 1988, just 15 years since the publication of *"The Baby Food Tragedy"* in 1973 (14), instead of simply attacking the aggressive marketing practices of the food industry, we may have learned the value of coming together: scientists, clinicians, academicians, activists, public agencies, and industry to address the underlying problems of population, poverty, malnutrition, lack of hygiene, safe water, and sewage disposal. As I have frequently stated: ''Everyone agrees that 'breast is best' but there are too many factors discouraging successful breast feeding for the first four to six months of life in the 'have' (or rich) societies; in the have-not societies failure to breast feed can be catastrophic.''

A complete analysis of the problems with some sort of a happy ending has recently been published (15) but I am certain there is more to be learned and more to be accomplished to ensure an optimum beginning for all of the world's infants and children.

ACKNOWLEDGMENTS

This work was partially supported by grants from the Carnation Company, Mead Johnson and Company, the Elizabeth and Carroll Boutell Fund, and the University of California San Diego Pediatric Immunology and Allergy Foundation. The assistance of Janice R. Turner, Linda Galbreath, Jill Gilbert, and Maria Ware is very much appreciated.

REFERENCES

1. May CD. Objective clinical and laboratory studies of immediate hypersensitivity reactions to foods in children. *J Allergy Clin Immunol* 1976;58:500–15.
2. Wilson N, Vickers H, Silverman M. Objective test for food sensitivity in asthmatic children. *Br Med J* 1982;284:1226–8.
3. Mellon M, Heller S, O'Connor RD, Hamburger RN, Zeiger R. Double blind food challenges in a prospective allergy prevention program for high risk infants. *J Allergy Clin Immunol* 1985;75:178.
4. Wraith DG, Merrett J, Roth A, Yman L, Merrett TG. Recognition of food-allergic patients and their allergens by the RAST technique and clinical investigation. *Clin Allergy* 1979;9:25–36.
5. Amlot PL, Urbanek R, Youlten LJF, Kemeny DM, Lessof MH. Type I allergy to egg and milk proteins: Comparison of skin prick tests with nasal, buccal and gastric provocation tests. *Int Arch Allergy Appl Immunol* 1985;77:171–9.
6. Hamburger RN, Cohen GA. *New and Promising Treatments*. In: Breneman JC, ed. *Handbook of Food Allergies*. New York and Basel: Marcel Dekker, Inc, 1987;271–8.
7. Schmidt E, Reinhardt D, Gerke R. The use of hypoallergenic milk formulas in newborns. *Der Kinderarzt* 1987;5:627–31.
8. Zabransky S, Zabransky M. Preliminary clinical experience with a hypoallergenic infant formula. *Extracta Paediatrica* 1987;11:10–2.
9. Businco L, et al. Anaphylaxis in cow's milk allergic infants due to hydrolyzed cow's milk formulas. *Ann Allergy (in press)*.
10. Grulee CG, Sanford HN. The influence of breast and artificial feeding on infantile eczema. *J Pediatr* 1936;9:223–35.
11. Zeiger RS, Heller S, Mellon MH, Forsythe AB, O'Connor RD, Hamburger RN, Schatz M. Effect of combined maternal and infant food allergen avoidance on development of atopy in early infancy: A randomized study. *J Allergy Clin Immunol (in press)*.
12. Hamburger RN, Casillas R, Johnson R, Mellon M, O'Connor RD, Zeiger R. Long-term studies in prevention of food allergy: Patterns of IgG anti-cow's milk antibody responses. *Ann Allergy* 1987;59:175–8.
13. Strapazon E. Introduction to the new Carnation Good Start H.A. formula. *this volume*.
14. Anonymous: *Action Now on Baby Foods*. New Internationalist, OXFAM and Christian Aid, Pub, Aug, 1973;1.
15. Dobbing J, ed. *Infant Feeding: Anatomy of a Controversy 1973–1984*. London, Berlin, Heidelberg: Springer-Verlag, 1988.

SUBJECT INDEX

A

Age
anaphylaxis and, 123
challenge testing and, 119
CMA and, 137,138–139,190,
221–222
cow's milk enteropathy and, 130,
159,190
food tolerance and, 3,86,105,110,
123–124,190–191
growth curves and, 259
infant serum motilin and,
179–181
intestinal blood loss and, 137,
138–139,159
iron deficiency and, 140,142
sleep problems and, 163,171
for solids feeding, 193–194,300

Allergens
additive effects, 4,219–220
casein as, 227–229,248
codfish model of, 14,15–16
concentration of, 288
cow's milk as, 11,73,121–122,
129–132,227–229, 273–276,
284–285
definition of, 9,37
dose effects, 4,23,26,28,33,207,
212,214–216,288
egg proteins as, 24–25,41,119
food additive effects, 4,5,76,146,
147,161
goat's milk as, 255
heat treatment of, 255–256
hydrolysis of, 256–257,293
IgE and, 1,2,3–4,37,59–60,62
in vitro tests of, 261–263,293
in vivo tests of, 259–261
β-lactoglobulin as, 25–27,41,73,
176–179,212–214
modified cow's milk as, 273–276
protein denaturation and, 12–13,41,
254–257,261–263
replacement of, 255

soybean proteins as, 223,224,
227–232
soy/protein formulas as, 230–232,
250,255
specificity of, 20
test system for, 273–276
wheat flour as, 11,26–27
whey proteins as, 260–261,
273–274,292,294

Allergic reactions
to breast milk proteins, 40–41,42
cord blood markers for, 95–99
definition of, 37
dose effects, 4,204–207,212,
214–216
drug effects, 94–95
to food additives, 161
genetic factors in, 93–94,105,283
HLA and, 94
IgE and, 1,2,3–4,37,83,105,107,
254,293
maternal-fetal factors in, 94–95
mucosal barrier and, 43,49–53,
69–70
peptide size and, 254
postnatal parameters in, 99–100
prevalence of, 93–94
prevention of, 93–94,292–293
risk due to, 93–94
use incidence, 119

Anaphylaxis response
age and, 123
to cow's milk, 7,129,159
cutaneous, 260–261
food allergy and, 83,87,123–124,
159,231
IgE and, 293
intestinal, 51,52,128–129
mechanisms in, 51,52
to soy protein formulations, 231
to whey proteins, 260–261

Antibodies
antigen binding and, 13–14
epitopes and, 13–14